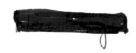

Surgery of the Lumbar Spine

Surgery of the Lumbar Spine

Sanford J. Larson, MD, PhD
Professor and Chairman
Department of Neurosurgery
Medical College of Wisconsin
Milwaukee, Wisconsin

Dennis J. Maiman, MD, PhD
Professor
Department of Neurosurgery
Medical College of Wisconsin
Froedtert Memorial Lutheran Hospital
Department of Veterans Affairs Medical Center
Milwaukee, Wisconsin

1999

Thieme
New York · Stuttgart

Thieme New York
333 Seventh Avenue
New York, NY 10001

Editor: Ave McCracken
Editorial Director: Ave McCracken
Editorial Assistant: Mindy Scalzetti
Developmental Editor: Kathleen Lyons
Director, Production & Manufacturing: Anne Vinnicombe
Production Editor: Janice G. Stangel
Marketing Director: Phyllis Gold
Sales Manager: David Bertelsen
Chief Financial Officer: Seth S. Fishman
President: Brian D. Scanlan
Cover Designer: Kevin Kall
Designer: Textbook Writers Associates, Inc.
Medical Illustrator: Robert Fenn
Compositor: Northeastern Graphic Services, Inc.
Printer: Maple-Vail Book Manufacturing Group

Library of Congress Cataloging-in-Publication Data

Larson, Sanford J.
    Surgery of the lumbar spine / Sanford J. Larson, Dennis Maiman.
      p.   cm.
    Includes bibliographical references and index.
    ISBN 0-86577-758-6
    1. Lumbar vertebrae—Surgery. 2. Backache—Surgery. I. Maiman,
Dennis. II. Title.
    [DNLM: 1. Lumbar Vertebrae—surgery. 2. Spinal Diseases—surgery.
WE 750 L334s 1999]
RD768.L37 1999
617.5′6059—dc21
DNLM/DLC
for Library of Congress   99-22441
                                                                                     CIP

Copyright © 1999 by Thieme Medical Publishers, Inc. This book, including all parts thereof, is legally protected by copyright. Any use, exploitation or commercialization outside the narrow limits set by copyright legislation, without the publisher's consent, is illegal and liable to prosecution. This applies in particular to photostat reproduction, copying, mimeographing or duplication of any kind, translating, preparation of microfilms, and electronic data processing and storage.

Important note: Medical knowledge is ever-changing. As new research and clinical experience broaden our knowledge, changes in treatment and drug therapy may be required. The authors and editors of the material herein have consulted sources believed to be reliable in their efforts to provide information that is complete and in accord with the standards accepted at the time of publication. However, in view of the possibility of human error by the authors, editors, or publisher of the work herein, or changes in medical knowledge, neither the authors, editors, publisher, nor any other party who has been involved in the preparation of this work, warrants that the information contained herein is in every respect accurate or complete, and they are not responsible for any errors or omissions or for the results obtained from use of such information. Readers are encouraged to confirm the information contained herein with other sources. For example, readers are advised to check the product information sheet included in the package of each drug they plan to administer to be certain that the information contained in this publication is accurate and that changes have not been made in the recommended dose or in the contraindications for administration. This recommendation is of particular importance in connection with new or infrequently used drugs.

Some of the product names, patents, and registered designs referred to in this book are in fact registered trademarks or proprietary names even though specific reference to this fact is not always made in the text. Therefore, the appearance of a name without designation as proprietary is not to be construed as a representation by the publisher that it is in the public domain.

Printed in the United States of America

5 4 3 2 1

TNY ISBN 0-86577-758-6
GTV ISBN 3-13-107991-6

To our residents and fellows.
*. . . Rabbi Chanina says. "Much have I learned from my teachers,
more than that from my colleagues, and from my students most of all . . . "*

Talmud, Tractate Ta'anis

Contents

	Foreword	ix
	Preface	xi
Chapter 1.	Lumbar Anatomy	1
Chapter 2.	Biomechanics of the Spine: Normal and Pathologic	13
Chapter 3.	Instability of the Vertebral Column	35
Chapter 4.	Metabolic Diseases of Bone	51
Chapter 5.	Disc Degeneration	79
Chapter 6.	Isthmic Spondylolisthesis	133
Chapter 7.	Infection	145
Chapter 8.	Trauma	157
Chapter 9.	Benign Tumors of the Spine	183
Chapter 10.	Primary Malignant Tumors	201
Chapter 11.	Metastatic Tumors of the Lumbar Spine	231
Chapter 12.	Bone Grafts and Orthoses	255
Chapter 13.	Surgical Approaches	267
	Index	325

Foreword

This book, written by two of the premier leaders of the modern spine surgery era, is a comprehensive treatise. It provides "everything you wanted to know" regarding the surgery of the lumbar spine. The authors have covered in great detail the anatomy and biomechanics of the lumbar spine, as well as its stability, and the management of instability. Fusion principles and surgical approaches are also covered in detail. In addition, it addresses a variety of lumbar spine-specific pathology, from an anatomical, clinical, and therapeutic point of view.

Drs. Larson and Maiman have pioneered both the study of the lumbar spine, as well as the surgical and nonsurgical management of lumbar spine pathology. Therefore, it is fitting that they have written this treatise on the subject. It parallels their clinical and laboratory work. This book clearly enhances the surgeon's ability to care for patients with lumbar spine pathology; and most importantly, it significantly advances the field.

I have been blessed with the uncommon and wonderful opportunity to have trained under the tutelage of Dr. Larson and with Dr. Maiman. It is wonderful to see, in written form, an expression of their life's work (to date). Please enjoy and absorb from this work its many facts, lessons, and pearls; for they will serve both you and your patients well.

Edward C. Benzel, MD
Professor and Chief
Division of Neurosurgery
University of New Mexico

Preface

When we decided to write this book several years ago, we first had to ask ourselves whether the world really needed another spine book. Indeed, while we were writing it, many new texts on the spine were brought to the public eye, but we were encouraged to continue by the words of Solomon in Ecclesiastes: "The making of many books is without limit."

When Thieme approached us about writing this book, we agreed, because we welcomed the opportunity to share our experience and philosophy, emphasizing the need to integrate biomechanics and clinical practice. Certainly, practices change, as do medications, techniques, and devices, but like the words of Solomon, principles do not.

We are grateful to our editors at Thieme for their patience and persistence, especially Avé McCracken, who brought this project to fruition; to our residents and fellows for their infectious enthusiasm, curiosity, and occasional quizzical stares; to Cheryl Mader, Sandi Wisniewski, and Cynthia Krafcheck for their editorial assistance; to Robert Fenn for his ability to depict the surgical procedures simply but beautifully; and to our families for their unfailing support. Most of all, we give thanks to the Author of the greatest Book for help in all things.

About the Cover
Finite element mesh of three lumbar vertebrae using brick elements. This mesh, based on one designed by Dr. Theo Smit of University Hospital Vrije Universiteit in Amsterdam, is adapted by permission. This state of the art model incorporates nonlinear material properties, and includes the spinal ligaments. The original images are available on the Internet at the ISB Finite Element Repository managed by the Istituti Ortopedici Rizzoli, Bologna, Italy.

Surgery of the Lumbar Spine

CHAPTER 1

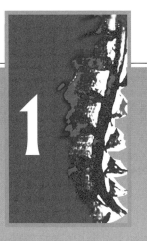

Lumbar Anatomy

Vertebral Body

Blood Supply to the Vertebrae

Nerve Supply to the Vertebrae

Lumbar Apophyseal Joints

Ligaments

Intervertebral Disc

Lumbar Anatomy

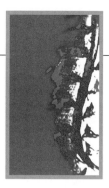

This chapter only briefly reviews anatomical considerations. A detailed and comprehensive presentation of lumbar anatomy can be found in the excellent book, *Clinical Anatomy at the Lumbar Spine*, by Bogduk and Twomey.[13]

Vertebral Body

The vertebral body develops from sclerotomal mesenchyme, which forms paired masses alongside the notochord separated by a fissure and by segmental arteries. The caudal half of each sclerotome becomes denser and joins the less dense cranial part of the next caudal sclerotome to form a primordial vertebra. The segmental artery now lies at the vertebral equator. Each pair grows medially around the notochord to form the vertebral body, dorsally around the neural tube to form the vertebral arch, and laterally to form the primitive costal arches. In the lumbar area, the costal arches eventually fuse with the transverse process to form its anterolateral portion, and it comprises the lateral portion of the sacrum and the inferior part of the ala. This contribution of the coastal arch to the lumbar vertebra explains the occasional unilateral or bilateral sacralization of the last lumbar vertebra. Fissures between the vertebral primordia develop into the intervertebral disc with the notochordal remnant persisting as the nucleus pulposus.

Chondrification develops from four centers, two in the vertebral body and one in each half of the arch. After the cartilaginous vertebra has been formed, ossification begins from three centers, one in the body and two in the vertebral arch. The vertebral arch centers form the pedicles, the laminae, and the dorsolateral parts of the vertebral bodies, along with costral ossification centers in the transverse processes. The neurocentral synchondroses between the junctions of the ossification centers persist until bony union occurs at about age 6. Secondary ossification centers begin in the tips of the spinous processes, in the transverse processes, and in the perimeter of the cranial and caudal surfaces of the vertebral body at about age 16 or 17. Union with underlying bone takes place by age 25. Before this occurs, the secondary ossification center in the perimeter of the end plate, the ring apophysis, may prolapse and cause symptoms (Fig. 1–1). The limbus vertebra probably represents either an ununited or detached anterior portion of the ring (Fig. 1–2).

Blood Supply to the Vertebrae

Arteries

From L1 to L4 the segmental artery leaves the aorta on either side, passing around the midportion of the vertebral body toward the root foramen. The artery for L5 is usually a branch of the first sacral artery. As each artery passes around the vertebral body, it gives off vertical ascending and descending branches on the surface of the vertebral body. Other branches penetrate the vertebral body, moving radially toward the center where they form a grid. On the way they give off ascending and descending vertical branches that are directed toward the end plates. As the main trunk reaches the interval between adjacent transverse processes, several branches leave it. The spinal branch breaks up into the postcentral artery to the vertebral arches, the anterior and posterior radicular arteries, and a

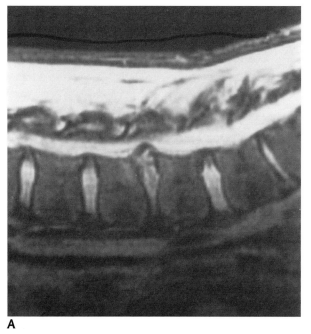

A

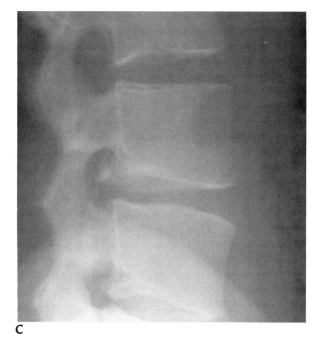

C

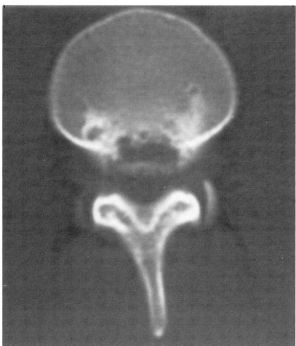

B

FIGURE 1-1
A Prolapsed ring apophysis at L3–4 in a 16-year-old male with back pain that followed intense athletic activity. **B** CT scan from same patient. The back pain subsided and he became a member of his high school and college swimming teams. **C** Lumbar spine film done 6 years later. The slipped ring apophysis has become a prominent osteophyte. He was fully active and had only occasional mild back discomfort.

branch that moves centrally on the floor of the spinal canal with vertical ascending and descending arteries moving radially into the vertebral body to meet the central grid. The muscular branch gives off an interarticular artery that moves medially over the posterior surface of the transverse process, giving off two superior articular arteries that proceed posteriorly around the superior lateral aspect of the joints and a communicating artery that crosses the posterior aspect of the transverse process, giving off an inferior articular artery before anastomosing with the next more caudal interarticular artery.[31] (The interarticular artery and its branches can be a source of annoying bleeding during the performance of a transverse process fusion.)

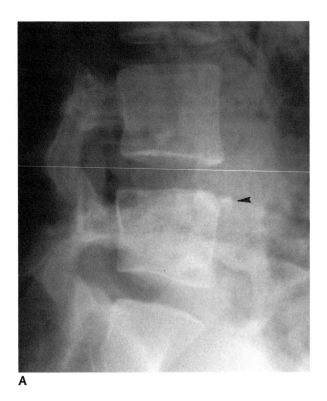 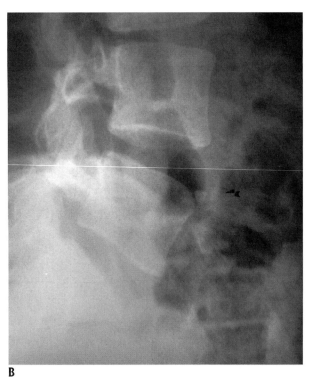

FIGURE 1–2 Limbus vertebra (*arrow*) during flexion **A** and extension **B** demonstrating detachment from vertebral body. This patient had significant back pain, but a causal relationship could not be established.

Veins

At the end plate a capillary bed is continuous across the disc bone interface and drains into venules, which then form a horizontal subchondral venous network, or into the marrow venous channels. These are organized into ascending and descending vessels that empty into the basivertebral vein.[18–20] The veins of the vertebral body drain into the internal and external venous plexuses. The internal venous plexus has two channels posterior to the dura and two channels anterior to it. The external venous plexus has two channels posterior to the lamina and two anterior to the vertebral body. All are valveless and freely anastomotic and empty into the intervertebral veins. These join the lumbar veins, which enter the vena cava and are also connected to the ascending lumbar veins. The latter give rise to the azygos and hemiazygos veins, which connect the inferior vena cava and the superior vena cava. In cadaver experiments, Batson[5] demonstrated that radiopaque material injected into the dorsal vein of the penis entered the vertebral venous plexuses, eventually reaching the cranial cavity. Radioactive material injected into the dorsal vein of the penis of an anesthetized monkey entered the inferior vena cava. However, when the Valsalva maneuver was simulated by tying a towel about the monkey's abdomen, the injected material entered the vertebral veins, suggesting diversion of blood from the caval system during raised intra-abdominal pressure. Batson considered this to be a mechanism for vertebral metastases.[5]

Nerve Supply to the Vertebrae

Distal to the dorsal root ganglion, the spinal nerve divides into an anterior ramus and a posterior ramus (Fig. 1–3). Before moving on to become part of the lumbosacral plexus, the anterior ramus gives direct branches to the posterior lateral aspect of the disc and communicating rami, which pass beneath and through the psoas to the sympathetic

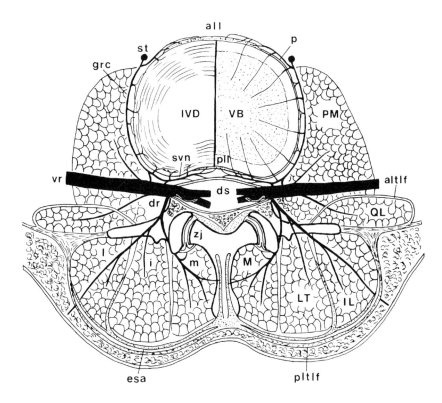

FIGURE 1–3 Lumbar cross section demonstrating nerve supply to structure that can be a source of pain. All, anterior longitudinal ligament; altlf, anterior layer of thoracolumbar fascia; dr, dorsal ramus; ds, dural sac; esa, erector spinae aponeurosis; grc, gray ramus communicans; i, intermediate branch; IL, iliocostalis lumborum; IVD, intervertebral disc; l, lateral branch; LT, longissimus thoracis; m, medial branch; pll, posterior longitudinal ligament; pltlf, posterior layer of thoracolumbar fascia; PM, psoas major; QL, quadratus lumborum; st, sympathetic trunk; sun, sinuventral nerve; VB, vertebral body; vr, ventral ramus; zj, zygapophyseal joint; (Reproduced by permission from Bogduk N, Twomey LT: Clinical Anatomy of the Lumbar Spine. Churchill Livingstone, Melbourne, pp. 197, 1991.)

ganglia. Along the way branches are given off to the lateral aspect of the disc and to the anterior longitudinal ligament.[14]

The posterior ramus gives a branch that is joined by one from the communicating ramus to form the sinuvertebral nerve.[41] The sinuvertebral nerve enters the spinal canal and breaks up into a smaller, caudally directed branch and a major branch that is directed rostrally parallel with the lateral border of the posterior longitudinal ligament. As it moves rostrally, branches leave it and pass deep to the posterior longitudinal ligament. The sinuvertebral nerve does not persist beyond the next most rostral disc. Smaller caudal branches are directed medially and caudally to supply the disc at the level of entry. The posterior ramus then divides into three major branches. The medial is directed dorsocaudally in the groove between the mamillary process and accessory process beneath the mamilloaccessory ligament. After leaving the groove, it gives rostral branches to the caudal aspect of the apophyseal joint and distal branches to the rostal aspect of the subjacent apophyseal joint before entering the multifidus. The intermediate branch is directed to the longissimus and the lateral branch to the iliocostalis.[15]

In the disc, the fibers terminate in the outer third to one-half of the annulus.[58] Free, nonencapsulated endings, some of which are simple and others more complicated, have been described in the annulus,[27,47] and encapsulated complicated endings have been found not only on the surface of the annulus but also within it. The anterior longitudinal ligament and the posterior longitudinal ligament have free nerve endings that are more numerous and more complicated in the posterior longitudinal ligament; in the anterior ligament, only a few single endings have been found. Encapsulated, complicated terminals are considered to be mechanoreceptors, and the nonencapsulated endings are thought to be nociceptors.[33,37] The supraspinous ligament, the interspinous ligament, the ligamentum flavum, and the lumbodorsal fascia also contain both free and mechanoreceptors.[27,41,44,56] In the fetus, nerve fibers have been found to enter bone in association with blood vessels and have also been found in association with vascular buds in the end plate.[41] Nerve fibers have been described in the marrow and in subchondral bone. Although these could be exclusively autonomic, some observations suggest that the fibers in subchondral bone are related to pain perception.[7]

Lumbar Apophyseal Joints

Coronally oriented in infants, the articular surfaces of the apophyseal joints gradually change to a biplanar configuration with the anterior portion more coronal and the larger posterior portion more sagittal.[50] The subchondral bone becomes thicker, reaching maximum thickness in the third and fourth decades. In subsequent decades, the subchondral bone becomes progressively thinner, with a corresponding loss of anticular cartilage. The increase in thickness of subchondral bone is more pronounced in the coronal than in the sagittal portion of the joint. The horizontal portion of the joints limits flexion, and the joint capsules provide 39% of the resistance to flexion.[4] When the erector spinae muscles become electrically silent in full flexion, the trunk is therefore supported to a significant degree by the joints.[28]

The sagittal component restricts the combined rotation of the lumbar vertebrae to about 10 to 15 degrees.[1] In the normal spine, rotational displacement of more than 1 mm has resulted in injury to articular cartilage. With degenerated discs, more rotation was allowed before failure.[1] The angle formed by the articular surfaces of the apophyseal joints is not always bilaterally symmetrical. Based on CT and MRI findings in patients less than 50 years of age, asymmetrical joints were associated with an increased incidence of disc degeneration.[38] In another study, based solely on CT scan with the assumption that discs without protrusion are normal, disc protrusion could not be correlated with joint asymmetry.[25]

The lumbar apophyseal joints contain meniscus-like invaginations from the joint capsules. These appear to be synovial reflections rather than cartilaginous. The theory that entrapment of a meniscus within a joint produces pain by exerting traction on the joint capsules has been invoked as the basis for manipulative therapy. However, the structure of the lumbar apophyseal menisci does not support this theory.[11,22]

Ligaments

In one study, the supraspinus ligament was found to end at L3 in 22% of specimens, at L4 in 75%, and at L5 in 5%.[45] Since the supraspinous ligament restricts flexion[4,21,23] and disc herniation is produced by flexion and compression,[2,3] it appears likely that the higher incidence of disc herniation at L4–L5 and L5–S1 is related to the absence of the ligament at those levels. The posterior longitudal ligament is restricted to the midsagittal portion of the lumbar canal, extending laterally over the intervertebral discs and blending with the annulus. The deep layer of the ligament bridges one motion segment, and the superficial layer extends over two to three levels. In the upper lumbar area the posterior longitudinal ligament is wider and has a loose central attachment, whereas it is narrower at lower levels. This may explain why central herniations are more frequent in the upper lumbar spine as opposed to more lateral herniations at lower levels.[40] As with the posterior longitudinal ligament, the deeper fibers of the anterior longitudinal ligament bridge one motion segment, whereas the more superficial fibers are longer.

Although not a true ligament, a peridural membrane corresponding to periosteum, which is absent in the spinal canal, covers the floor of the canal and is attached to the deep layer of the posterior longitudinal ligament.[55] The epidural veins are posterior to the membrane, penetrating it near the midline to form the basivertebral vein. The perivertebral membrane surrounds the spinal canal posteriorly, extending into the root formamina to cover the spinal nerves, but is absent over the annulus. It fixes the dura to the spinal canal as the nerve roots pass laterally from the main body of the dural sac into the vertebral foramen and exit from it. As with the posterior longtudinal ligament, the deeper fibers of the anterior longitudinal ligament bridge one motion segment whereas the more superficial fibers are longer.

In the lumbar area, the lumbodorsal fascia has a posterior and anterior layer. The posterior layer can be separated into two laminae. The superficial forms the origin of the latissimus dorsi, and the deep layer covers the erector spinae aponeurosis. The anterior layer runs from the tips of the transverse processes and intertransverse ligaments upon the quadratus lumborum to join the posterior layer at the lateral margin of the erector spinae. The raphe formed by this junction is the origin of the tranversus abdominus and part of the internal oblique. The orientation of the fibers of the posterior layers suggests that the lumbodorsal fascia can act in conjunction with the transversus abdominus to resist flexion.[12,24]

Intervertebral Disc

The intervertebral disc is made up of the nucleus pulposus, the annulus fibrosis, and the end plates. Degeneration of the intervertebral disc is related to loss of its normal biomechanical properties, and these properties are a function of its extracellular matrix. The extracellular matrix of the nucleus pulposus, annulus fibrosis, and the cartilaginous end plates is made up of collagen, water containing organic and inorganic solutes, and proteoglycans, formerly referred to as mucoproteins or mucopolysaccharides.[6,48]

Nucleus Pulposus

At birth, the nucleus pulposus consists of clumps of notochordal cells in a gelatinous matrix[39,51,52] that contains proteoglycans produced by the cells.[51] The line of demarcation is distinct between the notochordal nucleus derived from endoderm and the mesodermal cartilaginous end plate and annulus fibrosus. During the first 2 postnatal years, the number of notochordal cells increases and the nucleus pulposus enlarges. After the third year, the notochordal cells begin to disappear and are replaced by fibroblasts and by chondrocytes, which also produce proteoglycans. The line of demarcation between the nucleus and the perichordal components of the disc becomes progressively less distinct. By age 5 notochordal cells are no longer present and the nucleus pulposus is fibrocartilaginous.[52] The hydrostatic properties of the nucleus are, however, retained. During this time, significant changes also take place in the annulus fibrosus and the cartilaginous end plate.

Annulus Fibrosis

In infants, the outer one-third to one-half of the annulus contains blood vessels, but these decrease in number during childhood, and only a few persist in adults.[39] Arteries enter the spinal canal through the intervertebral foramina, penetrate the dorsal surface of the vertebral body, and branch within it, some entering the cartilaginous end plate. Other arteries ramify within the periosteum and move radially into the end plates at the cephalic and caudal ends of the vertebral body. Side branches are directed toward the nucleus pulposus and annulus fibrosus.[52] These vessels are most numerous at birth, gradually decreasing in number during the first 2 years of life, and more rapidly during the third year. The number of vessels then remains relatively constant during the remainder of the first decade.[51] A further reduction then occurs until, at skeletal maturity, blood vessels are seen only at the disc margin and where the marrow spaces are in contact with uncalcified portions of the end plate.[34]

The annulus fibrosis is made up of concentric lamellae of fibrocartilage oriented at approximately 60-degree angles. The outer layers are almost entirely fibrous and are inserted into the anterior and posterior longitudinal ligaments and into the edges of the vertebral body, whereas the inner and more cellular portion becomes fibrocartilaginous and its fibers are continuous with the collagenous fibers of the end plate.[52] Consequently, the nucleus pulposus is surrounded by a capsule of collagenous fibers contained within the annulus and cartilaginous end plate (Fig. 1–4). The nucleus pulposus holds the vertebral bodies apart, placing the fibers of the annulus under axial distractive tension. When an axial load is applied to the vertebral column, the annulus may bulge slightly but nevertheless serves as a hoop to restrain the nucleus pulposus. Similarly, the end plate, with its radially directed collagenous fibers, also has elasticity, allowing some bending into the

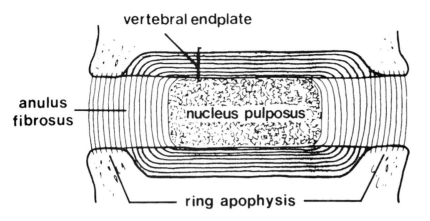

FIGURE 1-4
Intervertebral disc components. The exterior portion of the annulus is attached to the ring apophysis, and the internal portion forms a capsule for the nucleus pulposus. (Reproduced by permission from Bogduk N, Twomey LT: Clinical anatomy of the Lumbar Spine, Churchill Livingstone, Melbourne, pp. 197, 1991.)

vertebral body during an applied axial load. Degenerative changes in the annulus begin at about age 40 and become progressively more severe with advancing age.[10]

End Plates

The end plate of the intervertebral disc is made up of hyaline cartilage attached to underlying bone by a thin layer of calcium,[17] unlike the collagenous attachment of articular cartilage to underlying bone elsewhere in the body. At birth, the end plate is divided into an inner growth zone with columns of proliferating and hypertrophic cells and an articular region bordering on the nucleus pulposus. Collagen is found only in the articular region. The growth zone gradually diminishes, and at skeletal maturity only remnants persist. By the third and fourth decade, only articular cartilage remains. This layer is gradually resorbed and replaced by bone. By the sixth and seventh decades a narrow strip of articular cartilage remains with numerous collagenous fibers passing from the cartilage into what was the nucleus pulposus.[8] These collagen fibers are independent of the achoring fibers of the annulus (Fig. 1-5). Similar changes have been observed in the subhuman primate.[9]

Proteoglycans and Collagen

The adult intervertebral disc is nourished by diffusion across the cartilaginous end plate and to some extent across the annulus.[16] The matrix of the nucleus pulposus contains proteoglycans, which in the first 3 years of life are produced by notochordal cells and subsequently by the chondrocytes of the end plate and annulus. The chondrocytes also produce the collagen that with increasing age gradually forms much of the nucleus pulposus. The proteoglycans imbibe and retain water, and control diffusion of larger molecules into the nucleus pulposus.[6] The basic proteoglycan unit is the proteglycan monomer, made up of a protein core with glycosaminoglycan side chains. In the intervertebral disc, the side chains are chondroitin sulfate and keratin sulfate. Each chondroitin sulfate side chain is 50 nm long, with negatively charged groups repeating at 0.5-nm intervals. The shorter keratin sulfate side chains have similarly spaced negatively charged groups. Because of the negative charges, the side chains stand out stiffly at right angles like "bristles on a brush."[48] In the hyaline cartilage of the end plate and in the nucleus pulposus, some of the proteoglycans are linked in aggregates. Each consists of a hyaluronic acid chain to which the proteoglycan units are attached, with the union stabilized by a link protein attached to the hyaluronate and to the proteoglycan monomer. Because of the multitudinous negatively charged groups, the proteoglycan aggregates expand out stiffly in solution, occupying a much greater volume in vitro than in the end plate or nucleus, where the proteoglycans are constrained by the collagen fiber network.[48] When the end plates and nucleus pulposus are compressed, the proteoglycans are compacted and water is extruded. When compression is removed, water returns[54] and the proteoglycan aggregates expand until restrained by the collagen fibers. These cyclic changes give the cartilaginous end plate and the nucleus pulposus their elastic properties, and alterations from the normal values for these constituents of the extracellular matrix adversely affect elasticity. The proportion of proteoglycans present as aggregates is considerably greater in the end plate than in the nucleus pulposus,[35] and this may account for the relatively greater deformability of

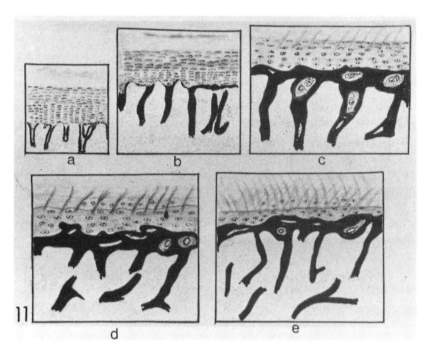

FIGURE 1–5 Changes in the intervertebral disc with increasing age. **a** Growth stage with an active growth cartilage zone characterized by columns of chondrocytes. **b** Maturation stage. The growth layer has become narrower and bone is beginning to seal off the cartilage border. **c** Growth stage is no longer present. Bone is now directly apposed to the articular cartilage, which is undergoing calcification. **d** Progressive replacement of articular cartilage by bone. **e** Only a thin layer of cartilage separates the bone from the disc and collagen fibers are more numerous. (Reproduced by permission from Bernick S, Cailliet R: Vertebral end-plate changes with aging of human vertebrae. Spine 7(2):97–102, 1982.)

the nucleus. The proportion and size of aggregated proteoglycans decrease with age. Although this appears to be inherent in the aging process,[35] it could be accelerated by other factors. The water content of the intervertebral disc decreases proportionately with the proteoglycan content.

In the intervertebral disc, the collagen content is greatest in the end plate and least within the nucleus pulposus, whereas water and proteoglycan content are least in the end plate and greatest in the nucleus.[46] The hydrostatic properties of the nucleus are dependent upon the proteoglycans, which are in turn dependent upon adequate nutrition of the chondrocytes. Reduced diffusion of nutrients can therefore be expected to adversely affect the extracellular matrix. Permeability decreases with age, partly because of the progressive ossification of the articular layer and perhaps, as water content decreases, because of precipitation of previously dissolved molecules within the proteglycan network. Nutrition of the disc is tenuous, as demonstrated by its hypocellularity compared to that of diarthrodial joints, which receive nutrients not only by diffusion from vertebral vessels but also from synovia and synovial fluid.

Ossification and Microfractures

Progressive ossification of the articular cartilage has been observed in humans,[8] subhuman primates,[9] and other species,[26] and therefore appears part of the aging process. Although the cartilaginous end plate is invaded by bone, it is not disrupted by it. However, penetration of disc material into the end plate is associated with local loss of chondrocytes and disruption of the end plate.[42,43,46] Loss of chondrocytes results in reduced production of proteoglycans and consequent loss of water from the disc. It has been shown that both water and proteoglycans are diminished in the immediate vicinity of these end plate fractures.[46] Contact between the avascular disc tissue and marrow produces an inflammatory response with locally increased vascularity that may thin and therefore weaken the bony end plate.[36] The disc tissue eventually ossifies,[43] further reducing the area available for diffusion. These microfractures can be considered traumatic events. Axial loading experiments have demonstrated that microfractures, which occur most frequently in the central, weaker portion of the end plate at loads of 2 to 10 kN, are not apparent on plain radiographs.[57] Radiographically demonstrable injury requires substantially greater forces. Microfractures also are more readily produced in degenerated than in normal disc.[57] They can occur at loads that are associated with at least some occupations, such as meat cutting, where average lifting loads are 4.9 kN.[32] Since stiffness is altered by cyclic loading, smaller forces not considered sufficient to produce structural damage might do so under repetitive loading. The relationship between repetitively applied loads and disruption of the end plate is supported by the increased incidence of back pain and of radiologically demonstrated abnormalities of the intervertebral disc in young athletes, particularly male gymnasts.[49]

Vertical Loads

The load on the intervertebral disc increases with the change from a supine to a more erect posture, and with application of force to the vertebral column. The vertical load on the annulus is least for a normal disc and substantially greater for one that is degenerated. In the normal intervertebral disc, part of a vertical load on the nucleus is resisted by the end plate, and part is distributed as a load perpendicular to the annulus. Since the annulus fibers are kept under distractive tension by the nucleus pulposus, they are consequently able to resist these forces. Although the end plate may bend inward and the annulus may bulge outward, neither is disrupted. As proteoglycan content decreases, water is lost, altering the hydrostatic and elastic properties of the nucleus and of the annulus fibrosus. The central portion of the disc then becomes less capable of withstanding vertical loads and may fail. The loads fall progressively on the annulus, which is not able to sustain them. In these circumstances it begins to bulge excessively, and eventually the lamelae develop fissures.[10] The annulus also undergoes cartilaginous metaplasia as a response to compressive forces.[46] The nucleus becomes more collgenous and the disc narrows, allowing relaxation of the apophyseal joint capsules. This, with relaxation of the annulus, permits abnormal translational movement of the vertebral bodies[29] and subsequent development of osteophytes.

The result of normal aging and the applied loads of occupation and avocation is the transformation of an intervertebral disc composed of clearly defined annulus fibrosus, cartilaginous end plate, and gelatinous nucleus pulposus into a largely collagenous structure with thin cartilaginous end plates and an ill-defined annulus that is not clearly distinguishable from the nucleus pulposus. A substantial factor in this process appears to be the progressively decreasing number of adequately nourished chondrocytes available to maintain the extracellular matrix.

REFERENCES

1. Adams M, Hutton W: The relevance of torsion to the mechanical derangement of the lumbar spine. Spine 6(3):241–248, 1981.

2. Adams M, Hutton WC: Prolapsed intervertebral disc: A hyperflexion injury. Spine 7(3):184–191, 1982.

3. Adams MA, Hutton WC: Gradual disc prolapse. Spine 10(6):524–531, 1985.

4. Adams MA, Hutton WC, Stott JRR: The resistance to flexion of the lumbar intervertebral joint. Spine 5(3):245–253, 1980.

5. Batson OV: The function of the vertebral veins and their role in the spread of metastases. Ann Surg 112(1):138–149, 1940.

6. Bayliss M, Johnstone B, O'Brien J: Proteoglycan synthesis in the human intervertebral disc. Spine 13:972–981, 1988.

7. Beaman DN, Graziano GP, Glover RA, et al: Substance P innervation of lumbar spine facet joints. Spine 18(8):1044–1049, 1993.

8. Bernick S, Cailliet R: Vertebral end-plate changes with aging of human vertebrae. Spine 7(2):97–102, 1982.

9. Bernick S, Cailliet R, Levy BM: The maturation and aging of the vertebrae of marmosets. Spine 5:519–524, 1980.

10. Bernick S, Walker JM, Paule WJ: Age changes to the annulus fibrosus in human intervertebral disc. Spine 16(5):520–524, 1991.

11. Bogduk N, Engel R: The menisci of the lumbar zygapophyseal joints: A review of their anatomy and clinical significance. Spine 9(5):454–460, 1984.

12. Bogduk N, Macintosh JE: The applied anatomy of the thoracolumbar fascia. Spine 9(2):164–170, 1984.

13. Bogduk N, Twomey LT: Clinical Anatomy of the Lumbar Spine. Churchill Livingstone, Melbourne, pp. 197, 1991.

14. Bogduk N, Tynan W, Wilson AS: The nerve supply to the human lumbar intervertebral disc. J Anat 132(1):39–56, 1981.

15. Bogduk N, Wilson AS, Tynam W: The human lumbar dorsal rami. J Anat 134(2):383–397, 1982.

16. Brown D, Tsaltas T: Studies on the permeability of the intervertebral disc during skeletal maturation. Spine 1:240–244, 1976.

17. Coventry M, Ghormley R, Kernohan J: The intervertebral disc. Its microscopic anatomy and pathology, Part I:Anatomy, development and physiology. J Bone Joint Surg 27:105–112, 1945.

18. Crock HV, Goldwasser M: Anatomic studies of the circulation in the region of the vertebral end-plate in adult greyhound dogs. Spine 9(7):702–706, 1984.

19. Crock HV, Yoshizawa H: The blood supply of the lumbar vertebral column. Clin Orthop 115:6–21, 1976.

20. Crock HV, Yoshizawa H, Kame SK: Observations on the venous drainage of the human vertebral body. J Bone Joint Surg 55B(3):528–533, 1973.

21. Cusick JF, Yoganandan N, Pintar FA, et al: Biomechanics of sequential posterior lumbar surgical alterations. J Neurosurg 76(May):805–811, 1992.

22. Engel R, Bogduk N: The menisci of the lumbar zygapophyseal joints. J Anat 135(4):795–809, 1982.

23. Goel VI, Fromknecht SJ, Nishiyama K, et al: The role of lumbar spinal elements in flexion. Spine 10(6):516–523, 1985.

24. Gracovetsky S, Farfan H, Helleur C: The abdominal mechanism. Spine 10(4):317–324, 1985.

25. Hagg O, Wallner A: Facet joint asymmetry and protrusion of the intervertebral disc. Spine 15(5):356–359, 1990.

26. Higuch M, Kaneda K, Abe K: Postnatal histiogenesis of the cartilage plate of the spinal column. Spine 7:89–96, 1982.

27. Jackson HC II, Winkelmann RK, Bickel WH: Nerve endings in the human lumbar spinal column and related structures. J Bone Joint Surg 48A(7):1272–1281, 1966.

28. Kippers V, Parker AW: Posture related to myoelectric silence of erectores spinae during trunk flexion. Spine 9(7):740–745, 1984.

29. Knutsson F: The instability associated with disk degeneration in the lumbar spine. Acta Radiol 25:593–609, 1944.

30. Leong JC, Luk KDK, Chow DHK, et al: The biomechanical functions of the iliolumbar ligament in maintaining stability of the lumbosacral junction. Spine 12(7):669–674, 1987.

31. Macnab I, Dall D: The blood supply of the lumbar spine and its application to the technique of intertransverse lumbar fusion. J Bone Joint Surg 53B(4):628–638, 1971.

32. Magnusson M, Granqvist M, Johnson F, et al: The loads on the lumbar spine during work at an assembly line. Spine 15:774–779, 1990.

33. Malinsky J: The ontogenetic development of nerve terminations in the intervertebral discs of man. Acta Anat 38:96–113, 1959.

34. Maroudas A, Stockwell R, Nachemson A, et al: Factors involved in the nutrition of the human intervertebral disc: Cellularity and diffusion of glucose in vitro. J Anat 120:113–130, 1975.

35. McDevitt C: Proteoglycans of the intervertebral disc. In The Biology of the Intervertebral Disc. CRC Press, Inc., Boca Raton, Florida, pp. 151–170, 1988.

36. McFadden K, Taylor J: End plate lesions of the lumbar spine. Spine 14:867–869, 1989.

37. Mendel T, Wink CS, Zimny ML: Neural elements in human cervical intervertebral discs. Spine 17(2):132–135, 1992.

38. Noren R, Trafimow J, Andersson GBJ, et al: The role of facet joint tropism and facet angle in disc degeneration. Spine 16(5)530–532, 1991.

39. Oda J, Tanaka H, Tsuzuki N: Intervertebral disc changes with aging of human cervical vertebra. Spine 13:1205–1211, 1988.

40. Ohshima H, Hirano N, Osada R, et al: Morphologic variation of lumbar posterior longitudinal ligament and the modality of disc herniation. Spine 18(16):2408–2411, 1993.

41. Pedersen HE, Blunck CFJ, Gardner E: The anatomy of lumbosacral posterior rami and meningeal branches of spinal nerves (sinu-vertebral nerves). J Bone Joint Surg 38A(2):377–391, 1956.

42. Pritzker K: Aging and degeneration in the lumbar intervertebral disc. Orthop Clin North Am 8:65–77, 1977.

43. Resnick D, Niwayama G: Intervertebral disk herniations: Cartilaginous (Schmorl's) nodes. Radiology 126:57–65, 1978.

44. Rhalmi S, Yahia LH, Newman N, et al: Immunohistochemical study of nerves in lumbar spine ligaments. Spine 18(2):264–267, 1993.

45. Rissanen PM: The surgical anatomy and pathology of the supraspinous and interspinous liga-

ments of the lumbar spine with special reference to ligament ruptures. Acta Orthop Scand Suppl 46:1–100, 1960.

46. Roberts S, Menage J, Urban JPG: Biochemical and structural properties of the cartilage end-plate and its relation to the intervertebral disc. Spine 14(2):166–174, 1989.

47. Roofe PG: Innervation of annulus fibrosus and posterior longitudinal ligament: Fourth and fifth lumbar level. Arch Neurol Psychiatry 44:100–103, 1940.

48. Rosenberg L: Structure and Function of Proteoglycans, ed. D.J. McCarty. Lea and Febiger, Philadelphia pp. 240–255, 1993.

49. Sward L, Hellstrom M, Jacobsson B, et al: Back pain and radiologic changes in the thoracolumbar spine of athletes. Spine 15:124–129, 1990.

50. Taylor JR, Twomey LT: Age changes in lumbar zygapophyseal joints: Observations on structure and fucntion. Spine 11(7):739–745, 1986.

51. Taylor J, Twomey L: The role of the notochord and blood vessels in vertebral column development and in the aetiology of Schmorl's nodes. In Modern Manual Therapy of the Vertebral Column, ed. G.G. Edinburgh. Churchill Livingstone, pp. 21–29, 1986.

52. Taylor J, Twomey L: The development of the human intervertebral disc. In The Biology of the Intervertebral Disc, ed. G. Ghosh. CRC Press, Cleveland, Ohio, 1987.

53. Transfeldt EE, Robertson D, Bradford DS: Ligaments of the lumbosacral spine and their role possible extraforaminal spinal nerve entrapment and tethering. J Spinal Disord 6(6):507–512, 1993.

54. Tyrell AR, Reilly T, Troup JDG: Circadian variation in stature and the effects of spinal loading. Spine 10(2):161–164, 1985.

55. Wiltse LL, Fonseca AS, Amster J, et al: Relationship of the dura, Hofmann's ligaments, Batson's plexus, and a fibrovascular membrane lying on the posterior surface of the vertebral bodies and attaching to the deep layer of the posterior longitudinal ligament: An anatomical, radiologic, and clinical study. Spine 18(8):1030–1043, 1993.

56. Yahia LH, Newman N, Rivard C-H: Neurohistology of lumbar spine ligaments. Acta Orthop Scand 59(5):508–512, 1988.

57. Yoganandan N, Maiman D, Pintar F, et al: Microtrauma in the lumbar spine. Neurosurgery 23:162–168, 1988.

58. Yoshizawa H, O'Brien JP, Smith WT, et al: The neuropathology of intervertebral discs removed for low-back pain. J Pathol 132:95–104, 1980.

CHAPTER 2

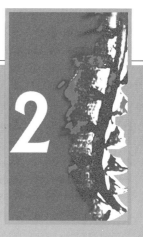

Biomechanics of the Spine: Normal and Pathologic

Spinal Stability

Biomechanics Research

Biomechanics of Spinal Elements

Functional Biomechanics of the Spine

Clinical Evaluation of Stability

Biomechanics of Treatment and Fixation

Future of Biomechanics of the Spine

Biomechanics of the Spine: Normal and Pathologic

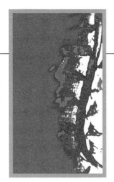

Biomechanics studies the consequences of external forces applied to a structure—in this case, the spine. Such forces may be normal (physiologic) or pathological. Even physiologic forces may be injurious to the structure and functional relationships of spinal structures, and thus produce degenerative disorders and trauma.

In this chapter, we present some technical considerations in biomechanics research and discuss their relevance to spine surgery. The reader is referred to basic works on the fundamentals of biomechanics, including terminology.[20,21,53,56,57,80,82,83,89,95,99] Instead, the interrelation between biologic structure and forces is presented, with an emphasis on the incorporation of biomechanics in clinical practice.

Spinal Stability

For the clinician, a unified theory of instability is important: such is suggested by the authors in Chapter 3. Any simple schematic should account for the development of degenerative changes and predict the outcome of treatment. Needless to say, this is difficult because of the heterogeneity of the spine and the variability of forces applied to it. Thus theories of spinal stability, important as they are, remain largely invalidated.

The classic clinical definition of spinal instability is the loss of the ability of the spine, under physiological loading, to maintain its displacement pattern, to prevent increased deformity and/or neurological deficit.[95] Protection of the spinal cord is a primary consideration, and abnormalities that do not produce major deformity or neurological deficit are not necessarily considered unstable. However, there are less dramatic biomechanical abnormalities that are mechanically significant, representing subclinical failure of multiple components of the spine.[1,13,24,42]

Neutral Zone Theory

The spine and its supporting structures are composed of three subsystems: the passive subsystem includes the vertebrae, ligaments, and disc and is acted upon by the active subsystem (which includes muscles and tendons that apply loads to to the spine). The neural subsystem incorporates the central and peripheral nervous systems and directs the active subsystem to maintain stability of the passive subsystem. Injury to the passive subsystem components can be compensated for by the neural subsystem; an example of this might be muscle spasm to protect a fractured spine.

Panjabi has presented a theory of spinal stability that reconciles the in vivo interrelationships between these spinal subsystems.[68–70] This hypothesis emphasizes the nonlinear nature of spinal loading. Loads delivered at the initiation of the load-deformation curve have different effects on deformation of the spine than those in the later, prefailure phases. There are two nonfailure components to the curve (Fig. 2–1), which together represent the normal range of the spine:

1. The *neutral zone* represents the portion of the ordinary physiologic motion of the spine measured from the neutral position, in which motion is produced with little internal resistance; that is, the spine is very flexible here.

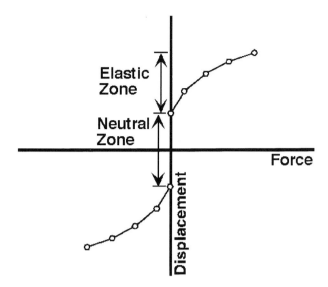

FIGURE 2-1 Schematic representation of "neutral zone." The neutral zone is the portion of the normal range of the spine measured from neutral position. In the "elastic zone," internal resistance to motion (for example, from muscles) exists; in order for the spine to continue bending, additional loads are required to overcome this resistance.

2. The *elastic zone* is still part of the physiologic loading of the structure, extending from the end of the neutral zone up to the end of physiologic loading, beyond which tissue injury occurs. Here motion is a consequence of overcoming internal resistance; thus the structure is usually at its maximal stiffness. Because tissue injury may occur at the upper margins of this stiffness curve, leading to later degenerative changes, this zone should not necessarily be considered part of the physiologic loading of the spine.

The neutral zone increases in spinal trauma and decreases in size after spinal fixation. Changes in the size of the neutral zone may be more significant than altered range of motion as predictors of injury, although measurement of the former may be difficult. Therefore, the clinical definition of instability mentioned at the beginning of this chapter has been modified to include the capacity of the spine to maintain the size of the neutral zone, as well as to prevent pain, deformity, and neurological deficit.

There appear to be clinical correlates for this theory. Preservation of a relatively normal neutral zone may be important to the integrity of the spine.

For example, the absence of a neutral zone as the result of a rigid fixation construct may be associated with pain, as we are only too aware.

Column Theories

Although theoretical constructs as described above are popular in the laboratory, clinicians tend to favor concepts of stability that can directly be applied to a given clinical situation. For example, Neumann et al conducted elegant investigations in an effort to determine radiographic criteria for instability in flexion-distraction (the "lap belt" injury). They concluded that, even in the absence of middle column injury, impending instability exists if there is kyphosis measuring more than 12 degrees at the level of injury, or more than 2 cm of distance between the spinous processes.[66] In our studies using dynamic loading, these findings were seen at the beginning of spine failure. Unfortunately, these criteria are only valid for a specific type of spinal injury. The authors are also careful to emphasize that these guidelines are not usable when there is substantial vertebral injury.[66]

The problem, of course, is that instability in injuries with obvious ligament injury (such as dislocation) is not difficult to determine. Rather, it is those cases where bone injury predominates that torture the clinician. Thus, the effort to develop theories of instability that emphasize visible structural injury: these include the "two-column" and "three-column" theories.

Two-Column Theory

Holdsworth held that the spine is composed of two "columns": the vertebral body, intervertebral disc, and its connecting ligaments constituting the anterior column, and the posterior elements and posterior ligamentous complex constituting the posterior column (Fig. 2–2).[37,38] Some argue that instability results from injury to the posterior ligamentous complex; most others, including us, assume that instability requires significant injury of either column and partial injury of the other. The two-column concept is validated by significant amounts of clinical data.[6,23,39,48,54,55,104]

The determination of stability using the two-column theory may be inaccurate: theoretically, a 50% or greater compression fracture with normal poste-

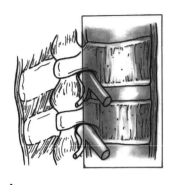
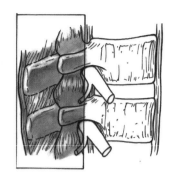

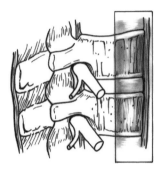
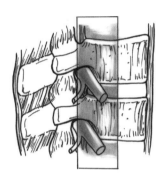
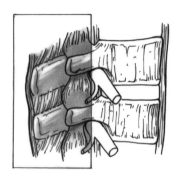

FIGURE 2–2 Two- and three-column concepts of stability. **A** Two-column theory. The anterior column (left) includes the vertebra, disc, and anterior and posterior longitudinal ligaments. The posterior column (right) includes the posterior elements and ligaments.[56,57]
B Three-column theory. The anterior column (left) includes the anterior longitudinal ligament, anterior disc, and vertebra. The middle column incorporates the posterior vertebra and disc, posterior longitudinal ligament, and (perhaps) the pedicle. The posterior column includes the posterior elements and ligaments.

rior ligaments is stable; however, in reality such a spine is at risk, as described below. However, significant anterior column injury without posterior element compromise is unlikely.[5,21,43,49,65,80,81]

Three-Column Theory

The most popular clinically based theory is probably that of Denis.[14] In this three-column model (Fig. 2–2), the posterior column includes the posterior ligamentous complex and arch. The middle column includes the posterior longitudinal ligament, the posterior aspect of the intervertebral disc and annulus, and the posterior aspect of the vertebral body. The anterior column is composed of the anterior vertebral body and disc and the anterior longitudinal ligament. The primary modification from Holsworth's two-column spine is assigning the posterior body and disc to prevent translation and anterior motion. Instability is graded on the basis of column injury and is assumed if two of the three spinal columns are injured. Thus the middle column becomes critical.

Transection of the posterior ligamentous complex *alone* does not produce instability.[31,75,79,92] When the posterior longitudinal ligament and posterior disc are also transected, biomechanical instability may result.[94] However, there is evidence that the most common type of spine loading, compression of the anterior and distraction of the posterior elements, produces posterior ligaments injury *prior* to vertebral body compression and is often unstable.[5,31,39,44,50,53] In these injuries, an additional load is placed on both vertebra and the middle column.

Panjabi et al have conducted biomechanical studies that have, to a significant degree, validated this concept of stability and have emphasized the role of the middle column in maintaining spinal stability. High-speed fractures were produced using pure axial loading or flexion-compression. Simply stated, column flexibility correlated most to middle-column injury.[72,73] Although important, this study ignores the effects of muscle forces and only partially incorporates the spinal ligaments.

The determination of ligament injury from static radiography is difficult. Studies of kinematics during spinal loading and fracture have shown significant variability in injuries produced with similar forces. As discussed later, partial injuries to structures such as the disc and body, as well as spinal ligaments, may allow pathologic motion, even if gross failure is not evident. Individuals with these injuries may be at risk for late deformity.

Continuum Concept

We prefer to consider experimental spinal stability as a continuum, with anatomic changes preceding physiologic abnormalities (i.e., pathologic motion).[101,105] Instability is not necessarily the product of destruction of spinal structures, but can be the product of partial injury to multiple components. Of particular concern is that over the spectrum of physiologic loading, one often reaches the margins of safe loading, defined by us as the physiologic loading region, and by Panjabi as the elastic zone.[70,71] During repeated loading in this region, microtrauma to spinal components may occur which is not radiographically apparent, but produces pain because of abnormal motion or alignment.

As can be observed from the force-deformation curve (Fig. 2-3), the traumatic loading zone does not represent the failure point of the spine; while anatomic injury is occurring, the spine is still resisting external loads, although less effectively than in the linear part of the curve.

Gross failure, defined as the point at which further loads are poorly resisted and the spine responds with increasing deformation, is easily determined. It is more difficult to determine the point at which injury to the spine is initiated, which may be more important in the area of degenerative diseases. For disc injury, our studies suggest that this point is reached when the end plates are injured.[101,103] However, even in trauma, the definition of instability must address the integrity of each spinal component.

In attempting to define spinal stability, then, several factors need to be considered. These include the force and mechanism of injury and the radiographic appearance of the lesion and structure involved. Results of biomechanical studies, as outlined below, should be incorporated into the

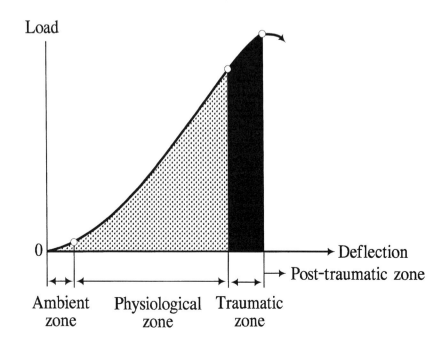

FIGURE 2-3
The continuum concept as described by Yoganandan et al.[101,102,108] This idealized force-deformation curve demonstrates four phases of loading. During the physiological zone, load/deformation behavior is almost linear. The critical phase is the traumatic zone, or the area of microtrauma. Here, although not grossly pathologic, injury to components of the column occurs, often not visible on radiography.

Biomechanics Research

This book concerns itself primarily with surgical treatment of disorders of the lumbar spine. However, surgeons need to have fundamental—and critical—understanding of research techniques in order to incorporate sound science into clinical practice. Biomechanics is a research-based discipline; deductive biomechanics should be rejected.

The spine should be considered as a modified column behaving in a non-linear manner rather than as a collection of motion segments, since the latter behave differently.

The smallest structure on which research regarding relationships between spinal components can be performed is the motion segment, composed of two vertebrae, the intermediate disc, and spinal ligaments. Motion segment research focuses on local structures such as the disc, as well as local effects of external forces, such as the pull-out strength of pedicle screws.[18,32] The behavior of the motion segment is a function of the relative proportions of its heterogeneous components, including ligaments (whose sizes vary from level to level), and spinal curvatures. For example, a thoracic motion segment behaves differently than one from the lumbar spine, even when both are subjected to similar loads.

Thus investigation of the macromodel (the spinal column itself) becomes critical. Although some have attempted to deduce column behavior in situations like trauma from motion segments, the use of an entire region has been shown to be more accurate. Not only can the biomechanics of the region be studied—for example, fracture biomechanics of the lumbar spine in response to pure-moment loading—but the effects of treatments such as fixation can be better predicted.

Studies of entire cadavers are particularly edifying for studying the relationships between the head and spine and between the spinal cord and the spine.[82,103] Such investigations are quite physiologic; the researcher can actually mimic what happens in the real trauma situations. However, experiments using full cadavers are rarely conducted because of difficulties in measuring and controlling the applied forces and in measuring the responses throughout the area of interest.

Loading Variables

Pure Moment and Complex Loading

Loading patterns also affect the nature and results of biomechanical studies. The simplest method of spinal loading is to use pure moments, i.e., to apply unidirectional forces around a single axis. These pure forces can be applied for each of the six possible moments (flexion, extension, right and left lateral bending, and right and left axial rotation); load magnitude can increase only to spine deformation (non-destructive loading) or to actual injury and failure.[11,26,33]

In pure moment loading, the amount of applied external force is controlled (load-control). The determination of load-deformation behavior, which is a primary consideration in spinal biomechanics, is probably best done using this type of loading. Pure moment loading has become increasingly popular over the last several years because it is more controllable than the alternatives.

A more complex technique for loading combines various forces, most commonly flexion and compression.[16,17] Although technically more difficult to perform and interpret, complex loading more effectively mimics the in vivo situation; for example, both clinical and some experimental studies have emphasized that thoracolumbar fractures are typically produced by complex loading (i.e., multimoment loading). In addition, translation and rotation can be easily applied in addition to flexion-compression, which may be critical clinically.

Why use complex loading if it is more technically difficult? Pure moment loading may introduce some inaccuracies if those data are extrapolated to the more complex clinical condition. For example, Edwards et al have shown that specimen stiffness is doubled by the addition of even small amounts of compression to pure moment loading.[17] Furthermore, lumbar motion segments are stiffer in flexion than in extension; the former are stiffer at high loads than at low loads.

Both loading options are valuable in the study of the spine: load-deformation behavior, determined by displacement control, is a fundamental biomechanical response. In creating clinical injury, complex loading or displacement control is critical. Pure moment loading may be best used to compare single variables: for example, pure moment loading of spines instrumented with fixation devices allows simple comparisons for each of the ordinary forces applied to the spine. However, cyclic loading with complex forces may provide accurate comparisons of the in vivo condition.[16] This controversy remains to be solved in the laboratory.

Quasistatic and Dynamic Loading

Loading rates can also be varied. The spine generally behaves as a viscoelastic structure and therefore responds differently to quasistatic (studying bodies at rest or being loaded at slow rates) and dynamic loading.[16,29,67,102] As is true for other variables in biomechanics research, the most controllable loading rate, quasistatic, is not always the most physiologic. More rapid dynamic techniques are necessary when evaluating most common injury-producing scenarios, but are much more difficult to control and monitor.

The spine is stiffer during dynamic loading, like a shock absorber whose compression is altered by the speed of loading. Data using dynamic loading have much more direct application to clinical injury than studies using static loading. Probably, quasistatic loading is best used for nondestructive loading and to provide information about material properties of spinal components; if failure mechanics are being studied, dynamic loading is more valuable.

For example, in our own quasistatic loading studies of thoracolumbar spinal columns taken to failure, the sequence of injury in the thoracolumbar spine is posterior element injury followed by vertebral body fracture. In dynamic loading, although the ultimate injuries may be similar, the sequence is altered, with vertebral compression sometimes occurring first.[52,53]

Others have studied this difference in loading rates and have considered the effect on neural injury. In one study, calf lumbar motion segments were used; transducers were placed in the spinal canal. Axial compression loads were applied at 20 msec or 400 msec. Spines loaded at the former had approximately 7% canal occlusion; for the higher loading rate groups, mean canal encroachment was over 47%. Not only is the severity of canal compromise different, but the authors hypothesized that the mechanism of fracture might even be different.[92]

Similarly, preloading (that is, aligning the spinal column in a given direction or with a small load on it prior to the major force application) is very important in quasistatic loading. If the spine is preloaded in flexion, for example, the major injury vector tends to be flexion, although intermediate column buckling may alter this phenomenon.[53] In dynamic loading, the effects of preloading are less predictable.

In a recent effort, motion segments were subjected to complex flexion-shear dynamic loading in order to produce injury, followed by static physiologic loading of the injured specimens to assess residual stability. In contradistinction to the results discussed above, bone density was the most important parameter in determining stability after trauma. Higher loading rates produced instability with less deformity, reflecting the increased stiffness of the motion segment during dynamic loading. Neumann et al recommend the use of complex loading, which they feel is more physiologic.[67] Indeed, efforts to produce complex dynamic loading are recognized as increasingly important: in a few short years, our understanding of the biomechanics of the thoracolumbar spine may radically change.

Biomechanics of Spinal Elements

Vertebra

The vertebral body resists tension better than compression.[100] With tension loading, failure is routinely observed at the disc end plate rather than in the body. Compression strength decreases more caudally in the lumbar spine and is a consequence of the orientation of the bony trabeculae and bone density.[27] The compressive strength of the vertebral body decreases about 50% at age 50.[9,27,43]

The articular processes are oriented to allow judicious motion of the spine and vary by region. From T1 to T10 the facets are almost coronal in orientation, but are sagittally directed at lower thoracic levels and in the lumbar spine. The particularly abrupt changes in the orientation of the facets at T11 render this transitional region susceptible to dislocation. The facets limit rotation more effectively than they resist translation.

The facets are important in normal loading of the spine, accepting over 20% of axial compression.[34] Loads are effectively distributed across the facets and vertebral body in the resting position; however, when loads are moved anteriorly by 5 mm in front of the center of the vertebra, strains increase in the vertebra as the facets are unloaded. Therefore, it is reasonable to assume that posterior element injury—often purely ligamentous—occurs with anterior loading. Especially in the case of degenerative changes associated with long-term loading at the upper part of the physiologic range, posterior element changes can be expected.

Intervertebral Disc

The biomechanics of the disc have been extensively studied, especially in compression. Many studies have suggested that end plate failure precedes disc failure; some have suggested that disc failure due to axial compression never occurs. This is partially because the normal nucleus pulposus acts hydrostatically during direct compressions, and pressures are uniformly distributed.[41] Actual failure in direct compression does not often occur without prior injury of the vertebra.[57] However, injury of the disc without gross bony failure certainly does occur.[65]

During all but direct compression, a portion of the disc is subjected to tension forces, under which the disc is less stiff. Torsion and bending loads are more dangerous to the disc than compression, with failure due to torsion with as little as 15 degrees of axial twist.[65] Roaf noted that bulging of the annulus occurs only on the concave side (away from the bending).[81] During torsion, shear stresses are seen principally at the peripheral aspect of the disc, with horizontal shear stiffness at 260 N/mm at failure.[58,65] This high load requirement suggests that disc failure due to pure shear loads is unlikely; instead, bending and/or torsion is necessary.[84]

As important as actual disruption of the disc may appear, degeneration of the disc as a function of repetitive loading may be a more significant phenomenon. Studies have shown that the disc is at its stiffest during physiologic elastic loading.[84,97,101] However, as loads increase, trauma to the disc occurs gradually, with microfailure—not often discernible on radiography—and with yielding of the disc. This is the point at which trauma has initiated. Eventually, with continued loading, stiffness decreases to zero, and gross failure occurs. The recognition that initiation of disc trauma can occur without visible changes is important clinically, representing the stage at which mechanical pain and osteophyte formation may begin. In addition, disc microtrauma may lead to increased loading of the facet joints and subsequent degeneration of these joints, even if the disc appears generally normal.

Spinal Ligaments

The spinal ligaments and joint capsules preserve the articulated nature of the spine, allowing restrained movement. For example, Sharma et al used finite element analysis to demonstrate that ligaments carry primary responsibility for resisting rotational forces and that retrospondylolisthesis and flexion-rotation instability do not occur without ligament injury.[85]

Anterior Longitudinal Ligament

The anterior longitudinal ligament (ALL) is composed primarily of longitudinally arranged collagen fibers aligned in interdigitating layers. The deepest of its three layers attaches to the edges of adjacent intervertebral discs; the middle layer binds to the bodies and discs over three levels, and the superficial fibers extend four to five layers. The ligament is thickest at the concavity of the vertebra, blending into the periosteum. Because of the high proportion of collagen in its composition and its firm bony attachments, the primary action of the anterior longitudinal ligament is to prevent hyperextension and overdistraction.

In tension, the mean breaking loads of the lumbar ALL averages 600 Newtons.[63,75,77] Although the breaking load values found for the anterior longitudinal ligament are approximately double those found for other ligaments (particularly the posterior longitudinal ligament), when one considers the values as a function of cross-sectional areas, breaking stresses are similar. As in most other studies, strength increases with loading rate.[102]

Posterior Longitudinal Ligament

The posterior longitudinal ligament (PLL) is located on the dorsum of the vertebral body from the axis to the sacrum. Like the ALL, this ligament consists of several layers, with the deep fibers extending to adjacent vertebrae and the stronger superficial fibers spanning several levels. The ligament closely adheres to the disc annulus, but only marginally to the vertebral body. This ligament is much thinner over the vertebral body than the disc, and is thickest overall in the thoracic region. It is substantially smaller in diameter (one-fourth to one-tenth) than the anterior longitudinal ligament.[75,77]

The PLL limits hyperflexion of the spine; in our clinical and experimental experience, it deforms less than the ALL. The tensile strength of the PLL ranges from 67 to 138 N.[77] Reliance on this relatively weak ligament to push bone fragments out of the spinal canal and back into the vertebral body during distraction may thus be unrealistic.

Ligamentum Flavum

The ligamentum flavum is a highly elastic paired ligament that arises from the ventral surface of the lower lamina and attaches to the dorsal border of the more cephalad lamina. The ligaments are discontinuous at midvertebral levels and in the midline, extend laterally to the joint capsules, and become confluent with them. They have their largest cross-sectional diameter in the lumbar spine.

Tensile strength of the ligamentum flavum is greatest at lower thoracic levels (mean = 300 N). Resting forces range from 18 N in the young to 5 N in the elderly, with proportional decrease in elasticity due to ligament fibrosis.[64] Certain types of degenerative pathology of the spine (lumbar stenosis, kyphosis) may increase the thickness of the ligament.[63]

The ligamentum flavum allows flexion of the spine with separation of the laminae and return of the laminae to their normal position. Because of both the elasticity of the ligament and the special extension seen in the resting state, a significant amount of extension can occur without permanent deformation of the ligament. White and Panjabi suggest that this characteristic is particularly important in preventing impingement on the spinal cord when the spine goes from flexion to extension (during which time the ligament is relaxed).[95]

Capsular Ligaments

The capsular ligaments and joint capsule attach to the vertebrae adjacent to the articular joints. The fibers tend to be taut and are perpendicular to the plane of the facets. Thus they serve primarily to limit distraction, and to a lesser degree to prevent translation. During anterior eccentric axial loading, these ligaments may be subjected to stretch. It is not very elastic and resists tension well. Preliminary studies showed tension failure occurring at 150 to 270 N in the thoracic region.[75,77]

Intertransverse Ligaments

The intertransverse ligaments are seen in the upper lumbar spine. They pass between the transverse processes and attach to the deep muscles of the back. Because of their large lever arms in lateral bending and axial rotation, these ligaments may have a disproportionate effect on the normal mechanics of the spine.[64]

Interspinous and Supraspinous Ligaments

The interspinous and supraspinous ligaments connect adjacent spinous processes. The former attach from the base to the tip of each spinous process, and the latter at their tips. The former ligament is most prominent in the lumbar region. These ligaments limit hyperflexion. We found that the interspinous ligament fails in tension at approximately one-third to one-half the values for the ALL.[75,77]

Instability

Failure patterns vary between ligaments. Indeed, the same ligaments may have different patterns at different levels. These differences relate to the geometry of the spine at different regions (i.e, the posterior elements are subjected to more tension during flexion than are the anterior ligaments). The type of attachment of the ligament to the spine is of importance: some ligaments are most likely to fail by avulsion from their bony insertions. The amount of deflection is related both to the proportion of elastic fibers composing the ligament, and also to the distance from the vertebral center of rotation.[3,44] As a result, for a given ligament, the strength tends to be greater on the convex side of curves than on concave surfaces.

These differences in failure patterns are of value in analyzing the traumatized spine. Although it is safe to assume that ligament rupture requires pathologic tension applied to the ligament itself, the same may not be true if failure is produced by avulsion from the spinal attachment.

In addition, all ligament injury may not consist of failure; there may be attenuation or partial disruption that causes weakening. Nachemson and Evans have shown that ligaments deform linearly; when they begin to fail, their curves become nonlinear.[65] Our data suggest that ligament injury occurs prior to spinal dislocation, not as a consequence of it,[53,103] and loss of ligament integrity produces loss of spinal alignment.

Functional Biomechanics of the Spine

Lumbar Spine Motion

Physiologic motion of the spine is both facilitated and inhibited by the musculature. Anterior muscle groups flex the spine. Oblique muscles, such as the abdominal obliques, cause spine rotation. Others, such as the psoas group, participate in lateral bending as well as rotation. Both superficial and deep posterior muscles promote extension of the spine; most muscles also are involved with rotation (such as the semispinalis) or lateral bending. The muscles found lateral to the spinal column are involved in lateral rotation as well as bending.

When considering the role of muscles in motion of the spine, one must recognize that typically several groups are simultaneously activated.[98] For example, maintenance of posture requires support of the weight of the torso. If the center of gravity of the torso is shifted, a counterbalancing force is required on the other side. Here, the longissimus dorsi muscles are generally active during standing. During rotation of the lumbar spine, the ipsilateral erector spinae and contralateral short rotators actively contract.

The extent of normal range of motion in the lumbar spine is of critical importance because of the extensive coupling, as well as the strong relationship of motion to the development of degenerative changes. In a sophisticated study by McGregor et al, normal volunteers underwent three-dimensional motion testing using a potentiometer-based system. Motion decreased as a function of age.[61] These differences may have implications in predicted outcomes from spinal surgery, and therefore have great value.

Overall, flexion measured 80 to 95 degrees in the younger population and about 60 degeees in the 60 to 70 group. Rotation was about 30 degrees in each direction, and lateral bending between 25 and 35 degrees, again decreasing in the oldest group.[74] Nonpublished studies from our group have found lumbar range of motion to be equal in younger populations undergoing successful fusion and postoperative rehabilitation with those treated nonoperatively. Older patients with excellent results following surgery had better range of motion in all directions than younger patients with continued pain and disability.

In per level measurements, flexion-extension increases caudally, from 12 to 14 degrees at L1 to 18 degrees at L5-S1. Lateral bending changes little, averaging 7 to 9 degrees throughout the lumbar spine. Similarly, rotation is consistent and extremely limited, averaging 3 degrees per level. In considering the little-studied area of translation (which is important in diagnosing degenerative instability), 2 mm is probably normal for the lumbar spine.

Coupling is an important phenomenon in the lumbar spine. The most clinically relevant pattern is that of axial rotation and lateral bending, again with strong relevance in the development of degenerative disc disease.[95,98] As discussed earlier, this pattern is paradoxical: the spinous process is directed in the same direction as the lateral bending; this is the opposite of that seen in the rest of the spine.

Biomechanics of Thoracic and Lumbar Spine Trauma

The Burst Fracture

The true burst fracture is produced primarily by axial loading. Several classical reports suggest that as the forces are directed through the vertebra, the intervertebral disc is traumatized, with fragments pushed into the vertebral body, creating at most a "two-column" injury. Typically, the end plate is injured by bulging of the disc; vertebral body fracture follows.[12,25,42,53,80] Continued loading pushes vertebral fragments into the spinal canal.

Theoretically, the burst fracture is stable in terms of the development of deformity, although the bone itself may have failed. Many authors have classified three-column injuries without deformity or ligament injury as burst fractures, focusing on the presumed mechanism of injury.[12,59,60] In biomechanical studies, however, disruption of the anterior and posterior longitudinal ligaments by disc herniation through the annulus is occasionally observed. The mechanism of this is uncertain: our efforts suggest that intermediate column buckling, with production of a flexion or extension bending moment and ligament injury, often occurs.[37] In addition, kinematic studies have also shown that some element of shear loading occurs during loading. In true experimental burst fractures, kinematic studies showed little movement of the targets in any direction; up to 80% compression of the vertebral body can occur in as little as 2 to 5 msec.[103]

Slosar et al created burst fractures in lumbar spinal segments using axial loads, and then subjected the injured segments to flexion, lateral bending, and axial rotation. Bilinear load-deformation curves, similar to those we've acquired for flexion-compression fractures, were observed with initial injury. When the spines were reloaded after fracture initial loss stiffness was seen with all subsequent nonpathologic loading (up to 10 Nm), and worst with axial loading. This corresponded to the weakness of the bone at the fracture site. Allowing the burst fracture to remain somewhat collapsed, rather than attempt physiologic reduction, provided more stability. As expected, the worst instability was seen with injury to the posterior elements: this did not include simple laminar fracture, which did not alter the behavior of the specimen.[87]

When fixated with pedicle screws one level above and one below the injured segment, stiffness was increased beyond that of the intact spine at lower loads (i.e., the first peak of the bimodal curve). At higher loads, in flexion, the column stiffness was similar to that of the intact specimen. If there was posterior element injury, so common in thoracolumbar fractures requiring stabilization, poor resistance to axial rotation was observed.

The authors conclude by emphasizing that the "behavior" of the fracture should determine treatment. That is, the premise is that stabilization reduces significant deformity and promotes fusion. However, correction of body collapse may be counterproductive, since this vertebral compression adds stability. Indeed, in our series of single-level (i.e., one above and one below) fixation for trauma, some collapse and loss of correction was always seen.

Flexion-Compression Injuries

Laboratory and clinical studies suggest that the majority of lumbar fractures are related to both compression of the vertebral body and multilevel distraction injuries of the posterior elements.[6,14,24,38,54,103]

In what we call flexion-compression loading, referring to what happens biomechanically rather than anatomically, a load is developed over the dorsum of the upper thoracic spine or through the base of the pelvis, with a lever arm developed at the eventual level of failure. The injury typically produced by this type of loading has also been termed the "Type C" burst fracture, or sometimes flexion-distraction injury.[60]

In the sitting position, the center of mass of the torso at the thoracolumbar junction is 4 cm anterior to the vertebra. Flexion of the thoracolumbar spine occurs during impact to the dorsum of the spine or up through the pelvis. Because of this flexion moment, distraction loads transmitted to the posterior elements may be more pronounced than the compression loads applied to the vertebrae. In intact cadaver and spinal column studies using quasistatic loading, early disruption of the posterior elements has been a consistent finding. Indeed, posterior ligamentous instability almost always occurs before vertebral fracture.[53,56] Findings may be different with dynamic loading, however. Here, injury of the posterior disc and posterior longitudinal ligament typically is the third part of the sequence, occurring after the vertebral fracture, although failure of the joint capsule occurs shortly after posterior ligament complex injury.[103]

Chance Fractures

We believe the Chance—or seat belt—fracture represents a modification of flexion-compression loading in which the predominant force is flexion, often incorporating some shear. The axis of loading is anterior to the spine, and progressive disruption of the posterior elements, followed by the disc and posterior longitudinal ligament, occurs. Typically, however, the load stops short of major compression of the vertebral body.

In the compression-flexion fracture with its prominent vertebral fracture, axial loading occurs simultaneously with the flexion moment, thus producing combined injury. In the seat belt injury, on the other hand, the top of the torso flexes over the fixed pelvis.[54,55]

Osteoporotic Fractures

These fractures are typically associated with trivial trauma, and may even occur with activities of normal living. Conventional thinking is that resorption of bone leads to decreased bone density and thinking of trabeculae. This effect is historically thought to be seen primarily in the horizontal trabeculae. Studies by Snyder et al have shown this not to be true, it appears that transverse trabeculae are less subject to resorption for unknown reasons.[89]

In a study using a finite element model, axial loading produced major tensile stresses at the cortical shell under the end plate. Reductions in both the trabecular and cortical bone moduli increased displacement but did not affect peak stress, but reducing the trabecular bone modulus by 50% increased peak stresses in the end plate. Elimination of the cortical shell reduced peak stress in the end plate by only 20%. With anterior compression, disproportionate modulus reductions in trabecular and cortical bone increases end plate and cortical shell stresses. This suggests that many osteoporatic fractures may have involved flexion forces applied to the anterior vertebra.[62] The typical preservation of the posterior elements may be related to this eccentric loading, or may be a consequence of the significantly increased proportion of cortical bone in the posterior elements, with its higher modulus.

Clinical Evaluation of Stability

One important consideration in the evaluation of the spine fracture is the degree of compression of the vertebral body. Vertebral body compression fractures of more than 50% are often considered unstable, although instability may be seen even with minimal compression, and isolated vertebral compression is rarely unstable. Evaluation of the posterior elements should include an overall view of spinal alignment. Increased distance between spinous processes often indicates disruption of the posterior ligamentous complex, presumably as the result of posterior distraction during flexion-compression loading. This picture suggests instability. Fractures of the pedicles and separation of the facets are of similar concern. Indeed, the best determination of thoracic and lumbar instability may come from the evaluation of pedicle status (interpedicular distance, fracture)[5] from the anteroposterior radiograph, as well as evidence of lateral translation. Certainly, fractures with deformity should be considered unstable.

Posterior element trauma can easily be missed on plain films because of the direction of the fracture line and because even severe ligament injury may not produce spinal dislocation at rest. Unfortunately, dynamic radiography such as is used in the cervical spine is rarely suitable. Thus one must evaluate the components of the fracture individually, as well as consider the nature of the forces producing trauma in making the determination of stability.

Biomechanics of Treatment and Fixation

Most studies of the biomechanical effects of treatment of spinal disorder have focused on the effects of spinal instrumentation on the stiffness of the spine. However, seemingly trivial treatment such as aggressive rehabilitation programs may positively affect spinal stability. Yet unpublished studies investigating spinal motion using motion analysis and internally measured forces (using thin-wire pressure transducers or flouroscopy) have suggested that such rehabilitation improves the range of motion to levels similar to lumbar fusion in patients with degenerative lumbar spine syndromes.

Surgical manipulations have an impact as well. Pediatric neurosurgeons have long known that laminectomy, particularly cervical, has an adverse mechanical effect on spinal alignment, causing kyphosis and deformity. In adults, scolosis may result from laminectomy in the patient with increased motion. Because of the heterogeneity of this phenomenon, however, cadaver studies are difficult.

Mathematical models have been proposed for studies of deformity.

Studies in the thoracolumbar spine indicate that biomechanical considerations are different than elsewhere in the spine. First, according to Denis,[14] the middle column acquires prominence. Second, loading factors are somewhat different, with larger bending moments delivered.[50] The following sections emphasize studies of transpedicular fixation, the "gold standard" of spinal fixation.

Intervertebral Fusion

Along with an increased clinical interest in anterior lumbar interbody and posterior lumbar interbody fusions is concern about the biomechanics of treatment. Tencer et al conducted extensive studies on intervertebral cages in cadaver and goat spines. Pure moment loading was used, and stiffness as well as neutral zone angles were measured. Orientation of placement did not affect stiffness except for torsional stiffness, which was decreased by posterior lumbar interbody fusion (PLIF) as a result of lamina and facet destruction. Cages decreased flexion and lateral bending as compared to the intact spine; cages were more effective in decreasing flexion than bony PLIF.[91]

Glazer et al recently compared two anterior interbody cages, lateral hollow Texas Scottish Rite Hospital (TSRH) interbody screws and anterior bone graft with anterior TSRH instrumentation. They found the cages to be comparable to TSRH instrumentation in axial rotation; stiffness was similar for the intervertebral screws and conventional instrumentation. The cages have significant benefit in their safety and in the direct promotion of fusion.[28]

In our yet unpublished studies on the biomechanics of cages, we have been exploring the ideal geometry of placement. In cadaver studies using pure moment loading, a single cage placed obliquely has been equivalent biomechanically to two cages placed in the traditional manner. This may be because of the preservation of a facet or because a single cage is simply adequate for stiffening the motion segment. The addition of spinous process wiring may increase stiffness even more.

Posterior Instrumentation

Several older studies investigated the biomechanics of Harrington distraction rodding. Jacobs et al determined years ago that a "tension band" is the best replacement for the incompetent ligaments in flexion injuries,[40] a principle that remains valid today.

Most investigators have found that Harrington distraction rods are effective in reducing dislocation but often disengage in flexion. Panjabi et al compared compression and distraction rods using three-point bending[69] and found distraction rods to be five times stiffer than compression rods. They recommended that distraction rods be used to reduce deformaties, and compression rods to improve stability.

Flexion loading has been used to compare Harrington distraction and compression rods and Roy-Camille plates fixed to the pedicles.[40] Distraction rods did not reduce deformaties well and failed easily. Compression rods fixated to the lamina and pedicle screw and plates fixed segmentally both performed well, failing at moments of 80 Nm with fractures at the fixation points. McAfee et al evaluated Harrington distraction rods and Luque rods in axial compression and rotation. The Luque rods provided the greatest stiffness and resistance to rotation.[59] In our own studies, Harrington distraction rods failed at low loads in flexion and were less stiff than sublaminar-wired Luque rods.[52] Further unpublished studies suggested that spinous process wiring improved the stiffness of Harrington rods, but that the hooks still were likely to fail in flexion.

"Universal" Instrumentation

In the early 1980s, the Cotrel-Dubousset "CD Universal Instrumentation" system was presented. Developed for scoliosis, it soon found applications in trauma, tumor, and degenerative disease. CD became quite popular, quite quickly, because of the flexibility in bone choices it offered and its quality of stabilization. Several competing systems of similar fundamental configuration have become available.

The biomechanics of universal instrumentation has been widely studied. Indeed, characteristics of the many different brands available are similar; differences are more related to the configuration of the construct.

An early biomechanical study of the Cotrel-Dubousset system comparing it to the more traditional segmentally wired Harrington distraction rods and Luque rods was carried out by Farcy et al.[22] Axial and rotational stiffness were determined for Cotrel-Dubousset at one and two levels above and below the "injured" vertebra, and compared with segmentally wired Harrington distraction rods and Luque rods placed two above and two below, using single-cycle quasistatic loading. Harrington rods demonstrated the lowest stiffness. In the calf spines, the single-level Cotrel-Dubousset was not stiffer axially than the other devices tested, but was more stable in torsion. However, as we have noted previously, most fractures are related to flexion-compression, and the forces that must be resisted for effective instrumentation are more related to axial configurations. Axial stability of two-level CD instrumentation was four times greater than Harrington distraction rods or single-level Coterl-Dubousset instrumentation.

In a related study by Kornblatt et al, translaminar facet fixation and Galveston/Luque pelvic fixation were compared in flexion and translation. Pelvic fixation was clearly stiffer than the other constructs tested. Although the authors' primary purpose in presenting this effort was to biomechanically validate transfacet screw fixation, which has not been popular in this country, it served well to point out the benefits of fixation to the pelvis.[45] Indeed, in performing repeat fusion in patients with persistent nonunion at L4–5 and L5–S1, fixation to the pelvis is valuable.

Pedicular Fixation In Trauma

Pedicle fixation is the most commonly used technique for stabilization of the traumatized lumbar spine (for good reason), and is commonly used to reverse subfailure resulting from degenerative disease and its treatment. Pedicle screw placement may provide three-column fixation, thereby allowing fewer segments to be incorporated.[2,8,15,30,36,90]

Geometry of Pedicle Fixation

Optimal geometry has been studied extensively. As important as studies on the effects of instrumentation are, surgeons require information on ideal geometry to assist them in developing constructs for given patients. These need to be configured for optimal stiffness, alignment, bone growth, and maximal patient comfort. Control of costs by eliminating nonessential components is also increasingly important. For example, Krag et al examined the effect of depth of screw insertion into the vertebral body, finding that depth into the body was significantly related to pull-out strength.[47]

In vitro evaluation to determine the role of transverse fixation and rod orientation on rotational stability has been performed.[78] Pedicle screws were mounted in polymethylmethacrylate molded to mimic lumbar vertebrae. Rod lengths of 6, 12, and 15 cm were used. In the rotation studies, twenty cycles were applied at loads of 15 Nm. Constructs were tested with medial or lateral rod placement, and with none, one, or two transverse fixators. In the flexion studies, loads of 120 N at 15 cm were applied to similar-length constructs incorporating Steffee plates or Isola rods.

With no transverse fixators, lateral rod placement was 20% stiffer in rotation than medial placement, particularly at the longer rod lengths. Although transverse fixators stiffened the medial rod constructs, they were still less than the lateral rods except at 18 cm. Except at longest lengths, one transverse was equal to two in rotation. Flexion studies failed to show any increased stiffness for any particular configuration. Most rotation occurred at the screw/vertebra interface, and such rotation was not decreased by placement of transverse fixators at the point of the screw. We concluded that lateral rod placement, with medially directed screws and with a single transverse fixator, may be the optimal configuration for short-segment fixation of the traumatized thoracolumbar spine. However, clinical considerations such as device fit and area for bone grafting have made this configuration impractical. In this same group of studies, we found Isola rod constructs to be as stiff as Luque plates.

Similar studies were carried out by Lin et al using cadaver spines. Nondestructive flexibility testing was done using three-dimensional motion analysis, followed by the development of a finite element model to determine the ideal transfixator position.[49] Since previous efforts, such as those of Slosar[87] cited earlier, indicate that transpedicular fixation is weakest in rotation, spines were subjected to a maximum rotational moment of 6.4 Nm. Transverse fixation resulted in significant improvement in rotational stiffness; if one was placed, the optimal position was at the proximal one-fourth of the rod. Their finding that two fixators were yet stiffer contradicts our data, although we agree that positions closer to the screw are optimal. However, in translating these data to the clinical condition, rotation is rarely a pathologic force after instrumentation: rather, it is principally flexion that is a problem and must be resisted.

Ashman et al[4] compared plate and rod systems in a corpectomy model using cyclic loading, measuring biomechanical strength characteristics for Zielke and AO Fixateur Internae rods[19] and Steffee plates. Axial and torsional stiffness values were similar for all. However, stresses were beyond the material endurance for the Steffee plates and the AO Fixateur Internae. Is this significant clinically? We suspect that these differences are not, since bone healing occurs long before fatigue of the screws, except in the case of nonunion.

Pedicle Fixation Construct

In an early clinical series, Whitesides and Shaw reported poor results in four of five patients with thoracolumbar fractures.[96] These patients suffered screw breakage, with recurrence of their deformities. The authors suggested that these failures could have been prevented with the use of anterior grafting, recognizing—clinically—the failure of rigid short-segment instrumentation to provide stability of the anterior column. This has been our clinical (as reported in Chapter 8) and laboratory experience.[57] Others have obtained satisfactory fusion, but with more deformity than seen with universal instrumentation.[39] Why?

Shea et al compared the performance of three stabilization systems: the Hartshill (wired) rectangle, the Steffee interpedicular screw and plate, and the Fixateur Internae. Constructs spanning two to four vertebral levels were compared for stabilization of the resected lumbar spine segments. The Steffee system with pedicular screws at L2–L5 allowed less distraction and sagittal rotation than the similarly affixed AO construct. There were no significant differences in stiffness across levels L3–L4 with the various implants.[86]

Gurr et al[35] used a calf model incorporating vertebrectomy and iliac crest grafting. Both posterior as well as anterior instrumentation systems were tested, among them Steffee plates inserted two levels above and below the osteotomy. The Steffee plates and anterior interbody graft behaved similarly to the intact spine and CD rods in axial loading. In rotation and flexion loading, the plates were as effective or more effective than the other devices tested, again using four-segment fixation and anterior graft. They suggested that the excellent resistance to pathologic forces resulting from pedicle fixation was related in part to anterior column fixation produced by the pedicle screw. The anterior devices resisted axial loading as well as posterior pedicle fixation; the model, however, did not include posterior element instability. In rotation, anterior fixation was the most efficient, followed by long-segment (four-level) pedicle fixation.

In the studies of Chang et al,[10] five-level posterior instrumentation was more effective in resisting rotational loads than a three-segment rod/screw system, a finding subsequently validated clinically. Three-segment fixation was more effective than other methods in resisting pure axial loads. In flexion, which may represent the most frequent loading responsible for failure of spinal instrumentation devices, the shorter system was not as effective as five-segment instrumentation. These studies may have clinical correlates in the development of deformity after instrumentation.

The effort of Slosar et al, discussed earlier, emphasized the failure of single-level transpedicular fixation to completely stabilize the traumatized spine. Although stiffness was improved in flexion, the results were less satisfactory for axial rotation and axial loading.[87] The ideal fixation of the reduced fracture, then, needs to be load-bearing. This implies that anterior column stiffening would be valuable. However, the question how this is best done—or even if it should be—remains to be answered. Indeed, Slosar et al observed that the minor collapse of the vertebral fracture provides stability: in the absence of neurological deficit, should a fractured vertebra best be left unaltered?

Stephens et al have made similar observations for short-segment fixation. They noted that with corpectomy there is no load sharing in the middle column. Three-level transpedicular fixation performed poorly in stiffening the porcine spine. Adding offset hooks at the superior level improved axial and torsional stiffness.[90] This conflicts with Ashman, who indeed did report significant stiffening, even with corpectomy.[4] Our biomechanical data confirm that stiffness is worse with short-segment fixation than with fixation supplemented with hooks, or an additional level cephalad to corpectomy.[51,53,107]

Recently, Bennett et al performed elegant biomechanical studies on lumbar spines of varying bone densities. Transpendicular fixation significantly reduced axial displacement and rotation after discectomy and facetectomy. Interbody fusion added an equal degree of stabilization; this was particularly the case in rotation in specimens with diminished bone density.[7]

Our series of patients undergoing pedicle fixation and fusion numbers about two thousand. We have found transpedicular fixation effective in decreasing motion and enhancing fusion rates; however, we have inferred the possibility of accelerated degenerative changes at adjacent segments, as suggested below.

Instrumentation Testing Methods

Historically we have employed entire thoracolumbar spinal segments, incorporating T11 to L5, in biomechanical studies, except when testing screw pull-out strength.[53] Three-dimensional motion analysis is an important component of instrumentation testing. A small amount of the anterior cortex of the vertebra in the middle of the spinal column is fractured using an osteotome to ensure fracture at an appropriate level. Each specimen is placed on a six-axis load cell that measures forces along the three anatomical directions and three respective moments (flexion, lateral flexion, and axial twist). If complex loading is to be used, the column is positioned in an electrohydraulic servo system with a slight flexion bending moment, and the spine is loaded to failure using compression and flexion under quasistatic loads. With the spine still under load, a lateral radiograph is obtained. The specimen is then reloaded (injury cycle) to the maximum deflection achieved at failure during the intact cycle. In pure moment nondestructive loading, the spine is mounted in a custom apparatus that carefully controls displacement and is loaded using the selected vector.

Following repeat radiography, fixation—for example, pedicle screw/rod fixation—is carried out at appropriate levels proximal and distal to the level of injury. The spine is then repositioned in the frame and following repeat radiography, reloaded (stabilized cycle) to the deformation experienced during the first run.

Results of Pedicle Fixation Studies

In our investigations, we determined that stiffness of the construct is quite high.[105] Following Steffee fixation, forces to deformation averaged 70% of control values, and deformations to failure were 166% higher than control values. Both the overall strength of the column and the ductility of the fixated spine were increased.

However, we observed little difference in the final stiffness values between the stabilized and injured columns, demonstrating that the fixated column responds the same as the unstable injured spine beyond a certain strain level. In the lumbar spine, instability is principally dictated by the decreased load-carrying capacity of the fractured vertebral body. We hypothesized that pedicle screw/rod fixation initially stiffens the posterior elements and enhances the strength of the injured spine. However, the failed vertebral column eventually cannot resist the additional load transmitted through it. Above some threshold, little stiffness is added to the lumbar spine.

Increased motion was observed at the discs outside the fixation, indicating increased flexibility at these levels and the potential for instability at adjacent segments. This observation has been made clinically but had not been previously demonstrated biomechanically. We also suggested that repetitive loading might affect the integrity of posterior fixation.[103,105]

Anterior Grafting Studies

The effects of anterior grafting on the strength of the fixated spine, in conjunction with partial corpectomy, have been investigated.[51] Two questions were addressed: does anterior grafting improve the biomechanics of pedicle fixation as discussed above; and what is the effect of corpectomy on the fixated spine?

Following partial vertebrectomy, a tricortical iliac crest graft was inserted. The specimens were then reloaded to failure deformation. Anterior vertebral height and Cobb angles were measured before, during, and after loading in each run. Force, deformation, stiffness, and energy were used to assess the strength characteristics of the specimen, and localized kinematics were obtained.

Differences in stiffness and loads between the intact and injury runs were significant. The fixated spines were almost as stiff as the intact spines. Maximum loads for the anterior graft trials were higher than those for the injured spine, but lower than those for the intact spinal column. In addition, they were lower than the values for the fixated column at the termination of loading.

In all instances, differences between preloading and postloading angles were significant. Cobb angles in the initial injury group increased from a preload value of 4 degrees to 16 degrees. Final Cobb angles in spines with pedicle fixation alone were not significantly different than those with anterior struts/pedicle fixation. However, anterior grafts plus posterior fixation maintained vertebral body height better than pedicle fixation alone.

We hypothesize that load sharing with the anterior graft occurs; another possibility is that the anterior graft, by better maintaining vertebral body height, allows loads to be more effectively transmitted though the instrumentation and normal vertebral loading paths. Concern still exists that pedicle fixation alone may be inadequate for stabilization: whether anterior strut grafting is associated with better alignment in the long-term remains a question.

The studies discussed here, although useful, have a significant problem: the single-cycle nature of the loading. Cyclic loading studies, as well as the multiaxis loading studies, are critical in determining the clinical utility of instrumentation devices.

Pedicular Fixation in Degenerative Disease

The information presented above is not as useful for nontraumatic instability. Typically, the spine rendered unstable due to degeneration has not failed, and some structural integrity is preserved. Single-cycle phenomena are not as critical as the impact of cyclic, or continuous, loading on the spine. Thus the characteristics of the systems used are very different: first of all, of course, they should provide increased stiffness. The question remains: how much stiffness is enough to maintain alignment and enhance bone healing (which is the desired outcome in all instrumentation)? Particularly in the absence of failure, dramatic increases in spinal stiffness are not only unnecessary but may actually be clinically undesirable.

There have been few investigations of pedicle fixation in the nonfailed lumbar spine. Panjabi et al have used an instability model consisting of removal of the posterior ligaments and injury of the disc at L5–S1. Three-dimensional vertebral motion was measured using a marker on each vertebra. Flexion, extension, lateral bending, and axial torque moments were applied to a maximum of 10 Nm to multiple commonly used systems. The authors found that flexion was reduced 50% from the intact state. Stiffness values were higher than the intact spine for all the devices. With extension loading, all the devices restored at least normal stiffness. In pure axial loading, all devices reduced motion to 50% to 75% of intact values, a statistically significant phenomenon.[68,69]

A great deal of work remains to be done to provide a rational, scientific basis for the use of spinal instrumentation. The costs, risks, and added technical difficulties of newer instrumentation types require biomechanical justification; utilization must be subject to the same careful scrutiny as that provided for drugs and other medical devices. Adequate studies on the fundamental properties of a given device, its effectiveness, and long-term biomechanics should be performed, disseminated, and studied before it is marketed and used by responsible surgeons. This area offers spine surgeons the opportunity to put objective information into the process of clinical decision making.

Future of Biomechanics of the Spine

Currently, there is a high level of interest in spinal biomechanics among spine surgeons because they recognize its importance in treatment. Although much of it is in relation to the mechanics of fixation, exciting work is being done—and is going to be done—in other areas as well. More investigation, particularly in trauma causation, will be performed using dynamic loading as we develop improved loading and measurement techniques. There is increasing interest in the pathophysiology of degenerative disease, which is critical for prevention as well as treatment. A better understanding of the spinal musculature and its role in maintaining the neutral zone of the spine will be valuable in understanding the nature of back pain.

Most exciting are efforts to physiologically replace injured spinal components, such as work on the artificial disc.[46] Although not discussed in this chapter, research on the biomechanics of the spinal cord itself needs to done, since this may have significant implications in our understanding of the pathophysiology of even common spinal disorders such as cervical myelopathy, lumbar stenosis, and spinal cord compression due to tumors.

An increasing emphasis on studies of spinal degeneration will be necessary. A scientifically rational basis for treatment is necessary: little is understood of the effects of chronic loading on the spine and on the development and progression of cervical and lumbar spondylosis.

Traditional biomechanics studies are carried out on spinal components as discussed above. However, in several centers an artificial spine is under development that may allow internal consistency (a significant problem in biomechanics research) as well as physiologic loading and injury patterns. Needless to say, these issues can be clarified only in the laboratory.

Further directions include improved use of digital technology for more accurate assessment of experimental data. Newer optical techniques, such as motion analysis, have expanded our capabilities in the important area of spinal kinematics greatly and hold great promise for the future. For instance, the motion of spinal segments adjacent to fixation points, the definition of unexpected injury adjacent to failure points in the spine, and the pathologic motion prior to the development of actual failure have been defined. Such information is unobtainable from force-deformation data and, in conjunction with stiffness data, has suggested further ideas for investigation.[103,106] In addition, mathematical modeling, particularly finite element analysis,[62] promises a nonlinear, nonexperimental means of extrapolating limited specimen data into comparisons of new fixation devices, and more importantly, into investigation of long-term changes not testable in tissue models.

In spite of the difficulties involved, it is imperative that our questions on the structure, function, and pathology of the spine be answered in the laboratory and that new treatments be subjected to biomechanical scrutiny. Although it is attractive to hypothesize on the basis of clinical experience and logic, it is unacceptable. Biomechanics is an experimental science, and its principles cannot be deducted. Theories and hypotheses must be studied and validated in the laboratory and then applied in the clinic and operating room. The surgeon's obligation is to ask the questions and use the information obtained for the benefit of his or her patients.

REFERENCES

1. Abumi K, Panjabi MM, Kramer KM, et al: Biomechanical evaluation of lumbar spinal stability after graded facetectomies. Spine 15:1142–1147, 1990.
2. Aebi M, Etter C, Kehl T, et al: The internal skeletal fixation system: A new treatment of thoracolumbar fractures and other spinal disorders. Clin Orthop 227:30–43, 1988.
3. Andriacchi TP, Schultz AB, Belytscko TB, et al: A model for studies of mechanical interactions between the human spine and rib cage. J Biomech 7:497–508, 1974.
4. Ashman RB, Galpin RD, Corin JD, et al: Biomechanical analysis of pedicle screw instrumentation systems in a corpectomy model. Spine 14:1398–1405, 1989.
5. Atlas SW, Regenbogen V, et al: The radiographic characterization of burst fractures of the spine. Am J Radiography 147:575–582, 1986.
6. Bedbrook GM: Treatment of thoracolumbar dislocation and fractures with paraplegia. Clin Orthop 112:27–43, 1975.
7. Bennett GJ, Serhan HA, Sorini PM, et al: An experimental study of lumbar stabilization: Restabilization and bone density. Spine 22:1448–1453, 1997.
8. Carl AL, Tromanhauser SG, Roger DJ: Pedicle screw instrumentation for thoracolumbar burst fractures and fracture-dislocation. Spine 17:S317–324, 1992.
9. Carter DR, Hayes WC: Bone compressive strength: The influence of density and strain rate. Science 194:1174–1176, 1976.
10. Chang KW, Dewei Z, McAfee PC, et al: A comparative biomechanical study of spinal fixation using the combination spinal rod-plate and transpedicular screw fixation system. J Spinal Disorders 1:257–266, 1989.
11. Coe JD, Warden KE, Sutterlin CE III, et al: Biomechanical evaluation of cervical spinal stabilization methods in a human cadaveric model. Spine 14:1122–1131, 1989.
12. Cotterill PC, Kostuik JP, Wilson JA, et al: Production of a reproducible spinal burst fracture for use in biomechanical testing. J Orthop Res 5:462–465, 1987.
13. Cusick JF, Yoganandan N, Pintar FA, et al: Biomechanics of sequential lumbar posterior surgical alteration. J Neurosurg 76:805–811, 1992.
14. Denis F: Spinal instability as defined by the three-column concept in acute spine trauma. Clin Orthop 189:65–76, 1984.
15. Dick W, Kluger P, Magerl F, et al: A new device for internal fixation of thoracolumbar and lumbar spine fractures: The 'fixateur interne'. Paraplegia 23:225–232, 1985.
16. Edwards WT: Biomechanics of posterior lumbar fixation: Analysis of testing methodologies. Spine 16:1224–1232, 1991.
17. Edwards WT, Hayes WC, Posner I, et al: Variation of

lumbar spine stiffness with load. J Biomech Eng 109:35–42, 1987.

18. El Hagediab A, Yoganandan N, Pintar FA, et al: Biomechanical model of a lumbar intervertebral joint: A systems approach. In Mechanics Computing in 1990s. Adeli H, and Sierakowski R, (ed.): New York, Beyond, Vol 1, American Soc of Civil Engineers, 1991, pp 569–573.

19. Esses SI: The AO spinal internal fixator. Spine 14:373–388, 1989.

20. Evans FG: Mechanical Properties of Bones. Charles C. Thomas Publishers. Springfield, IL, 1973, 332 pp.

21. Ewing CL, Thomas DJ, Sances A Jr, Larson SJ (ed.): Impact Injury of the Head and Spine. Charles C. Thomas Publishers, Springfield, IL, 1983, 654 pp.

22. Farcy JP, Weidenbaum M, Michelsen CB, et al: A comparative biomechanical study of spinal fixation using Cotrel-Dubousset instrumentation. Spine 12:877–881, 1987.

23. Farfan HF: The torsional injury of the lumbar spine. Spine 9:53–59, 1984.

24. Ferguson RL, Tencer AF, Woodard P, et al: Biomechanical comparisons of spinal fracture models and the stabilizing effects of posterior instrumentation. Spine 13:453–460, 1988.

25. Frederickson BE, Edwards WT, Rauschning W, et al: Vertebral burst fractures: An experimental, morphologic, and radiographic study. Spine 17:1012–1021, 1992.

26. Gaines RW, Carson WL, Satterlee CC, et al: Experimental evaluation of seven different spinal fracture fixation devices using nonfailure stability testing. Spine 16:902–911, 1991.

27. Galante JO, Rostoker W, Ray RD: Physical properties of trabecular bone. Cal Tiss Res 5:236–246, 1970.

28. Glazer PA, Colliou O, Klish SM, et al: Biomechanical analysis of multilevel fixation methods in the lumbar spine. Spine 22:171–182, 1997.

29. Goel VK, Lim TH, Gwon J, et al: Effects of rigidity of an internal fixation device: A comprehensive biomechanical investigation. Spine 162: 155–161, 1991.

30. Goel VK, Pope MH: Biomechanics of fusion and stabilization. Spine 20S: 85–99, 1995.

31. Goel VK, Voo LM, Weinstein JN, et al: Response of the ligamentous lumbar spine to cyclic bending loads. Spine 13:294–300, 1988.

32. Goel VJ, Winterbottom JM, Weinstein JN: A method for the fatigue testing of pedicle screw fixation devices. J. Biomech 27:1383–1388, 1994.

33. Goel VK, Wilder DG, Pope MH, et al: Biomechanical testing of the spine:Load-controlled versus displacement controlled analysis. Spine 20:2354–2357, 1995.

34. Gregerson GC, Lucas DB: An in vivo study of the axial rotation of the human thoracolumbar spine . J Bone Joint Surg 49A:247–262, 1967.

35. Gurr KR, McAfee PC, Shih CM: Biomechanical analysis of anterior and posterior instrumentation systems after corpectomy. J Bone Joint Surg 70:1182–1191, 1988.

36. Gwon JK, Chen J, Lim TH, et al: In vitro comparative biomechanical analysis of transpedicular screw instrumentation in the lumbar region of the lumbar spine. J Spinal Disorders 4:437–443, 1991.

37. Holdworth FW: Fractures, dislocations, and fracture/dislocations of the spine. J Bone Joint Surg 45B:6–20, 1963.

38. Holdsworth F: Review article. Fractures, dislocations, and fracture dislocations of the spine. J Bone Joint Surg 52:1534–1551, 1970.

39. Hollowell JP, Maiman DJ: Management of thoracic and thoracolumbar spine trauma. In Rea GL and Miller CA (ed.): Spinal Trauma: Current Evaluation and Treatment, Park Ridge, IL: Am Assoc Neurol Surgeons, pp 127–156, 1993.

40. Jacobs RR, Nordwall A, Nachemson A: Stability and strength provided by internal fixation systems for dorso-lumbar spinal injuries. J Biomech 13:802–807, 1980.

41. Johnstone B, Bayliss MT: The large proteoglycan of the human intervertebral disc. Spine 20:674–684, 1995

42. Kaigle AM, Holm SH, Hansson TH: Experimental instability in the lumbar spine. Spine 20:421–430, 1995.

43. Kazarian L, Graves GA: Compression strength characteristics of the human vertebral centrum. Spine 2:1–14, 1977.

44. King AI, Vulcan AP: Elastic deformation characteristics of the spine. J Biomech 4:413–429, 1971.

45. Kornblatt MD, Casey MP, Jacobs RR: Internal fixation in lumbosacral spine fusion: A biomechanical and clinical study. Clin Orthop 203:141–150, 1985.

46. Kostuick JP: Intervertebral disc replacement: Experimental study. Clin Orthop 337:27–41, 1997.

47. Krag MH, Beynnon BD, Pope MH, et al: Depth of insertion of transpedicular vertebral screws into human vertebrae: Effect upon screw-vertebra interface strength. J Spinal Disorders 1:287–294, 1989.

48. Larson SJ: Unstable thoracic fractures: Treatment alternatives and the role of the neurosurgeon. Clin Neurosurg 27:624–640, 1980.

49. Lin TH, Eck JC, An HS, et al: Biomechanics of transfixation in pedicle screw instrumentation. Spine 21:2224–2229, 1996.

50. Lucas DB, Bresler B: Experimental and theoretical study of spine stability. J Bone Joint Surg 37A:411–412, 1955.

51. Maiman DJ, Pintar FA, Yoganandan N, et al: Effects of anterior vertebral grafting on the traumatized lumbar spine following pedicle screw-plate fixation. Spine 18:2423–2430, 1993.

52. Maiman DJ, Sances A Jr, Larson SJ, et al: Biomechanical analysis of spinal fixation devices. Neurosurgery 17:574–580, 1985.

53. Maiman DJ, Sances A Jr, Mykelbust JB, et al: Experimental trauma of the thoracolumbar spine. In Sances A Jr., Thomas DJ, et al (eds.): Mechanisms of Head and Spine Injury. Goshen NY: Aloray Publishers, 1986, pp 489–504.

54. Maiman DJ, Sypert GW: Management of trauma of the thoracolumbar junction: Part I. Contemp Neurosurg 11:1–6, 1989.

55. Maiman DJ, Sypert GW: Management of trauma of the thoracolumbar junction. Part II. Contemp Neurosurg 11:7–12, 1989.

56. Maiman DJ: Anatomy and clinical biomechanics of the thoracic spine. Clin Neurosurg 38:296–324, 1992.

57. Maiman DJ, Yoganandan N: The biomechanics of spinal instrumentation. In E Benzel (ed.): Spinal Instrumentation Chicago: American Assoc Neurologic Surgeons, 1994, pp 11–30.

58. Markolf KL, Morris JM: The structural components of the intervertebral disc. J Bone Joint Surg 56A:675–687, 1974.

59. McAfee PC, Werner FW, Glisson RR: A biomechanical analysis of spinal instrumentation systems in thoracolumbar fractures. Spine 10:204–216, 1985.

60. McAfee PC, Yuan HA, Lasda NA: The unstable burst fracture. Spine 7:365–373, 1982.

61. McGregor AH, McCarthy ID, Hughes SP: Motion characteristics of the lumbar spine in the normal population. Spine 20:2421–2428, 1995.

62. Mizrahi J, Silva MJ, Keaveny TM, et al: Finite-element stress analysis of the normal and osteoporotic lumbar vertebral body. Spine 18:2088–2096, 1993.

63. Myklebust JB, Pintar F, Yoganandan N, et al: Tensile strength of spinal ligaments. Spine 13:526–531, 1988.

64. Nachemson A, Evans J: Some mechanical properties of the third lumbar interlaminar (ligamentum flavum) ligament. J Biomech 1:211–220, 1968.

65. Nachemson A: The load on lumbar discs in different positions of the body. Clin Orthop 45:107–122, 1966.

66. Neumann P, Nordwall A, Osvalder AL: Traumatic instability of the lumbar spine: A dynamic in-vitro study of flexion-distraction injury. Spine 20:1111–1121, 1995.

67. Neumann P, Osvalder AL, Hansson TH, et al: Flexion-distraction injury of the lumbar spine: Influence of load, loading rate, and vertebral mineral content. J Spinal Disord 9:89–102, 1996.

68. Panjabi MM, Yamamoto I, Oxland TR, et al: Biomechanical stability of five pedicle screw fixation systems in a human lumbar spine instability model. Clin Biomech 6:97–205, 1991.

69. Panjabi MM: Biomechanical evaluation of spinal fixation devices: A conceptual framework. Spine 13:1129–1134, 1988.

70. Panjabi MM: The stabilizing system of the spine: Part I. Function, dysfunction, adaptation and enhancement. J Spinal Disord 5:383–389, 1992.

71. Panjabi MM: The stabilizing system of the spine: part II. Neutral zone and instability hypothesis. J Spinal Disord 5:390–397, 1992.

72. Panjabi MM, Oxland TR, Lim RM, et al: Thoracolumbar burst fracture. A biomechanical investigation of its multidirectional flexibility. Spine 19:578–585, 1994.

73. Panjabi MM, Oxland TR, Kifune M, et al: Validity of the three-column theory of thoracolumbar fractures. Spine 20:1122–1127, 1995.

74. Pearcy MC, Tibrewal SB: Axial rotation and lateral bending in the normal lumbar spine measured by three-dimensional radiography. Spine 9:582–591, 1984.

75. Pintar F, Myklebust JB, Yoganandan N, et al: Biomechanics of human spinal ligaments. In Sances A Jr, Thomas DJ. Mechanisms of Head and Spine Trauma. Aloray Publishers, Ewing CL, Larson SJ, Unterharnscheidt F (eds.): Goshen, NY: pp 505–530, 1986.

76. Pintar FA, Cusick JF, Yoganandan N, et al: Biomechanics of lumbar facetectomy under flexion-compression. Spine 17:804–810, 1992.

77. Pintar FA, Yoganandan N, Myers T, et al: Biomechanical properties of human lumbar spine ligaments. J Biomech 25:1351–1356, 1992.

78. Pintar FA, Maiman DJ, Yoganandan N, et al: Rotational stiffness of a lumbar spinal pedicle screw/rod system. J Spinal Disord 8:49–55, 1995.

79. Pope MH, Novotny JE: Spinal biomechanics. J Biomech 115:569–574, 1993.

80. Rauschning W: Anatomy of the normal and traumatized spine. In Mechanisms of Head and Spine Trauma, A. Sances Jr, DJ Thomas, CL Ewing, SJ Larson, F Unterharnscheidt (eds.): Aloray Publishers, Goshen, NY, 1986, pp. 531–564.

81. Road R: A study of the mechanics of spinal injuries. J Bone Joint Surg 42B:810–823, 1960.

82. Sances A Jr, Myklebust JB, Maiman DJ, et al: The biomechanics of spinal injuries. CRC Crit Rev Bioeng 11(1):1–76, 1984.

83. Sances A Jr, Thomas DJ, Ewing CL, et al (eds.): Mechanisms of Head and Spine Trauma, Aloray Publisher, Goshen, NY, 1986, 746 pp.

84. Seligman JV, Gertzbein SD, Tile M, et al: Computer analysis of spinal segment motion in degenerative disc disease with or without axial loading. Spine 9: 566–573, 1984.

85. Sharma M, Langrana NA, Rodriguez J: Role of ligaments and facets in lumbar spinal stability. Spine 20: 887–900, 1995

86. Shea M, Edwards WT, Clothiaux PL, et al: Three-dimensional load displacement properties of posterior lumbar fixation. J Orthop Trauma 5: 420–427, 1991.

87. Slosar PJ, Patwardhan AG, Lorenz M, et al: Instability of the lumbar burst fracture and limitations of transpedicular instrumentation. Spine 20: 1452–1461, 1995.

88. Snyder BD, Piazza S, Edwards WT, et al: Role of trabecular morphology in the etiology of age-related vertebral fractures. Calc Tiss Int 53 S1:14–22, 1993.

89. Sonoda T: Studies on the strength for compression, tension, and torsion of the human vertebral column. J Kyoto Pref Med Univ 71:659–702, 1962.

90. Stephens GC, Devito DP, McNamara MJ, et al: Short segment transpedicular Cotrel-Dubousset instrumentation: A porcine corpectomy model. J Spinal Disord 6:252–255, 1993.

91. Tencer AF, Hampton D, Eddy S: Biomechanical properties of threaded inserts for lumbar interbody spinal fusion. Spine 20: 2408–2414, 1995.

92. Tran NT, Watson NA, Tencer AF, et al: Mechanism of the burst fracture in the thoracolumbar spine. Spine 20:1984–1988, 1995.

93. Tkaczuk H: Tensile properties of human lumbar longitudinal ligaments. Acta Orthop Scand (Suppl) 115:1–69, 1968.

94. White AA, Hirsch C: The significance of the vertebral posterior elements in the mechanics of the thoracic spine. Clin Orthop 81:2–14, 1971.

95. White AA, Panjabi MM: Clinical Biomechanics of the Spine. 2nd Edition, Philadelphia, JB Lippincott Co. p. 722.

96. Whitesides TE, Shaw SGA: On the management of unstable fractures of thoracolumbar spine: Rationale for use of anterior decompression and fusion and posterior stabilization. Spine 1:99–107, 1976.

97. Weinhoffer SL, Guyer RD, Herbert M, et al: Intradiscal pressure measurements above an instrumented fusion. Spine 20:526–531, 1995

98. Wilke HJ, Wolf S, Claes LE, et al: Stability increase of the lumbar spine with different muscle groups. Spine 20:192–198, 1995.

99. Yamada H: Strength of Biological Materials. Robert E Krieger Publishers, Huntington, NY, 1973 p. 197.

100. Yoganandan N, Myklebust JB, Cusick JF, et al: Functional biomechanics of the thoracolumbar vertebral cortex. Clin Biomech 3:11–18, 1988.

101. Yoganandan N, Maiman DJ, Pintar F, et al: microtrauma in the lumbar spine: A cause of low back pain. Neurosurgery 23:162–168, 1988.

102. Yoganandan N, Pintar F, Butler J, et al: Dynamic response of human cervical spine ligaments. Spine 14:1102–1110, 1989.

103. Yoganandan N, Pintar F, Sances A Jr: Biomechanical investigations of the human thoracolumbar spine. SAE Transactions 97:676–684, 1989.

104. Yoganandan N, Haffner M, Maiman DJ, et al: Epidemiology and injury biomechanics of motor vehicle related trauma to the human spine. SAE Transactions 98:1790–1807, 1990.

105. Yoganandan N, Larson SJ, Pintar FA, et al: Biomechanics of lumbar pedicle screw/plate fixation in trauma. Neurosurgery 27:873–881, 1990.

106. Yoganandan N, Pintar FA, Sances A Jr, et al: Strength and kinematic response of dynamic cervical spine injuries. Spine 16:S511–S517, 1991.

107. Yoganandan N, Maiman DJ, Pintar FA, et al: Kinematics of the lumbar spine following pedicle screw plate fixation. Spine 18:504–512, 1993.

108. Yoganandan N, Maiman DJ, Pintar FA, et al: Biomechanical effects of laminectomy on thoracic spine stability. Neurosurgery 32:604–610, 1993.

CHAPTER 3

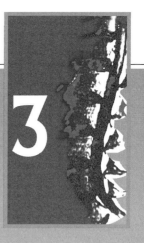

Instability of the Vertebral Column

Normal Functioning

Abnormal Functioning

Instability of Chronic Vertebral Trauma

Instability of Acute Vertebral Trauma

Summary

Instability of the Vertebral Column

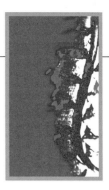

A major problem in the consideration of instability of the vertebral column is arriving at a definition of instability. The definitions that have been published vary widely.[8,11,19,-21,32,39] Instability has been defined in anatomical terms, in clinical terms, and in a combination of both including pain and neurological dysfunction.

Although neurological function is obviously important, it is not a factor in vertebral column stability. One person may have an unstable spine and be neurologically normal and without symptoms, whereas another may have an abnormal but stable vertebral column with significant symptoms or neurological dysfunction or both. Therefore, instability should be defined in anatomical terms, and the implications of instability can then be applied to the clinical situation.

Normal Functioning

The normal vertebral column is mobile in flexion-extension, axial rotation, lateral bending, and translation. The range of normal vertebral motion has been studied using several techniques.[9,16,23,30,31,37] Although this motion varies and decreases with age it is always symmetrical. The range and direction of movement are limited by the orientation of the articular processes and the characteristics of the ligamentous structures and the intervertebral discs. Normal motion is always coupled: that is, motion about one axis is always accompanied by motion about at least one other axis. Since primary and coupled motions are limited by anatomical constraints, the pertinent anatomical factors are briefly reviewed.

In the cervical region, the supraspinous ligament is represented by the ligamentum nuchae, which is connected to the cervical spinous processes by fibrous strands; the other ligaments and the intervertebral disc are relatively weak compared to corresponding structures in other portions of the column. The forward slope of the articular surfaces allows for substantial range of motion from extension to flexion, and is accompanied by a normal translational movement that becomes greater at each level from C7 to C2, with 3.5 mm suggested as the upper limit of normal.[12] Because the articular surfaces also have a medial orientation, rotation and lateral flexion are coupled. For example, rotation to the left causes lateral bending to the left, and lateral bending to the left causes rotation to the left.

The rostral caudal orientation of the articular processes of the thoracic vertebrae are in the coronal plane, nearly parallel to the long axis of the vertebral column. The configuration inhibits flexion, which is also limited by the costovertebral and costotransverse articulations and related ligaments. Extension is restricted by contact between the inferior articular processes and the subjacent laminae. The superior articular processes of T1 to T11 are directed dorsally and laterally, and the inferior articular processes of T1 to T10 are directed medially and ventrally. This configuration permits rotation, which is the major motion in the thoracic spinal column. The 2nd through the 9th ribs are attached to two vertebral bodies. These costovertebral articulations with the related radiate ligaments provide substantial support to the vertebral column, as do the costotransverse joints and intertransverse ligaments. The 11th and 12th vertebrae do not have a costotransverse articulation, and the configuration of the 11th and 12th thoracic vertebral bodies is similar to that of the upper lumbar.

The 11th or sometimes the 12th vertebra is transitional, with coronally oriented superior articular processes and sagittally oriented inferior processes.

The lumbar ligaments, joint capsules, and intervertebral discs are stronger than those of the thoracic and cervical regions, and the vertebral bodies are bulkier. The articular surfaces of the apophyseal joints are more vertically oriented, permitting flexion, extension, and lateral bending, but limiting axial rotation. As in the cervical vertebrae, rotation and lateral bending are coupled. Translational movement occurs in association with flexion but is normally less than 3 mm[11,34] because of the resistance to shear by the intervertebral disc and the coronally oriented anterior portion of the superior articular processes.

Abnormal Functioning

With regard to stationary objects, instability can be defined as not stationary, or not steady in position, and movements are unstable if they are unsteady or irregular. Since the vertebral columns is in one sense stationary and in another mobile, both features should be incorporated in the definition of stability and instability. The stable spinal column is symmetrical in movement, and its configuration, whether normal or abnormal, does not change with time. The unstable spinal column may be asymmetrical in movement, its configuration may change with time, or both may occur.

The transition from the predominant cervical flexion-extension and axial rotation to axial rotation in the thoracic portion of the column to flexion-extension in the lumbar region is relatively smooth, as are changes in coupled movement. In contrast, the unstable spinal column displays asymmetrical motion. This may be asymmetrical angular motion without abnormal coupling (Fig. 3–1), asymmetrical motion with abnormal coupling (Fig. 3–2), or abnormal coupling without asymmetrical angular movement. For example, at an unstable motion segment, flexion and extension may be restricted while associated translational movement is greater than normal (Fig. 3–3A). The limits of normal translation were established by in vitro experiments in which restriction of flexion and extension was not a factor.[34] Because coupling is proportional to the primary movement, the translation associ-

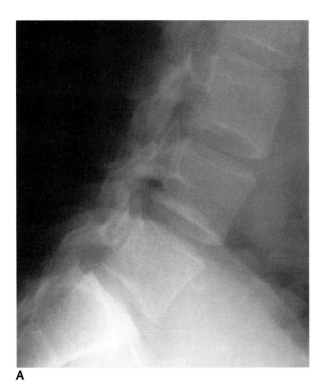
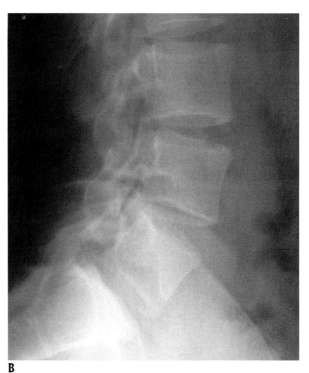

A   B

FIGURE 3–1 Films during flexion **A** and extension **B** demonstrate greater angular motion at L4–L5 than at L3–L4 or L5–S1.

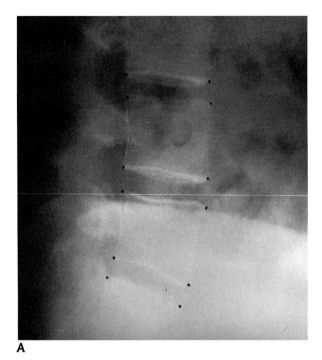 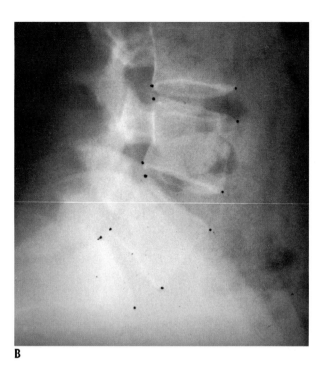

FIGURE 3–2 Films during flexion **A** and extension **B** showing retrolisthesis in extension at L4–L5 with greater angular motion at L4–L5 than at L3–L4 or L5–S1.

ated with flexion or extension may be within normal limits if these movements are restricted by pain. Therefore, translational movement at a motion segment that is greater than that at adjacent segments can be considered evidence of instability even if it falls within established values for normal. Even if asymmetrical translational movement cannot be demonstrated on bending films, it can be implied from the development of traction spurs (see Fig. 3–3B). In the patient pictured in Figure 3–3B, minimal angular movement occurred during flexion and extension because of the severe pain associated with attempts at bending. Similarly, structural injury to the vertebral column or pain may inhibit voluntary movement, but permit progressive deformity under physiological loads. Occasionally asymmetrical translational movement may occur during lateral bending as well as during flexion and extension (see Fig. 5–18, Ch. 5). Instability may also occur in the long axis of the vertebral column (Fig. 3–4). The 20-year-old patient in Figure 3–4 had back pain that was relieved by lying down and precipitated by standing and sitting.

Instability may develop slowly as a result of the chronic trauma of ordinary activity, or abruptly from an acute traumatic event. In general, the instability of chronic trauma is primarily related to change in soft tissue with slowly developing secondary changes in bone and in alignment. Treatment is usually directed toward relief of pain. In contrast, the instability of acute trauma can be secondary to either ligamentous injury without change in bone, or concurrent injury to bone and soft tissue, with change in alignment occurring more rapidly. Treatment is primarily directed toward correcting or preventing neurological deficit. Therefore, although the same structures are involved, it is more convenient to consider the instability of chronic and acute trauma separately.

Instability of Chronic Vertebral Trauma

The instability of chronic vertebral trauma is primarily related to degenerative changes beginning in the nucleus pulposus. In the normal motion unit, the vertebral body glides back and forth over the nucleus pulposus, and the apophyseal joints are not subjected to axial load except during extension.[1,2]

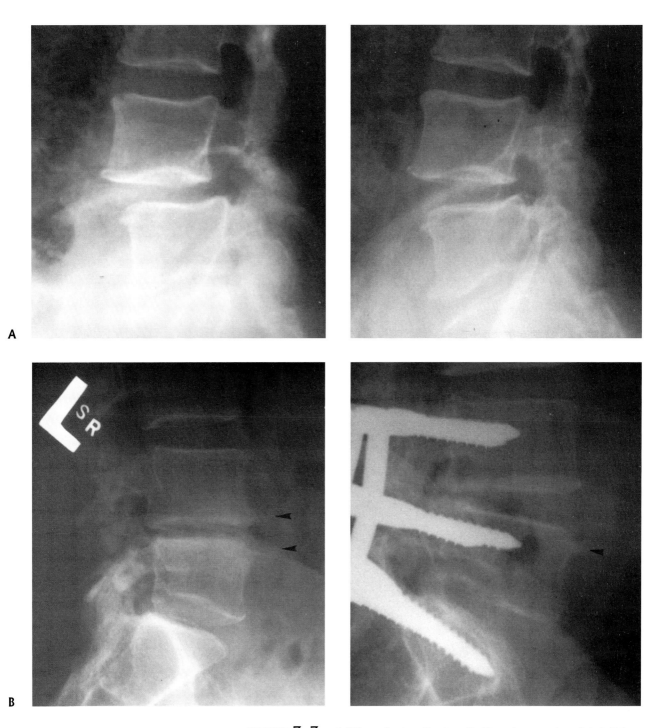

FIGURE 3-3 **A** Films during flexion (*left*) and extension (*right*) demonstrating anterolisthesis at L4–L5. **B** Traction spurs (*arrows*) on L4 and L5 before (*left*) and 6 months after (*right*) fusion. The L4 spur is no longer present, and that on L5 is smaller.

With degeneration of the nucleus, the annulus, which does not effectively withstand compressive loads, bulges, and resistance of the disc to shear is reduced. Consequently, vertebral motion becomes more parallel. Also, as the degenerating disc narrows, the apophyseal joints come under pressure even in flexion, with the area of maximum pressure increasing and moving posteriorly with extension.[10] Narrowing of the disc also leads to laxity of the joint capsules, permitting greater movement of

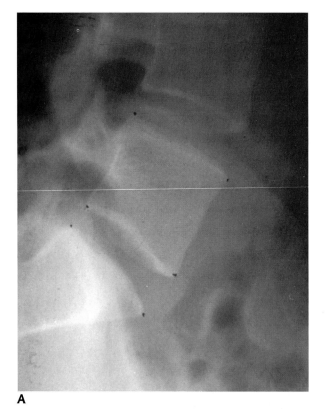
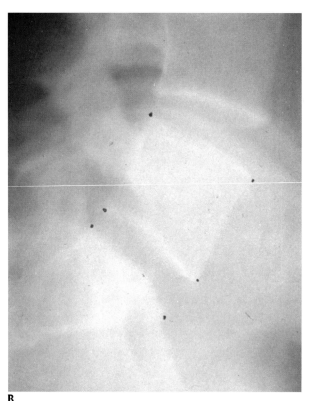
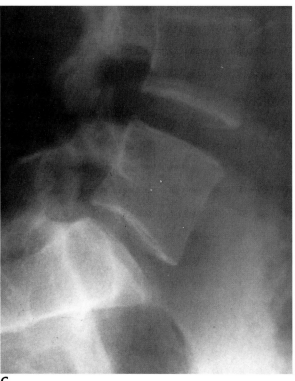

FIGURE 3-4
A Lateral film taken while supine. **B** Film taken with patient standing, demonstrating 25% reduction in disc height. **C** Film taken 1 year later, demonstrating narrowing at L5–S1.

the articular processes than is normally possible. Decreased resistance of the disc to shear, the abnormally increased freedom of movement in the apophyseal joints, and the increased pressure on the articular surfaces lead to structural changes. These include degeneration of articular cartilage, eburnation and thickening of the subchrondral bone, hypertrophic changes in the apophyseal joint, degeneration and thickening of the capsular portion of the ligamentum flavum, degeneration of the synovial folds, loose bodies in the apophyseal joints, hypertrophy of the pedicles, the development of sclerotic ridges on the vertebral margins, and increased translational movement and displacement of the vertebral body anteriorly, posteriorly, or laterally.

Radiographic Evaluation

Although instability can be suspected on clinical grounds, it can only be demonstrated radiographically.[11,15,17,22,33,35,40] In clinical practice this is accomplished by singe-plane radiography. In the normal motion segment, the vertebral body has a rocking movement over the nucleus pulposus, and the center of rotation is located in the posterior portion of the disc, moving backward and forward with flexion and extension and from side to side with lateral bending. Abnormal movement at a motion segment is associated with displacement of the center of rotation. Consequently, identification of the center of rotation can effectively determine whether the motion segment is stable or unstable.[6,13,14,31,32] Gertzbein introduced the concept of the centrode, defined as the locus of centers of rotation measured at increments of motion from full extension to full flexion.[14] The in vitro experiments demonstrated that in a normal motion segment the centrode remains in the posterior portion of the intervertebral disc. However, in degenerated discs, the centrodes became more complex, moving out of the disc. The most complex centrodes were found in discs with minor degeneration, and the least complex but most displaced were found in those that were severely degenerated, suggesting that the major abnormality early in the development of instability is erratic rather than excessive movement.

Despite the limitations of single-plane radiography (see discussion below) Knutsson[22] reported a deviation from normal patterns of movements in patients with low back pain, and similar observations have been made by others. Pennal[32] demonstrated that the center of rotation could be identified with reasonable accuracy by single-plane radiography, and Dupuis et al[11] have shown that abnormal coupled motion can be satisfactorily demonstrated by function films in frontal and lateral planes. In the normal lumbar motion segment during lateral bending, the spinous processes move toward the concavity and shear is not demonstrated. In the unstable motion segment during lateral bending, the spinous process may move toward the convexity, lateral shear may be demonstrated, or both may occur.[11]

Anatomical-clinical correlation remains a major problem, as in the patient who develops acute and disabling pain with restriction of movement and whose spine films appear normal. Various explanations have been advanced for this, including entrapment of the meniscus-like invaginations of the joint capsule or of loose bodies in the joint. Loose bodies, however, are observed very infrequently on CT scans, and entrapment of the capsular invaginations does not appear to be a likely cause.[4] It is possible that the more complicated techniques, such as analysis of the centrode, may detect changes in the pattern of motion that might explain the clinical picture. The ligamentum flavum, supraspinous ligament, and joint capsule contain nerve endings, and injection of hypertonic saline into these structures is associated with pain similar in character and distribution to that described by patients with low back syndromes.[18]

Conversely, abnormality of movement and alignment may not necessarily be associated with pain or abnormal physical findings. Spondylolisthesis has been demonstrated in 1.5% of asymptomatic individuals.[38] The flexion-extension films shown in Figure 3–5 demonstrate abnormality of movement from L3 to the sacrum. The patient's symptoms were aggravated by extension, decreased by flexion, and relieved by transverse process fusion from L4 to the sacrum. The L3–4 motion segment is unstable, but apparently not a source of pain. Consequently, persistence of pain following fusion of an unstable motion segment may only mean that the patient's symptoms were not related to the radiographically demonstrated instability.

Limitations

Single-plane radiography has limitations because the x-ray tube acts as a point source with unavoidable magnification and distortion secondary to

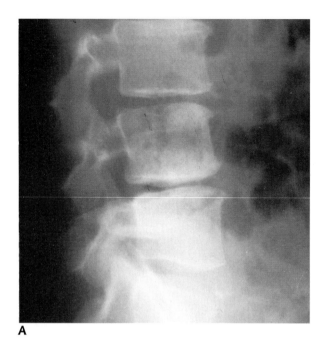 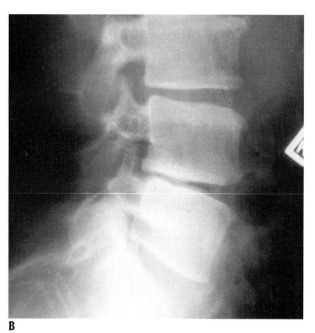

FIGURE 3–5 **A** Anterolisthesis at L3–L4 during flexion. **B** Retrolisthesis at L4–L5 during extension.

beam divergence. Additional distortion may be introduced by movement that may not always be monoplanar in flexion-extension, and is never confined to a single plane in lateral bending. Consequently, identification of relatively small translational movements may be difficult, and large errors can be introduced into the identification of the center of rotation.[28,29,31]

The identification of the center of rotation in vivo can be difficult, requiring specialized techniques.[5,26,27,34,36] Large errors in the location of the center of rotation may result from relatively small errors in the measurement of input coordinates.[28,29] This effect increases with decreasing values for range of rotation, and the error becomes substantial with angles of rotation less than 5°.[28]

Another criticism of single-plane radiography is that it does not provide a three-dimensional description of vertebral geometry. To achieve this, methods using biplanar radiography and computer analysis have been developed.[5] These too have been considered inadequate, and methods for the analysis of primary and coupled movement using stereo radiography have been developed. In these techniques, landmarks are identified on each vertebra, digitized, and computer-analyzed. The most precise method is roentgen stereophotogrammetry, where tantalum spheres with a diameter of 0.8 mm are placed percutaneously into the spinous processes, neural arches, and transverse processes of the motion segments analyzed.[26,27] This method requires specialized equipment and computer analysis.

Instability of Acute Vertebral Trauma

The instability associated with acute trauma can be defined as osseous or ligamentous injury sufficient to allow progressive vertebral malalignment under physiological loads. Nicoll[25] analyzed fractures of the thoracolumbar junction and observed that progressive deformity did not occur unless the posterior ligamentous complex had been disrupted. Holdsworth[19,20] pointed out that except for the first two cervical vertebrae and the sacrum, all vertebrae articulate through the intervertebral disc and the apophyseal joints. Motion between the vertebral bodies is limited by the intervertebral disc and longitudinal ligaments. Movement at the apophyseal joints is limited by the joint capsule, the ligamenta flava, the interspinous ligament, and the supraspinous ligament, which Holdsworth called the posterior ligamentous complex.[19,20] Holdsworth confirmed Nicoll's observations and expanded the concept to include the entire vertebral column. He

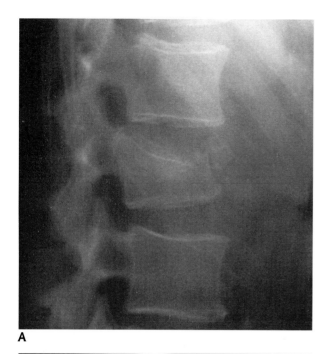
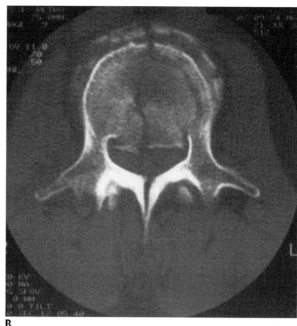
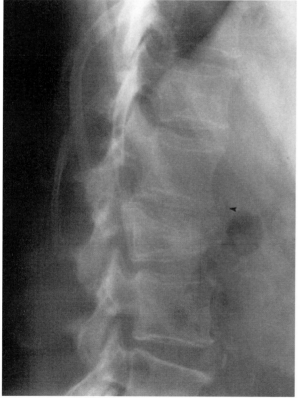

FIGURE 3-6
A Axial load fracture of L3. **B** CT scan from the same patient, who had minimal and transient neurological deficit. The posterior elements are intact, except for a sagittal laminar fracture, which does not affect stability. **C** The same patient 1 year later. Bony union has occurred with slight angulation secondary to disc resorption and consequent displacement of the detached anterior portion of the vertebral body.

concluded that "after injury, it is on the integrity or otherwise of this posterior complex that the stability of the spine depends." Although this was made in the context of concomitant injury to the vertebral body, the statement has been made that "he insisted that rupture of the posterior column was sufficient to create instability of the spine."[8] Because experimental evidence was available demonstrating that instability did not occur after division of the posterior ligamentous complex until the posterior longitudinal ligament and the annulus fibrosis had been cut,[3] a three-column system was pro-

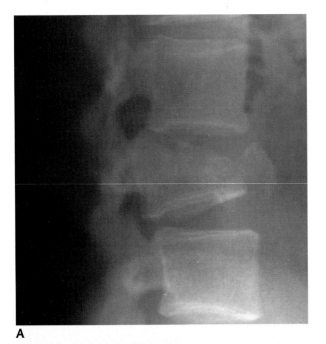
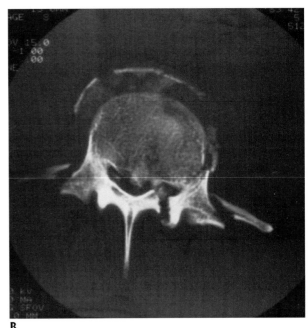
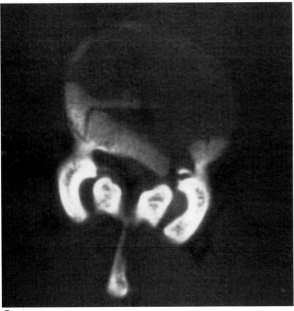

FIGURE 3-7

A Vertebral body configuration after a flexion compression injury. **B** Both pedicles are fractured. Although the fracture of the right pedicle is not clearly seen, it can be inferred from the angle of the pedicle with the vertebral body. This should be considered an unstable fracture. **C** Same patient demonstrating joint disruption.

posed.[7,8] In this system, the anterior column is made up of the anterior longitudinal ligament, the anterior portion of the annulus fibrosis, and the anterior part of the vertebral body. The posterior column is the neural arch and related ligaments. The middle column consists of the posterior longitudinal ligament, the posterior portion of the vertebral body, and the posterior portion of the annulus fibrosis. However, experiments involving sequential division of ligaments and of the annulus are not applicable to the clinical situation. Cutting is not the same as ripping. Cutting disconnects, whereas ripping separates. If the spinous processes are pulled apart sufficient to tear the posterior ligaments, the separation must of necessity disrupt the posterior longitudinal ligament and annulus or produce a fracture of the vertebral body. Furthermore, in the three-column system, midline laminar fractures that may occur in association with the lateral displacement of the apophyseal joints and pedicles in the axial load or burst fractures are considered indicators of potential instability. This, however, does not appear valid, since the ligaments and joint capsules would not be disrupted by this type of

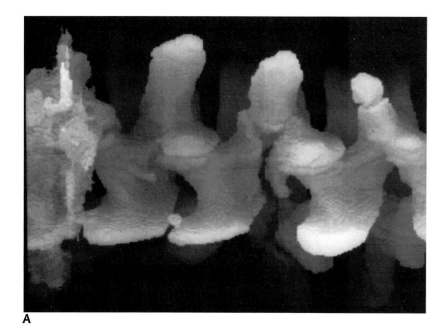
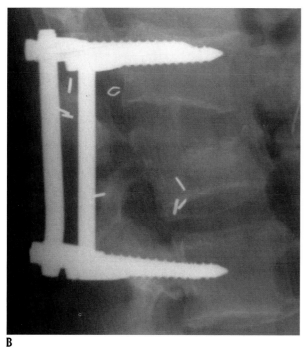
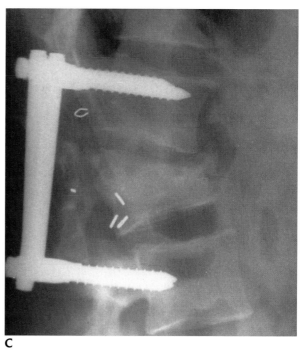

FIGURE 3-8
A Three-dimensional CT scan demonstrating posterior disruption in a patient with flexion-compression injury and incomplete neurological deficit. **B** Immediate postoperative film in the same patient. Neurological recovery was complete. **C** Film taken 1 year later. Deformity has decreased despite pedicle fixation. The lower screws have partially pulled out, and vertebral height has decreased anteriorly. Deformity probably would have been greater if pedicle fixation had not been done.

injury. Although McAcfee et al[24] used the three-column system, they found that burst fractures with intact posterior elements were stable, whereas fractures with similar vertebral body comminution but with disrupted posterior elements were not. The three-column system also appears artificial, since the neural arch is organized around the neural tube and the vertebral body around the notochord.

As Holdsworth[19,20] pointed out, the deformity produced depends upon the direction in which the force is applied to the vertebral column. If the compressive force is applied axially with the vertebral bodies aligned in a relatively straight column, the load is absorbed by the vertebral body, narrowing it vertically and expanding it circumferentially. The posterior elements are not significantly affected, and therefore further deformity would not be anticipated unless another load were applied that exceeds that producing the original injury (Fig. 3-6).

In flexion and compression the force is not distributed uniformly but is concentrated anteri-

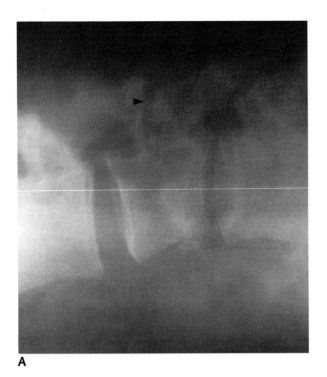
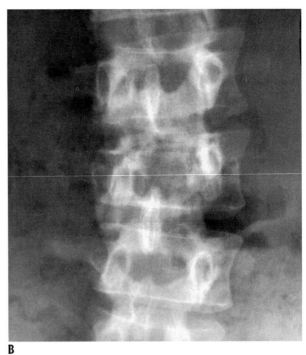

FIGURE 3–9 **A** Flexion distraction injury. The pedicle is split vertically (*arrow*). **B** AP film from the same patient demonstrating separation of the spinous processes.

orly, producing anterior wedging of the vertebral body (Fig. 3–7). A portion of the vertebral body may be displaced posteriorly into the spinal canal. If the posterior elements remain intact, further deformity should not occur under physiological loads and the fracture can be considered stable. However, if the axis of rotation is location more anteriorly in the vertebral body, there may be distraction posteriorly with disruption of the neural arch (Fig. 3–8). If the posterior elements are disrupted, then progressive deformity can be anticipated since flexion is not adequately opposed.

Flexion-distraction injuries produce the *Chance fracture* and its variants. The separation begins posteriorly in the spinous process or interspinous ligament and moves anteriorly through the pedicles and vertebral bodies or disc (Fig. 3–9). The Chance fracture is an unstable lesion because flexion forces will not be adequately resisted.

In the thoracolumbar area, rotation produces the *slice fracture*.[19,20] This fracture usually occurs in the vicinity of the transitional vertebra, which has a horizontal thoracic–type superior articular process and a more vertical lumbar–type inferior process. The transitional vertebra is usually either the 11th or the 12th thoracic vertebra. Rotational movement of the transitional vertebra is blocked by contact between its vertically oriented inferior articular process and the superior facet of the vertebra below it. With sufficient force, a fracture occurs either through the pedicle or sometimes through the vertebral body with displacement of the facet and transverse process of the inferior vertebra laterally. Usually the superior portion of the inferior vertebra remains attached to the rotating transitional vertebra (Fig. 3–10). Because disruption is circumferential, this is a particularly unstable lesion, even though alignment may appear good initially.

Summary

In summary, instability occurs when both the vertebral body and the neural arch or related soft tissue elements are disrupted. Under these conditions, progressive deformity and malalignment can be anticipated, with the possibility of neurological deficit in previously normal patients, or further loss of

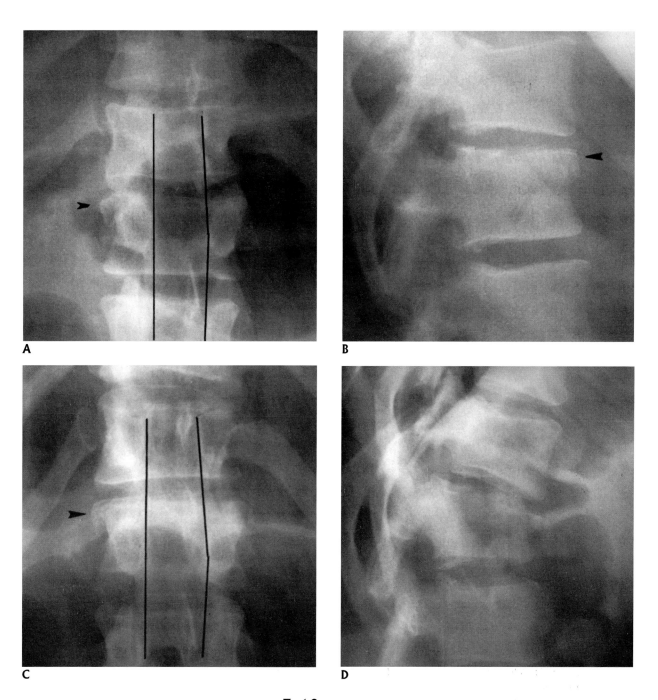

FIGURE 3–10 **A,B** Films demonstrate attachment of the superior portion of the lower vertebrae to the rotating vertebra and lateral displacement of its pedicle. **C,D** Films taken several days later demonstrating increased deformity. The patient had been kept recumbent during the entire time.

function in those with incomplete deficit. Consequently, instability must be identified so that the neural elements can be protected during necessary surgical procedures such as laparotomy and thoracotomy and until the vertebral lesion can be treated definitively.

REFERENCES

1. Adams JA, Hutton WC: The effect of posture on the role of the apophyseal joints in resisting intervertebral compressive forces. J Bone Joint Surg 62-B(3):358–362, 1980.

2. Adams M, Hutton, W: The mechanical function of the lumbar apophyseal joints. Spine 8(3);327–330, 1983.

3. Bedbrook G: Stability of spinal fractures and fracture dislocations. Paraplegia 9:23–32, 1971.

4. Bogduk N, Engel R: The menisci of the lumbar zygapophyseal joints: A review of their anatomy and clinical significance. Spine 9(5):454–460, 1984

5. Brown R, Burstein A, Nash C, et al: Spinal analysis using a three-dimensional radiographic technique. J Biomech 9:355–365, 1976.

6. Cossette J, Farfan H, Robertson G, et al: The instantaneous center of rotation of the third lumbar intervertebral joint. J Biomech 4:149–153, 1971.

7. Denis F, Armstrong G: Compression fractures versus burst fractures in the lumbar and thoracic spine. J Bone Joint Surg 63B(3):462, 1981.

8. Denis F: The three column spine and its significance in the classification of acute thoracolumbar spinal injuries. Spine 8(8):817–831, 1983.

9. Dimnet J, Fischer L, Gonon G, et al: Cervical spine motion in the sagittal plane: Kinematic and geometric parameters. J Biomech 15(12):959–969, 1982.

10. Dunlop R, Adam M, Hutton W: Disc space narrowing and the lumbar facet joints. J Bone Joint Surg 66B(5):706–710, 1984.

11. Dupuis PR, Yong-Hing K, Casssidy JD, et al: Radiologic diagnosis of degenerative lumbar spinal instability. Spine 10(3):262–276, 1985.

12. Fielding J: Normal and selected abnormal motion of the cervical spine from the second cervical vertebra to the seventh cervical vertebra based on cineroentgenography. J Bone Joint Surg 46A(8):1779–1781, 1964.

13. Gertsbein S, Holtby R, Tile M, et al: Determination of the locus of instantaneous centers of rotation of the lumbar disc by Moire fringes: A new technique. Spine 9(4):409–413, 1984.

14. Gertzbein SD, Seligman J, Holtby R, et al: Centrode patterns and segmental instability in degenerative disc disease. Spine 10(3):257–261, 1985.

15. Gianturco C: A roentgen analysis of the motion of the lower lumbar vertebrae in normal individuals and in patients with low back pain. Am J Roentgen 52(3):261–268, 1944.

16. Gregersen G, Lucas D: An *in-vivo* study of the axial rotation of the human thoracolumbar spine. J Bone Joint Surg 49A(2):247–262, 1967.

17. Hanley EN Jr, Matteri RE, Frymoyer JW: Accurate roentgenographic determination of lumbar flexion-extension. Clin Orthop 115:145–148, 1976.

18. Hirsch C, Ingelmark B, Miller M: The anatomical basis for low back pain. Acta Orthop Scand 33:1–17, 1963.

19. Holdsworth F: Fractures, dislocations and fracture dislocations of the spine. J Bone Joint Surg 45B(1):6–20, 1963.

20. Holdsworth F: Review article: Fractures, disclocations, and fracture-dislocations of the spine. J Bone Joint Surg 52A(8):1534–1551, 1970.

21. KIrkaldy-Willis W, Farfan H: Instability of the lumbar spine. Clin Orthop 165:110–123, 1982.

22. Knutsson F: The instability associated with disk degeneration in the lumbar spine. Acta Radiol 25:593–609, 1944.

23. Lindahl O: Determination of the sagittal mobility of the lumbar spine: A clinical method. Acta Orthop Scand 37:241–254, 1966.

24. McAfee P, Yuan H, Lasda N: The unstable burst fracture. Spine 7(4):365–373, 1982.

25. Nicoll E: Fractures of the dorsolumbar spine. J Bone Joint Surg 31B(3):276–394, 1949.

26. Olsson TH, Selvik G, Willner S: Kinematic analysis of spinal fusions. Invest Radiol 11:202–209, 1976.

27. Olsson T, Selvik G, Willner S: Mobility in the lumbosacral spine after fusion studies with the aid of roentgen stereophotogrammetery. Clin Orthop 129:181–190, 1977.

28. Panjabi M: Centers and angles of rotation of body joints: A study of errors and optimization. J Biomech 12:911–920, 1979.

29. Panjabi M, Goel V, Walter S: Errors in kinematic parameters of a planar joint: Guidelines for optimal experimental design. J Biomech 15(7):537–544, 1982.

30. Panjabi M, Krag M, Goel V: A technique for measurement and description of three-dimensional six degree-of-freedom motion of a body joint with an application to the human spine. J Biomech 14:447–460, 1981.

31. Panjabi M, White AI: A mathematical approach for three-dimensional analysis of the mechanics of the spine. J Biomech 4:203–211, 1971.

32. Pennal G, Conn G, McDonald G, et al: Motion studies of the lumbar spine: A preliminary report. J Bone Joint Surg 54B(3):442–452, 1972.

33. Penning L, Blickman JR: Instability in lumbar spondylolisthesis: A radiologic study of several concepts. Am J Roentgenol 134 (February):293–301, 1980.

34. Posner I, White AA, Edwards WT, et al: A biomechanical analysis of the clinical stability of the lumbar and lumbosacral spine. Spine 7(4):374–388, 1982.

35. Stokes IAF, Wilder DG, Frymoyer JW, et al: Assessment of patients with low-back pain by biplanar radiographic measurement of intervertebral motion. Spine 6:(3):233–240, 1981.

36. Suh C: The fundamentals of computer aided x-ray analysis of the spine. J Biomech 7:161–169, 1994.
37. Taylor J, Twomey L: Sagittal and horizontal plane movement of the human lumbar vertebral column in cadavers and in the living. Rheumatol Rehabil 19:223–232, 1980.
38. Torgerson WR, Dotter WE: Comparative roentgenographic study of the asymptomatic and symptomatic lumbar spine. J Bone Joint Surg Am 58-A(6):850–853, 1976.
39. White AI, Panjabi M: The problem of clinical instability in the human spine: A systematic approach. Part 4: The lumbar spine (L2-L5). In Clinical Biomechanics of the Spine, M.P. AA White III. JB Lippincott, Philadelphia, pp. 251–264, 1978.

CHAPTER 4

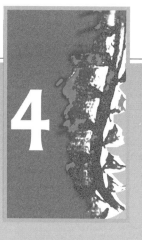

Metabolic Diseases of Bone

Osteitis Deformans

Osteoporosis

Ankylosing Spondylitis of the Lumbar Spine

Metabolic Diseases of Bone

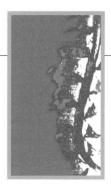

A wide spectrum of metabolic diseases affects the lumbar spine, often acting like neoplasms. A detailed discussion of these is beyond the scope of this book; rather a summary of interest to the surgeon is presented.

Osteitis Deformans

Osteitis deformans, better known as Paget's disease, is the most common exogenously stimulated (i.e., attributable to an external cause) metabolic bone disease.[7] There is a predilection for involvement of the lumbar spine.[59] Although the etiology remains uncertain, most evidence points to slow virus infection: commonly seen are nuclear inclusions in osteoblasts.[77] In addition, recent studies have shown proteinaceous viruslike structures within affected osteoclast nuclei and cytoplasm.[76] Because slow viruses are known to induce neoplasms, many question whether Paget's disease is a metabolic disease or a true benign tumor.[103] The incidence of Paget's disease has increased over the last few decades: it is seen in approximately five percent of European adults over the age of 50, making it second only to osteoporosis in incidence of spinal diseases.[82]

Pathology

The fundamental pathologic process in Paget's disease is a cyclic process of abnormal bone resorption and subsequent growth.[59] In the first stage of the disease, abnormal multinucleated osteoclasts cause focal resorption and cavity formation in affected bone. This is known as the *osteolytic phase*, and weakness in the vertebral body at this time may produce collapse.[71]

In the second stage, *lamellar bone formation* occurs at the edges of the cavities produced by bone resorption. This new bone is exuberant and typically disorganized and even appears to be woven, in contrast to the typical lamellae seen in healthy bone.[71] The compressive strength of this bone is marginal. Over time, this woven bone will be replaced by more calcified tissue, producing typically the first radiographic abnormalities. Connective tissue growth also occurs within the marrow cavity and around the bone at this stage. There is a high degree of vascularization of the new bone and connective tissue, which may cause vascular steal, as discussed later. One of the unique pathologic events of Paget's disease is the *late increase in bone density*, with continued production of bone followed by a loss of osteoblastic activity and marked bony sclerosis.[71]

Clinical Presentation

The majority of patients with spinal involvement are asymptomatic. However, symptoms of the disorder may range from low back pain to severe myelopathy and even paraplegia. Back pain may be a consequence of widening and decreased height of affected vertebral bodies and vertebral body collapse.[96] Clinical studies have indicated that the back pain in Paget's disease is often more related to secondary changes.[2] For example, decreased vertebral body height or widening of the vertebral body will lead to accelerated osteoarthritis in the facet joints and hypertrophy of the posterior elements. The latter may cause spinal cord and/or nerve root compression.

The most common neurologic manifestation of long-standing Paget's disease of the lumbar spine is lumbar stenosis, which is not necessarily compressive in nature.[23,59] On occasion, the hypervascularity within involved posterior elements produces actual vascular steal from the nerve roots, dural sac, and even the spinal cord. This may occur early in the disease and be out of proportion to the bony changes (Fig. 4–1).[42] Typically, mechanical back pain occurs in the later sclerotic phases. Deformities may also occur due to remolding of vertebral bodies. Although this typically occurs in the thoracic spine, it has been reported in the upper lumbar spine as well.[96]

As the spinal canal is narrowed by the continued development of disorganized new bone, slowly progressive cauda equina syndrome may develop. This is probably the most common serious neurological manifestation of Paget's disease. The lumbar stenosis of Paget's disease is somewhat unusual in that it often includes the more proximal lumbar nerve roots, along with claudication (both vascular and mechanical) and sphincter disturbances.[35] Typically, patients complain of more back pain than in other types of lumbar stenosis.

Patients with advanced spinal Paget's disease may also suffer from hearing loss due to narrowing of the eighth cranial nerve canal, and cerebellar abnormalities. High-output cardiac failure due to vasodilatation and increased vascular flow is common. Malignant degeneration of Paget's disease, while well known and properly feared, is extremely uncommon. Chondrosarcomas have been occasionally observed (Fig. 4–2). These are more common in long bones than in the spine and appear as calcified matrix in a destructive lesion, usually at long bone joints.[9] While quite unusual, osteosarcomas may arise from involved vertebra. These tend to be extremely aggressive, even for sarcomas.[96] The osteosarcoma of Paget's disease is highly malignant. It presents most typically as an exophytic mass with vertebral compression (Fig. 4–3).[34] Occasionally, however, cauda equina syndrome with canal stenosis will be the first manifestation.[13]

Diagnosis

The diagnosis is made radiographically. During the osteolytic phase, cavities may occasionally be identified within vertebral bodies. Changes in vertebral geometry, including loss of vertebral body height, will occur because of collapse and remodeling (Fig 4–4).[59] Enlargement of the pedicles and masses of poorly calcified osteoid tissue extending laterally may be seen during the late osteolytic period. Scalloping of the dorsal aspect of the vertebral body is quite common. This is largely due to collapse within the middle of the body.

During the stage of lamellar bone formation, when osteoblast activity is at its height, the classic picture of Paget's disease appears. The longitudinal and vertical cortical shells undergo widening with marked sclerosis at the periphery, creating a very sclerotic triangle. The center of the vertebra will often appear almost hollow. Later, exuberant soft tissue extending from the bone is often seen; this is incompletely calcified.[59]

Imaging beyond plain radiography is indicated only the presence of neurological deficit. Computed tomography (CT) is ideal for identifying foraminal narrowing. Magnetic resonance imaging (MRI) is important to distinguish between pathologic soft tissue producing nerve and spinal cord compression and normal structures. Canal studies, regardless of the type used, may inaccurately determine the amount of neural compromise, since symptoms may be due to ischemia from vascular steal rather than compression.[42] Angiography is occasionally used in presurgical planning to identify hypervascular bone.[52] On occasion, we have used preoperative embolization prior to vertebral resection.

Because Paget's disease is often multifocal, nuclear scanning should be routinely employed. Preoperatively, it will often demonstrate vertebral involvement prior to radiographic abnormalities, and may also show multifocal states. The success of nonsurgical treatment can be measured by serial scanning: decreasing uptake indicates improvement.[99] Quantitative bone scanning can be particularly valuable in evaluating the results of treatment.[83]

The biochemical changes associated with Paget's disease can be useful in determining the stage and severity of the disorder, although neither serum nor urine testing can be used for initial diagnosis. Hydroxyproline and hydroxylysine (which form much of the collagen matrix of bone) are excreted in the urine. Measurement of urinary hydroxyproline can be performed but is difficult, expensive, and often inaccurate. It is therefore an impractical tool for monitoring clinical status. There is little change in serum calcium because the losses are counteracted by osteoblastic activity. Serum alkaline phosphatase levels are elevated, and loosely correlate with osteoblast activity.[59] Enzyme levels will accurately reflect reactive osteoblastic bone synthesis and can be used to monitor medical

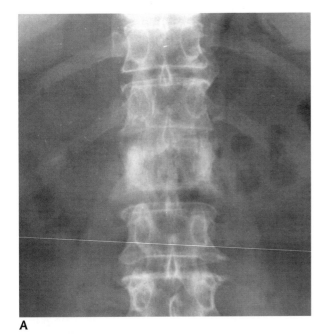
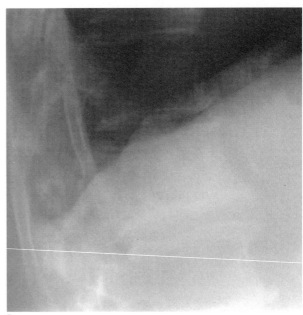
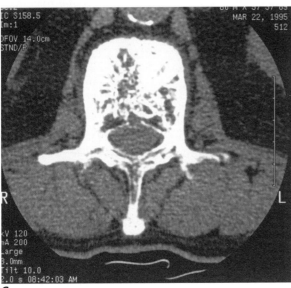
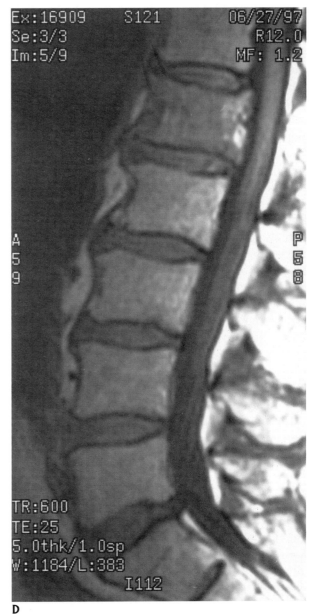

FIGURE 4–1

Fifty-one-year-old male with a 4-year history of neurogenic claudication. **A** and **B** Anteroposterior (AP) and lateral radiographs demonstrate typical striations in the L1 vertebral body. There is thickened cortical bone at margins of the vertebra. **C** An axial computed tomogram demonstrating lamellar bone formation. **D** Sagittal MR image demonstrates no significant canal compromise, a finding verified at laminectomy. Symptoms improved following surgery. **E** Microscopic section (100×) demonstrating typical pathologic lamellar bone formation.

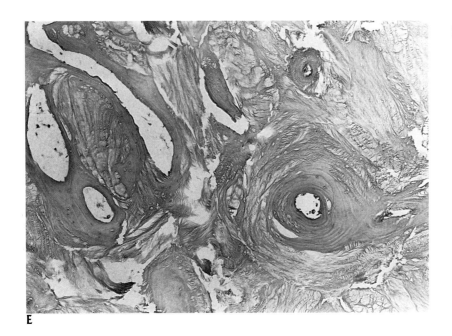

FIGURE 4–1 E

treatment. Hyperuricemia is common and may correlate with the severity of the disease. Indeed, almost 20% of patients with both Paget's disease and hyperuricemia have clinical gout.[59]

Management

Although the names of some of the drugs are different, little else has changed in the management of Paget's disease since our report almost a decade ago.[70] Most patients will require only occasional follow-up, since the majority demonstrating spinal involvement remain asymptomatic. Minor back pain can be managed with anti-inflammatory agents and minor analgesics in the absence of progression of bony pathology. For more significant pain and progressive osteolysis, three major agents are available.

Drug Therapy

Historically, *calcitonin* has been the mainstay of drug treatment. It is obtained from the parafollicular thyroid cells, and consistently inhibits osteoblastic changes immediately following parenteral administration. Over 80% of patients respond, often for one or more years following several months of treatment. Decreased uptake characteristic of improvement will be observed on bone scans; such may be seen on radiography as well.

Unfortunately, the effects sometimes do not last beyond the administration of the drug, and a significant percentage of patients will develop blocking antibodies: these patients require (extremely expensive) human calcitonin formulation.[70,88]

The *diphosphonates* represent the second pharmaceutical level of attack. These drugs inhibit bone resorption, and thus slow new bone formation.[27] *Etidronate* is especially effective in relieving bone pain at low doses; high doses may actually increase pain. The major advantage of etidronate over calcitonin lies in its oral administration and lack of antibody development.[70] On occasion, the two drugs can be given together with synergistic activity. Unfortunately, in inhibiting bone regrowth, the use of diphosphonates can lead to weakened bones and increased risk of osteoporotic fracture.[21,27]

A newly developed biphosphonate which shows significant promise is *alendronate*, recently approved by the FDA for treatment of osteoporosis and Paget's disease.[89] A recent multicenter study demonstrated marked decrease in alkaline phosphatase levels as compared to patients treated with etidronate.[104] Patients were much more likely to revert to normal osteoblast activity. Additionally, bone mineralization was vastly superior to that seen with other drugs.

Long-term treatment with other biphosphonates such as *pamidronate* occasionally will reverse neurologic deficits due to stenosis and steal.[113] Reported side effects of biphosphonates are limited to gastrointestinal abnormalities, typically managed

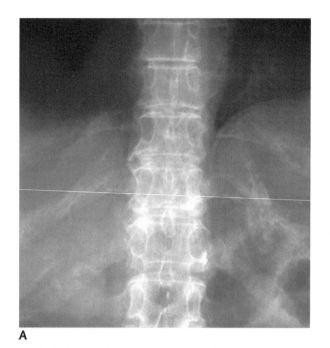
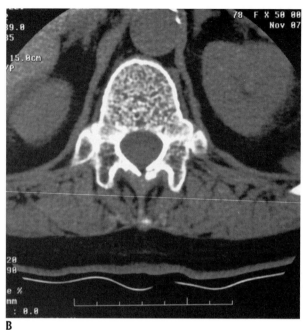
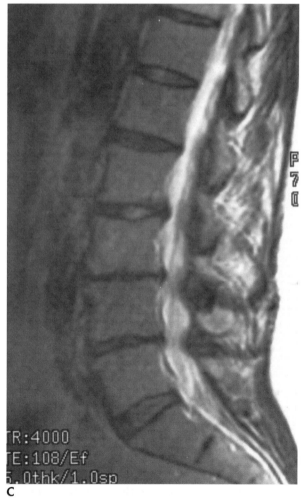

FIGURE 4–2

Chondrosarcoma of the spine arising from Pagetic spine in 60-year-old male with back pain. Plain radiographs **A** computed tomography **B** and MRI **C and D** demonstrated involvement at T11 and minor involvement of L4 **E and F** Repeat MRI performed 6 months later showed progression in T11 and L4. Pathology proved to be chondrosarcoma, and widespread metastases were found within 3 months.

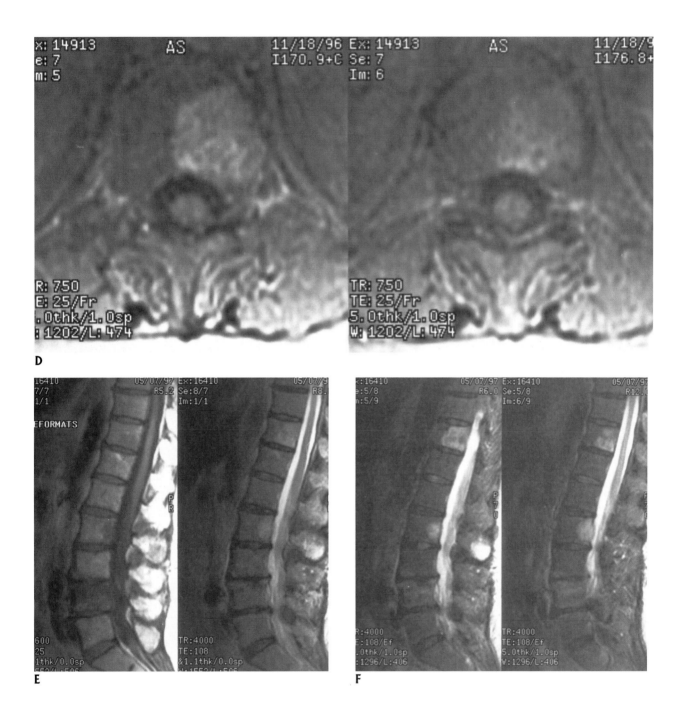

successfully by altering the schedule of the drug. Unfortunately, the drugs remain more expensive than other agents.

Mithramycin has been used in Paget's disease as well. Mithramycin functions by inhibiting DNA-dependent osteosynthesis and is toxic to osteoclasts.[52] It is particularly effective in the management of bone pain. Unfortunately, it has reported significant side effects, including thrombocytopenia and nephrotoxicity. Thus it is generally reserved for those who do not respond to other agents.

Surgical Treatment

Surgical indications are the same as those for any other type of spinal disorder. Operative treatment for back pain is rarely necessary, even in the presence of vertebral body fracture. The more common surgical indication is the treatment of bony overgrowth causing spinal cord, cauda equina, or nerve root compression.[23] Generally, hypertrophic laminae and vascular steal will cause apparent lumbar stenosis, as defined earlier.[35,118] Paget's involving the laminae-even without neural compres-

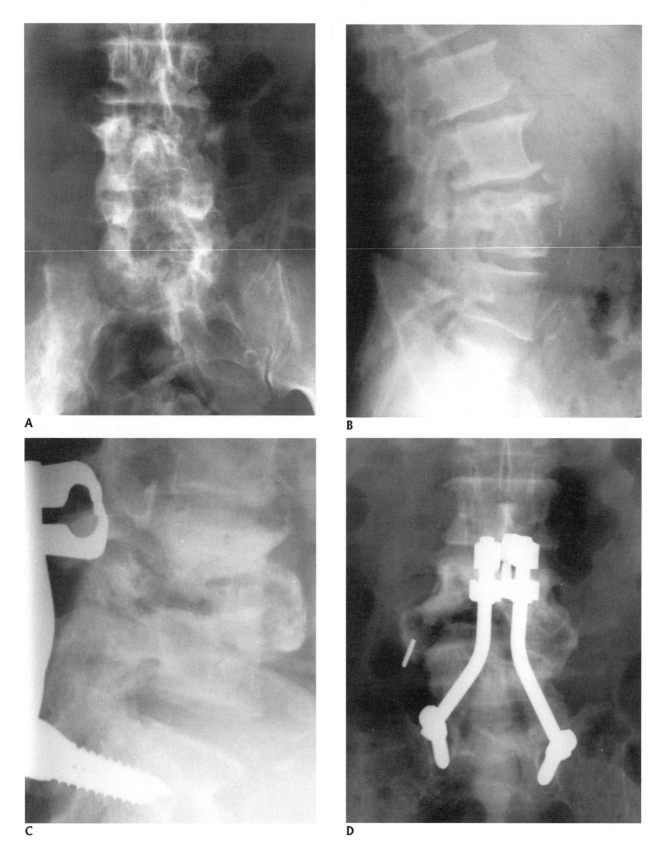

FIGURE 4-3 Osteosarcoma in a 68-year-old male with 18-year history of Paget's. **A and B** AP and lateral radiographs following complaints of lumbar stenosis with classis late picture and exuberant ossified soft tissue. Plain radiographs **C and D** and myelogram **E** performed 20 months after laminectomy and fusion, for cauda equina syndrome. During anterior decompression and fusion, the exuberant mass was resected, proving benign. Instrumentation was also removed. **F** Two years later, a mass had recurred. **G** MRI demonstrates extensive vertebral involvement and a prevertebral lesion. **H** Following angiography and embolization, the vascular mass was resected. Pathology showed "low-grade" osteosarcoma. Patient is recurrence-free 14 months later.

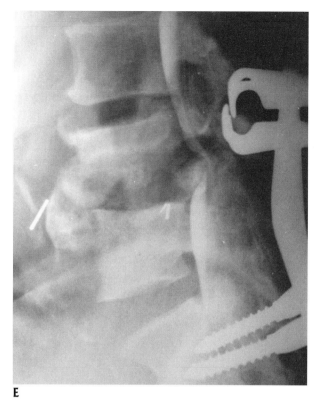

E

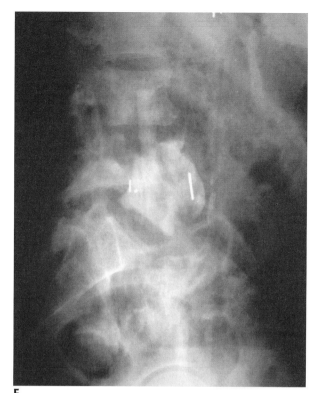

F

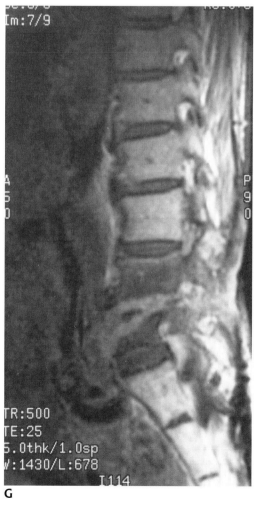

G

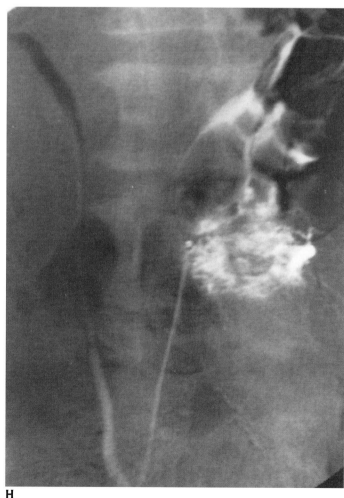

H

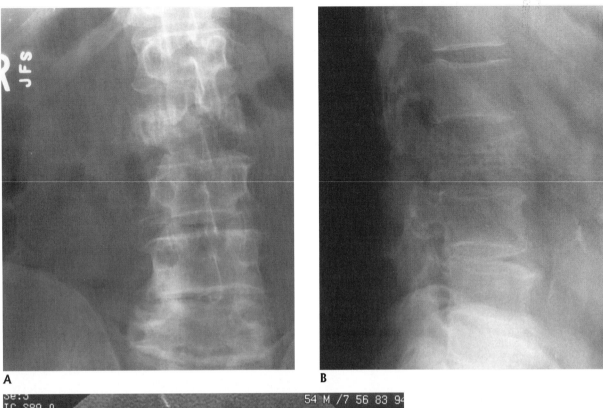
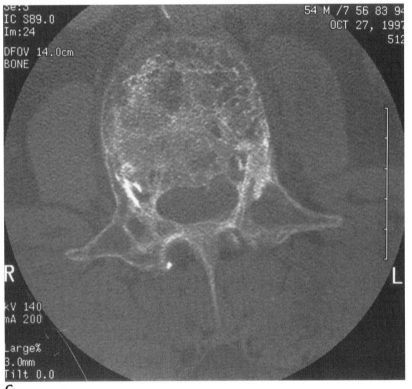

FIGURE 4–4
L2 fracture in Paget's disease. **A and B** AP and lateral radiographs show decreased body height with typical appearance. **C** Computed tomogram with central cavities. There is little marginal hypertrophy of the cortex. **D and E** MRI shows marked canal compromise. Patient refused surgery and has a partial cauda equina syndrome.

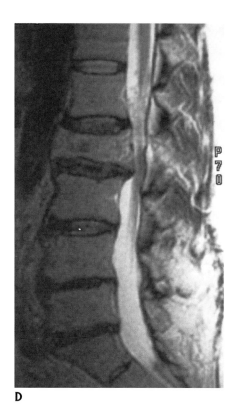
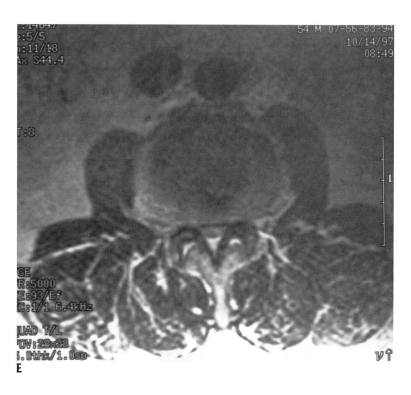

sion—may require surgical treatment if the patient fails to respond to medication and demonstrates intractable neurogenic claudication due to steal.[53,118] The selection of operative procedures should be based on the extent and location of the pathology.

Drug treatment should precede elective surgery to decrease the hypervascularity of pathologic bone, prevent postoperative hypercalcemia, and foster healing and bone fusion.[70,88] (Etidronate is not appropriate for this purpose, however, since it may slow down fusion of normal bone, as well.) In addition, the risk of high-output cardiac failure will be lessened by drug use prior to surgery.

Surgical procedures will likely be complicated by significant bleeding. Spinal angiography is often useful: when local arterial feeders are evident, embolization will often decrease intraoperative hemorrhage. Other risks include intraoperative and immediate postoperative cardiac failure and elevated serum calcium.[70] Generally, the surgeon should avoid removing involved bone that is not producing clinical symptoms, since progression is not the rule; rather, only the pathology producing the clinical syndrome should be addressed.

Removal of a normal lamina to decompress a neural sac compressed by a fractured vertebral body is no more acceptable than with neoplasms.

The residual vertebral body is significantly weakened and deformity can be expected to occur. Therefore, as is the case with tumors or trauma, surgical attention must be directed to the pathology. We consider Paget's disease to be a neoplasm and therefore pathologic bone should be surgically manipulated as such. The use of instrumentation with deformity or for immobilization purposes is often important in vertebral body involvement. Fixation devices should not be placed into levels or structures with known Pagetic involvement.

If the diagnosis of sarcoma can be made radiographically, biopsy should not be performed, since the tumor is quite vascular. Rather, the goals of surgery are radical extirpation, including appropriate stabilization.[70] Chemotherapy and radiation therapy should follow. In spite of aggressive treatment, long-term survival is uncommon.[44]

Osteoporosis

Osteoporosis refers to decreased calcification of the spine. Although a more precise definition would be preferable, even an NIH consensus conference in 1984 recommended that primary osteoporosis be defined as an "idiopathic age-related disorder characterized by decreasing bone mass and resultant increased susceptibility to fracture."[56,60a] It is clearly related to decreased endogenous estrogen, impaired Vitamin D metabolism, cigarette use, decreased vascularity of bone as a consequence of sedentary lifestyle, excessive consumption of caffeine and alcohol, and decreased serum calcium.[19] The use of exogenous corticosteroid is a well-known cause of osteoporosis. Some patients have benefited from the simultaneous prophylactic use of biphosphonates.[41]

With almost 10% of the population demonstrating decreased bone density (and an increasing incidence), osteoporosis represents an epidemic problem for every physician treating spinal disorders.[56] It is most commonly seen in the elderly and in postmenopausal women, where incidence has been reported to be as high as 40 to 50%.[5] Almost one million vertebral body fractures will occur annually, mostly in the thoracic and lumbar spine;[49] 40% of women over 60 years old suffer vertebral body fractures due to decreased bone density.[68,114]

Overall, women are much more likely to suffer vertebral body fractures secondary to osteoporosis than men, although the incidence is similar before age 65.[68] Studies have shown that this is the case even in individuals whose bone densities are the same. In a recent investigation, the question of why osteoporotic fractures were more likely to occur in women was investigated. Gilsanz et al found that the cross-sectional diameter of vertebrae in women with fractures was 5 to 11% smaller, and the moment arm of spinal musculature 3 to 7% shorter in women with fractures.[30] This suggests that the mechanical stresses in intact vertebrae are significantly higher in women with fractures than in those without, for equivalent loads. Thus women with smaller spines are more likely to suffer vertebral fractures due to osteoporosis.[64,68,78]

An interesting observation is that the incidence of osteoporotic fractures in males is increasing, particularly in those with stroke and other neurologic disease. Unpublished data from our institution in patients with Brown-Sequard syndrome has demonstrated that decreased bone density not uncommonly occurs on the weak side. However, the degree of calcium loss is not as dramatic as it often is in a truly paraplegic population, suggesting that weight bearing, physical activity, and other movement-related risk factors are not as significant as metabolic ones. This suggests that there may be additional etiologic factors in the neurologically impaired population yet to be determined.

Pathology

As a consequence of reduced bone mass, impaired strength of the spine results from osteoporosis. Historically, some have argued that osteoporosis is primarily a consequence of demineralization of the trabeculae. Ritzel et al have performed elegant histomorphometric studies demonstrating that the cortical bone is as severely involved as the trabeculae.[94] Because the thickness of the cortex is maximal in the lower thoracic and lumbar spine, loss of bone mass in this region may explain why spinal fractures are more likely to occur here than elsewhere in the spine.

Clinical Presentation

Osteoporosis is most commonly asymptomatic. When symptomatic, it typically presents as pain, usually due to fracture. Such pain will result from even normal activity or minimal falls. Pain is rarely radicular, and neurological deficit is uncommon; the fractured osteoporotic vertebral body has diminished capacity to compress the spinal cord. When neurological deficit does occur, it is typically in the mid-thoracic spine where the canal is already marginal. The pain of vertebral body fracture is typically exacerbated by physical activity and is decreased by bracing. Ultimately it will improve with successful healing of the fracture, which will be quite slow.

Some have suggested that the increased bone density associated with osteoarthritis decreases the risk of osteoporotic fracture. A major recent study proved this not to be the case.[50] Patients with osteoarthritis did indeed demonstrate higher bone density in the lumbar spine. However, they also had higher body sway and lower quadriceps strength, with an increased risk of falling, and thus fracture.[45]

On occasion, multiple vertebral body fractures will occur either simultaneously or in sequence with the development of deformity as a result. Typically seen in the thoracic spine, these are often best treated nonoperatively.

Diagnosis

The diagnosis of osteoporosis is best made radiographically. Plain radiographs will demonstrate decreased bone calcification. CT may suggest trabecular loss as well as cortical bone remodeling. However, in the presence of actual vertebral collapse, the distinction between osteoporosis and malignancy may be difficult (Fig. 4–5). Laredo et all identified certain characteristics for benign osteoporotic fractures using computed tomography: fractures of the cortical bone without destruction, intravertebral vacuum sign, and bone retropulsion into the spinal canal. Malignancies were likely associated with cortical destruction, pedicle involvement, and epidural or large extravertebral soft tissue masses.[61]

MRI with gadolinium enhancement is often helpful. In a study by Cuenod, preservation of normal signal intensity on T1-weighted images and isodense images on T2 were suggestive of osteoporosis. Malignancy was characterized by epidural masses, a convex posterior vertebral cortex, and altered signals within the pedicles and in the vertebra following contrast.[16] Rupp et al questioned these findings in a recent report. Several patients with vertebral fractures underwent MRI and bone biopsy. Decreased T1 signals on routine imaging and increased T2 signals were sensitive for tumor, and normal bone marrow suggested metabolic disease. Only pedicle involvement and soft tissue masses consistently identified tumor.[95]

Dual photon absorption (DPA) techniques for bone densitometry measure both cortical and medullary density with a high degree of reliability.[97,98] DPA can be helpful in assessing the preoperative patient for pathologic degrees of decreased bone density, but this information is advisory at best. DPA can also be of benefit in decision making regarding use of spinal instrumentation. Unfortunately, absolute DPA criteria that can be used to define treatment risks do not exist.[97]

Laboratory tests for readily treatable causes of osteoporosis, including erythrocyte sedimentation rate (ESR), eletrophoresis, thyroid function, estrogen levels, and vitamin D, can be performed. Early myeloma may result in widespread osteoporosis. Often rheumatologists will recommend an iliac crest bone biopsy to distinguish bone volume mineralization and bone turnover. Unfortunately, no reliable and readily measurable markers of bone turnover exist.[20]

Management

Treatment is quite varied. Cigarette smoking is bad for the spine in general; it is particularly dangerous for those with osteoporosis.[18] At least as important in the prevention of osteoporosis is an active exercise program to maintain bone mass.[105] Weight-bearing exercises such as walking performed two to three times weekly will improve bone mineral content in the spine. Muscle mass seems to be directly correlated to bone mass.[17] Isometric strength of the back extensors is inversely related to compression fractures. Therefore, it would seem logical to promote lumbar stabilization rehabilitation programs to patients with early osteoporosis. However, aggressive spine flexion/rotation and extension may cause fractures de novo.[102]

Dietary Supplements

Increased dietary calcium may be of value by protecting or increasing bone mass. Riggs et al[91] recommended that premenopausal women receive a supplemental 1.2 grams of calcium as a daily supplement, and postmenopausal women 1.5 grams. Vitamin D from 400 to 800 units is recommended. This is particularly important in the elderly, who are at additional risk of osteoporosis, and who have decreased metabolism of vitamin D. Following treatment with vitamin D daily and an exercise program, premenopausal and postmenopausal women demonstrated improved bone mass as measured by DPA.[91]

The studies of Ettinger[24] and Riis[93] cast some doubt on the usefulness of vitamin D and calcium. In these two double-blind studies, 1.5 to 2.0 grams of calcium alone failed to decrease the rate of bone loss in the early postmenopausal period. In spite of the controversy, considering the low morbidity of the treatment, elemental calcium plus Vitamin D appears appropriate in people with evidence of osteoporosis and in all postmenopausal women.[73,93]

Sodium fluoride has been shown to increase bone mass.[38] The density of bone thus stimulated remains to be determined. In one of the initial studies of fluoride treatment, Riggs et al found that fluoride had a strong synergistic effect with calcium on vertebral body fractures. This was further increased by treatment with estrogen.[90,92] Indeed,

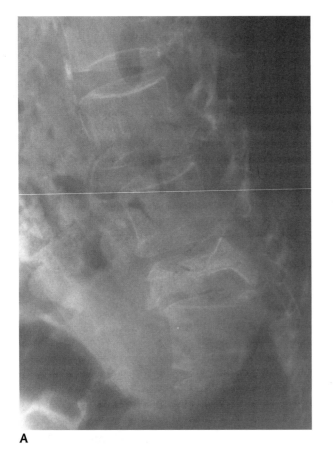
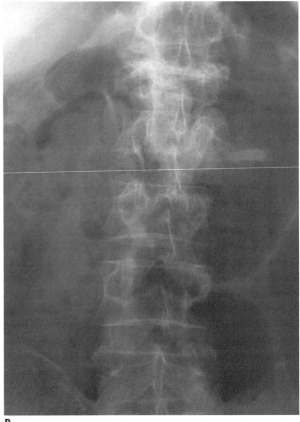
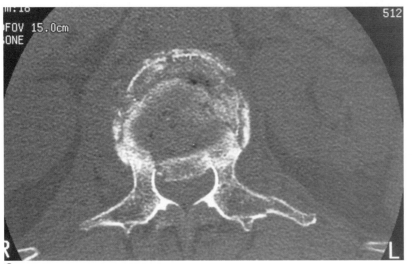

FIGURE 4–5
Fifty-year-old woman with history of osteoporosis and cancer with severe L1 vertebral collapse. **A and B** Plain radiographs suggest canal compromise, thought by some to be indicative of cancer. **C and D** CT demonstrates canal compromise and the unusual finding of gas within the disc space, diagnostic of avascular necrosis.
E On MRI a more consistent picture of osteoporotic fracture is seen.

Lane et al demonstrated that the use of calcium fluoride and vitamin D dramatically decreased spinal fracture.[60a,60b] Unfortunately, the use of fluoride has not achieved wide acceptance. Fluoride therapy without calcium produces weakly mineralized bone and may increase trabecular formation while weakening the cortex.[10,25]

Drug Therapy

Estrogen replacement is commonly used in post menopausal women. Although given almost universally in past years, use has been decreasing somewhat because of the increased risk of estrogen-sensitive cancers (particular breast), hypertension,

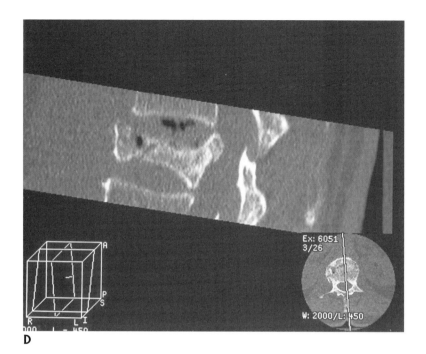
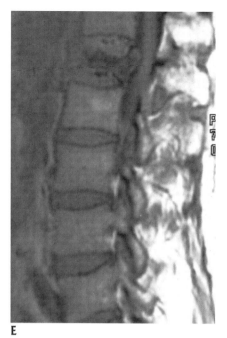

D

E

and liver disease.⁶ The NIH consensus report recommended combination hormonal therapy for all women under the age of 60.⁸¹ Others recommend starting estrogen therapy in any individual with bone mass one or more standard deviations below normal, with accelerated bone density loss defined as more than 3% per year while receiving calcium, vitamin D, and exercise. Estrogens do not improve calcification of bone, but do slow bone loss. Therefore, some feel this therapy should be initiated immediately following menopause and not wait for actual fractures to occur, in spite of the risks of treatment.⁷⁵ Recently, estrogen patches have become increasingly popular because of their improved drug delivery.

The use of *biphosphonates*, for the treatment of postmenopausal osteoporosis has recently become quite popular. Early biphosphonates, such as etidronate, have been shown to significantly decrease vertebral fractures by preserving bone mass.¹¹⁵

A new drug, *alendronate*, is rapidly replacing other agents in the treatment of severe osteoporosis. This drug is an extremely potent inhibitor of bone resorption. It does not affect mineralization, and therefore is a better drug for most patients than etidronate, which negatively impacts bone mineralization. Alendronate functions by inhibiting osteoclast-mediated resorption of bone. In two recent multicenter studies, the drug was compared to placebo with all groups getting calcium. Bone mineral density was improved over the calcium-only group. The drug has a low incidence of side effects, primarily gastrointestinal in nature. Increased bone density is significant and lasts for at least a year after the drug is stopped. Unfortunately, long-term safety and efficacy remain unproven.⁵⁴,⁶⁶

Surgical Treatment

We are primarily concerned with the surgical implications of this pandemic medical disorder. Unfortunately, fractures producing intractable pain commonly occur in this disorder. Fortunately, few of these need surgical treatment. A significant percentage of patients with lumbar stenosis, degenerative scoliosis, and radiculopathy will be shown to have associated osteoporosis. Indeed, the two may actually be related. Margulies et al⁷² recently investigated 294 patients with lumbar spine degeneration and suspected osteoporosis. Peripheral osteoporosis correlated with severe degenerative changes in the discs and facets as well as osteoporosis of the lumbar spine. This has implications for those with osteoporosis: they are at increased risk for the accelerated development of degenerative changes. Although the authors do not investigate this, it may well be that the aggressive treatment of early osteoporosis may prevent accelerated development of degenarative changes in the lumbar spine.

Generally speaking, surgery is to be avoided when possible, because of poor healing and additional surgical morbidity.[85] At times, neurological deficit and deformity will make operative intervention appropriate.[58,107] When neurological deficit does occur, it is often the result of progressive collapse of the fractured vertebra.[4] This deficit is preceded by increasing radicular complaints.[40]

Kumano et al found that patients with less than 100 mg/mm bone mineral density are no less likely to fuse than those with higher bone mineral density.[60] Radiographic grading of osteoporosis, however, did not correlate well to bone mineral density. They concluded that pedicle fixation could be used in spinal canal stenosis with single-level fusions in patients with mild to moderate osteoporosis. Furthermore, they found bone mineral density testing to be more sensitive than radiography to measure osteoporosis and recommended its use in surgical planning.

It has been our practice to use the lateral extracavitary approach for decompression if deformity is present, or a transpedicular approach if anterior fusion is not necessary. If the major anterior mass compressing the cord can be resected through a transpedicular approach, significant blood loss will be avoided.[4] Fusion rates are clearly lower in patients with osteoporosis, and thus anterior fusion is less likely to be successful.[64]

Instrumentation carries with it significant risk as well. Transpedicular fixation, to a significant degree, relies on the integrity of the trabecular bone for maintenance of screw integrity. Pull-out strength is significantly decreased in patients with osteoporosis, and is proportional to bone density. In addition, "screw wobble" is increased with decreased bone density. On the other hand, cortical bone, although weakened as well, is still more suitable as a fixation point.[85] Therefore, it is our preference to use instrumentation techniques that rely equally upon the cortex and cancellous bone.

In posterior instrumentation, where neutral fixation of the spine is to be maintained, our preferred approach is to use sublaminar and spinous process wiring of L-rods or segmental instrumentation placed with minimal laminar stress.

Commonly, we will apply Galveston rods to the spine with double wiring at each level (Fig. 4–6). Alternatively, a simple segmental universal instrumentation-type rod will be applied with claws at the ends and sublaminar wiring in between at the critical junctures. Surgical procedures are discussed in later chapters.

Transpedicular fixation should be avoided. This has not been the experience of Baba et al, however, who reported 27 cases of anterior or posterior treatment for osteoporotic vertebral collapse. In almost all patients, there was progression of both bone collapse and neurological deficit due to retropulsed fragments. Their favorite surgical technique was transpedicular decompression and transpedicular screw fixation. Their argument was that the minimal morbidity and time factor for this type of surgery outweigh the risks of the osteoporotic spine.[4] Unfortunately, our experience has been much less satisfactory.

Halvorson et al performed biomechanical studies comparing a combination of pedicle screws and laminar hooks with screw placement in normal and osteoporotic spines.[37] They found pedicle screw pull-out strength to be directly related to bone density as well as to surgical preparation, and recommended that tapping be minimized in patients with osteoporosis. Okuyama et al add that bone mineral density should be assessed preoperatively in osteoporotic patients to ensure the safety of transpedicular fixation, without providing absolute criteria.[79] The use of laminar hooks in conjunction with pedicle screws improved pull-out strength. The latter was studied by Hasegawa et al in cadaver spines.[39] Construct stiffness was much greater with the combination, irrespective of mineral bone density. Our experience with this technique in four cases has been unsatisfactory: screw pull-out with laminar fracture occurred in two while the patients were immobilized in orthoses.

Ankylosing Spondylitis of the Lumbar Spine

Ankylosing spondylitis (AS) and its resulting deformities represent a significant challenge to the spinal surgeon. The incidence of AS is approximately 1 to 2% in the normal population. The typical age of onset is 30 to 50 years.[51] Although the clinical picture is similar in both men and women, the disease seems less severe in the latter.[48] A particular human leukocyte antigen (HLA) encoded on genes in the sixth chromosome is seen 8% of the Caucasian population but in almost 90% of Caucasians with AS.[22] The pathophysiology of ankylosing spondylitis appears to be an inflammatory disorder which is presumably stimulated by inflammatory or infectious agents in hosts with the HLA-B27 antigen. Recently, the peptide felt responsible for

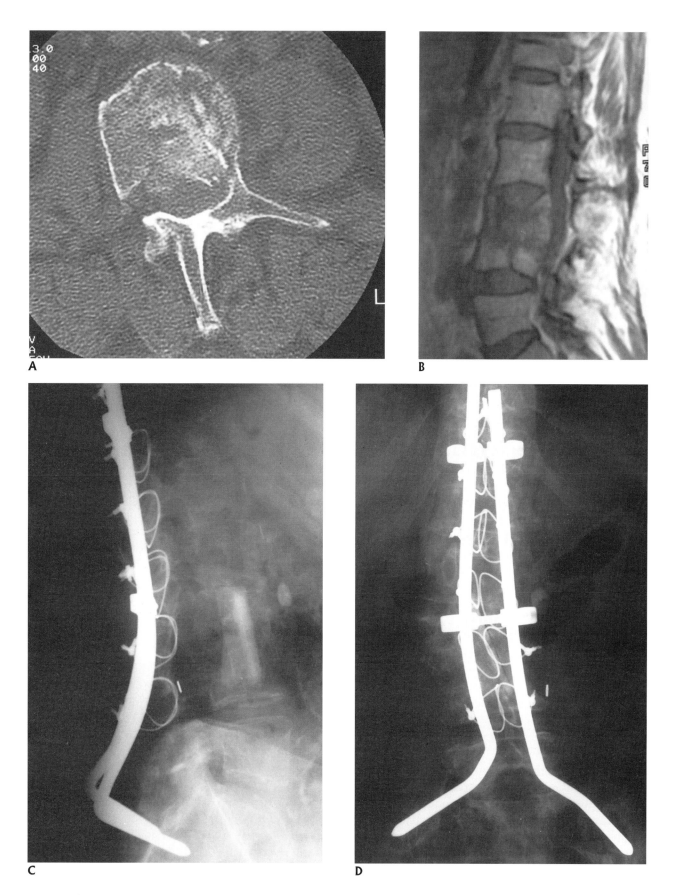

FIGURE 4–6 L3 fracture secondary to osteoporosis with cauda equina syndrome. **A** Canal compromise and "convexity" of dorsal vertebra evident on CT. **B** MRI confirms canal compromise; there is no uptake in the body with contrast. **C and D** Following an extracavitary approach to the spine with interbody fusion and Galveston pelvic fixation the patient made an excellent recovery.

stimulating the response has been found to be of bacterial origin.[69] This antigen can be used to identify risk populations.

Pathology

The pathology is characteristic. Inflammation, bone changes and erosion, and subsequent ankylosis are ubiquitous. Particularly common is a lymphocytic inflammatory infiltrate at the annulus of the disc and end plate. The inflammation and its subsequent ossification lead to the classic ankylosed bamboo spine. Deformity is a consequence of asymmetric loss of disc height during the inflammatory process, to some extent a result of spinal loading.[51,70,82,101]

Clinical Presentation

Clinical presentation is variable. Most patients present during young adulthood with low back pain. Progressive deformity then develops in more severe cases of spinal involvement. Peripheral arthritis usually coincides with spinal problems. Uveitis is not uncommon; it is much more common in HLA 27–positive patients with advanced disease than in others.[67] Most functional losses occur in the first 10 years, followed by a plateau without improvement.[33]

In a recent longitudinal study by Lee et al,[65] a group of men were followed with radiography, bone mineral density, bone turnover assessment, and bone biopsy. Individuals with early disease, identified as sacroiliitis alone, had more normal bone densities that did not change. The converse was true in late disease, with widespread spinal involvement. There were no consistent histologic changes in bone biopsies. In spite of medical treatment resulting in decreased pain and increased activity, laboratory values and bone density did not improve. Thus the severe osteopenia typically seen in spinal involvement cannot be attributed to inactivity or specific hormonal abnormality.

Marked lumbar stenosislike complaints may occur. These symptoms are improved by exercise and are worsened by being in the supine position.[28] Rarely is the syndrome progressive, however, and cauda equina syndrome has been only occasionally observed.[100] Dural ectasia with laminar erosion is usually seen on magnetic resonance imaging in these individuals.[57]

As a result of the deformity as well as the ankylosis, the mechanical integrity of the spine is significantly altered. Although it appears stiff, the strength in shear and in flexion loading is decreased because of the brittleness of the spine. Furthermore, because of the loss of mobile segments, forces applied to the spine are absorbed only by a rigid column, and thus fracture may occur even with trivial injury. Osteopenia is quite severe in many cases as well.[55,110] The thoracolumbar spine is particularly at risk, presumably because of loading factors. In a cohort study performed in Rochester, Minnesota, patients with AS were far more likely to suffer thoracolumbar fractures, although limb fractures occurred at the same rate as in the control cohort population.[12]

Diagnosis

Evaluation of the ankylosing spondylitis patient is best made radiographically in the individual who is at risk and has the typical pain syndrome (Fig. 4–7). Indeed, extent of disease in patients with sacroiliac joint and lumbar spine involvement on radiography correlates quite well with a battery of range-of-motion testing.[112] HLA-B27 typing is best limited to patients with atypical radiographic findings. Patients with radiographic evidence of ankylosing spondylitis in the spine should also undergo radiography of the hips and other joints. Plain radiographs should be adequate for that purpose, although some have recommended radionuclide studies because of their sensitivity. Indeed, the latter have been shown to be predictive in demonstrating changes long before radiography, particularly pseudoarthrosis in advanced disease.[84] MRI is extremely sensitive for the inflammatory changes, but since the results of MRI are unlikely to alter treatment, the utility is limited. Indeed, the nonoperative treatment of ankylosing spondylitis is typically unchanged by the radiographic extent of the disorder.

In patients with pulmonary complaints, high-resolution CT is valuable. Whereas chest radiographs are typically normal, computed tomography often demonstrates interstitial lung disease, bronchiectasis, and emphysema. Thus, although most AS patients with respiratory difficulties have chest wall constriction due to deformity, a sig-

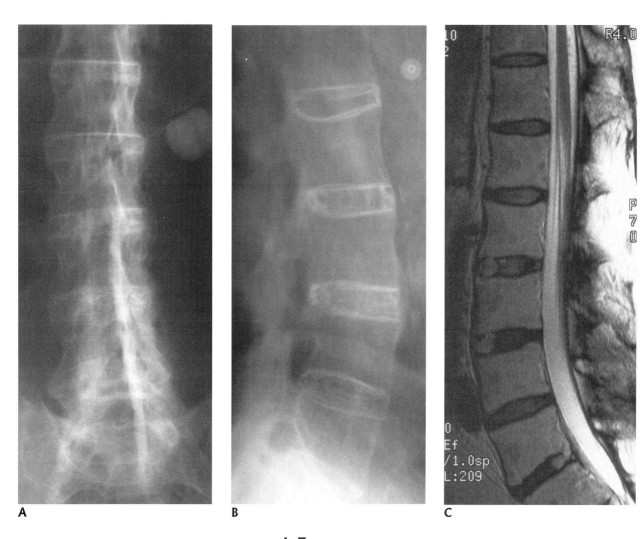

FIGURE 4–7 Classic ankylosing spondylitis in 43-year-old man with severe back pain. **A and B** AP and lateral radiographs show "bamboo spine" **C** MRI shows calcification within affected disc spaces.

nificant percentage will suffer primary pulmonary disease.[26]

Management

Drug Therapy

The value of drug therapy is inconsistent. *Antiinflammatory agents* will decrease symptoms, especially in earlier stages of the disease, but do not reverse or prevent the progression of structural abnormalities.[87] Some have suggested more aggressive pharmacotherapy, including antibiotics and therapy with drugs such a methotrexate and cyclosporine as well as other *anti-autoimmune agents*. Although Creemers et al have reported significant clinical improvement,[14] the long-term value of this agent remains to be proven.[15]

Physical Therapy and Exercise

Physical therapy is critical in ankylosing spondylitis for preservation of residual spine mobility and range of motion of joints. A recreational exercise program is particularly valuable, including swimming. Cross country skiing is valuable because of its extension of the paravertebral muscles.[43]

Nonoperative Treatment of Fractures

Our preference is to treat fractures nonoperatively using rigid orthoses for four to six months and longer, although many use posterior stabilization and fusion even in the absence of neurological deficit or deformity.[32] Healing rates have been satisfactory in that environment. Nonunions may occasionally be seen in the lumbar spine: these appear as end plate sclerosis and need not be associated with actual deformity. They are often quite painful and are best treated by posterior fusion with instrumentation.[86] Healing rates with or without surgery parallel those of the general population.

Surgical Treatment of Fractures

Apple and Anson demonstrated that nonoperative treatment can maintain spinal alignment quite effectively.[3] In a multicenter concurrent study, 22 patients were treated operatively and 37 nonoperatively. Patients in the latter group had fewer complications, shorter lengths of stay, and similar neurological outcomes to those treated operatively. Thus surgery is best reserved for patients with acute traumatic deformity, cord compression with progressive neurological deficit due to changes in the spine, and pseudoarthrosis.

Olerud et al take a much more aggressive approach treating fractures, in spite of a very high surgical complication rate.[80] They treat most cervical fractures with anterior/posterior procedures. In a recent series, most thoracolumbar injuries were treated with posterior decompression/fixation alone. They now recommend circumferential decompression/fusion here as well. Their principal argument for surgery is the prevention of neurological deterioration resulting from motion of the ankylosed sections, which increases thecal sac compression.

Surgical Treatment of Deformity

Ankylosing Spondylitis
Surgery is occasionally indicated for decompression of stenotic segments with resulting neurologic compromise.[28,100,111] In these instances, simple decompression and maintenance in an orthosis for 3 to 4 months will likely lead to improvement rates similar to those expected in individuals without AS.

In recent years there has been major interest in the correction of the severe deformities that are common in the disorder. These are quite challenging procedures and require prolonged patient interaction through potentially multiple operations, long periods of immobilization, and intense patient and family education.

Indications are both local (i.e., spinal) and systemic. Most commonly, patients undergo surgical treatment of deformity to improve posture, ambulation, and daily activity. However, occasionally thoracic kyphosis will be severe enough to cause restrictive pulmonary disease and abdominal problems.[29,31]

Before surgery, careful attention to the patient's general status is critical. Restrictive pulmonary disease should be evaluated preoperatively and managed aggressively. Intubation often represents a particular problem; thus many surgeons have operated under local anesthetic, which may be difficult in a major spine procedure. Before correcting a lumbar deformity, it is prudent to evaluate and treat the very common hip flexion deformity. Correcting a complex spine deformity with rigidly flexed hips will rarely be productive. Cardiac complications of ankylosing spondylitis are not uncommon, and rigorous monitoring and judicious management of fluids are mandatory.

Procedures for correction of AS deformity are very similar to those used for the correction of other abnormalities, and may incorporate both anterior and posterior approaches. Although some surgeons prefer to perform their surgeries at separate settings, most will now use two-incision anterior and posterior operations. In our institution we have had significant success with the extracavitary approach to the spine for simultaneous decompression, stabilization, and reduction of local thoracic and lumbar deformity. Since the general surgical procedures are presented in Chapter 13, only specifics for ankylosing spondylitis are discussed later.

In correcting lumbar deformity, attention is ideally diverted directly to the apex of the pathology. However, that is often not possible in AS, because there will be multiple deformities over the length of the spine. Furthermore, in correcting lumbar deformities, it is critical that the surgeon remember the effects of spine manipulation on the vascular structures and abdominal contents. Attempting to completely correct a major deformity at a single level may be hazardous.

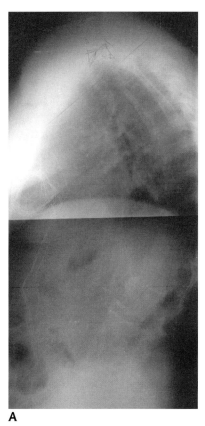
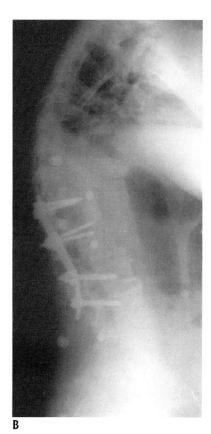
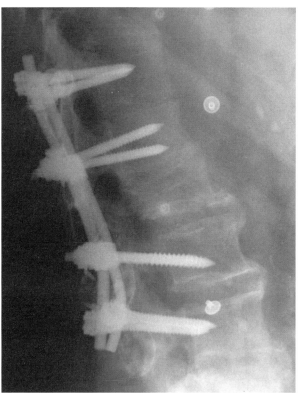
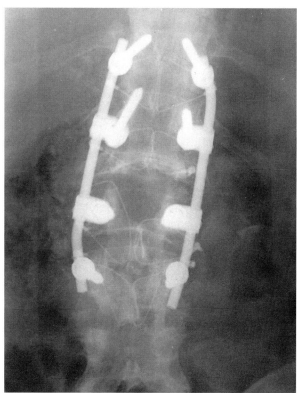

FIGURE 4–8
A AS with severe chin/chest deformity. **B** Patient realized 29° improvement in kyphosis from extension osteotomy. **C and D** Transpedicular fixation and sublaminar wiring were used for instrumentation.

Most commonly, lumbar surgery is used as the first stage in the correction of thoracic deformity or chin-chest deformity. In this circumstance, wide laminectomy and wedge osteotomy can lead to gratifying improvement in alignment, quality of life, and often pulmonary status.[1,8,11,47] Indeed, in some patients in whom staged procedures are planned, no further surgeries will be necessary beyond the first (Fig. 4–8). Therefore, in most instances of deformity, the results of the lumbar procedure are assessed over several weeks prior to consideration of more morbid thoracic or cervical reconstruction.

Lumbar Wedge Osteotomy We recommend the use of a spine frame if the deformity allows. This permits the patient to be appropriately positioned, while allowing the table to be rotated for radiography and for most effective performance of the wedge osteotomy. Furthermore, the Jackson frame allows one to maintain maximum appropriate lordosis. Under certain circumstances, correction results spontaneously after wedge osteotomy as a function of gravity. Other surgeons prefer to use the operating room table because of the potential for active hyperflexion of the spine, which aids in reduction following osteotomy.[62] Our preference is to use spinal instrumentation, not the table, to assist in this effort. Although we do not routinely use evoked potential monitoring for spinal procedures, we find it valuable in protecting neural function during the elective correction of a deformity: certainly, most surgeons would settle for less than full correction of a deformity in the face of neurophysiologic changes. Similarly, fluoroscopy has great value in monitoring reduction.

The osteotomy is performed at the level immediately below the conus. Following appropriate exposure, a generous laminectomy is performed for both decompression of the stenotic lumbar canal and exposure of the dural sac (Fig. 4–9A). Excision of the lamina and joints using osteotomes and a high-speed drill will make the spine somewhat mobile. Pedicle reduction or removal is important, as well a wide foraminotomies.[74,108,109] Attention is then turned to the vertebral body, where a wedge osteotomy is performed in the midst of the vertebral body see (Fig. 4–9B) using narrow osteotomes directed sequentially and radially to the midline (see Fig. 4–9C, D). In our experience, a 15 to 20-mm osteotomy in midbody can be safely accomplished and will comfortably allow 25 to 35 degrees of eventual spine extension, although we do not "break" the spine at this point.

Attention is then turned to posterior fixation. In the past, we preferred sublaminar wiring and Luque rodding for fixation. However, several clinical studies have emphasized the superiority of transpedicular fixation in maintaining correction.[116] As a result, in recent years we have begun using transpedicular fixation in spite of the relative osteopenia present. We currently use multilevel fixation (at least two above and two below, and more commonly three levels) for correction. Because of concern about screw pull-out, we typically add sublaminar wiring if the spinal canal diameter allows. Compression across the inner pedicle screws followed by tightening of the wires leads to the desired compression of the residual vertebral body and extension of the lumbar spine (see Fig. 4–9E). We do not perform in situ rod bending because of the osteopenia. Radiograpic confirmation is followed by placement of a posterior bone graft on the decorticated residual lamina and transverse processes.

Occasionally, the surgeon will want more correction than can safely be obtained through a single level procedure. Excessive extension at a single level risks catastrophic injury to the spinal cord and great vessels. In these instances, multilevel posterior closure osteotomy can be accomplished. However, we do not recommend performing this procedure at more than two adjacent levels. For two or more levels, the lateral extracavitary approach can also be used to avoid anterior/posterior procedures.

Patients are mobilized the day of surgery in an extended thoracolumbar orthosis. Many require extensive rehabilitation, even in the absence of complications, because of the change in gait and visual cues for ambulation. Typically, some correction will be lost over the healing period, but improvement in overall head/thoracic/lumbar alignment may be as high as 25 to 35 degrees with minimal risk. Result are gratifying in successful cases.

Halm et al have applied a modified Arthritis Impact Measurement Scale to a large series of patients with AS who underwent correction of deformity.[36] The overwhelming majority reported significant improvement in mobility, physical activity, pain, ability to work, and self-image. This effectively eliminates the oft-quoted societal argument that such correction is largely cosmetic. We find that most patients who obtain good results from lumbar osteotomy decline further deformity correction.

In Lazennec et al's series of lumbar osteotomies performed for AS, osteoclasty was used rather than osteotomy.[63] That is, the osteotomy is limited to the lateral vertebral body, and medial bone is not removed under the assumption that vertebral compression will occur. Pedicle fixation is then used for

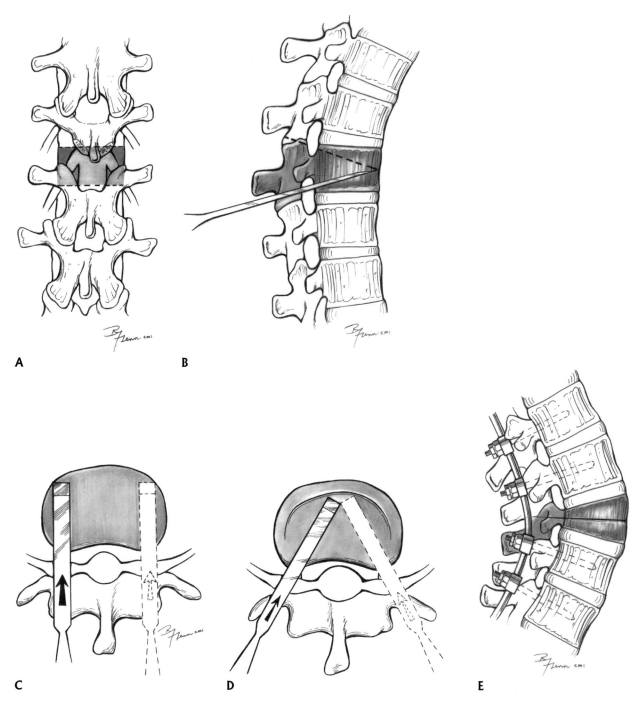

FIGURE 4–9 Technique of wedge osteotomy. **A** A wide laminectomy is performed at the level of the osteotomy, usually below the conus. The facet joints are resected and the pedicle drilled flush with the canal. Wide foraminotomies are important. **B** The margins for the osteotomy are marked. If desired, Steinman pins can be placed for radiographic confirmation. Osteotomes are used to make the vertebral incision, starting laterally **C** and moving medially, **D** at both the superior and inferior margins of the osteotomy. We discourage manipulation of the thecal sac; working as described will allow generous body removal. The loose bone is removed with Kerrison rongeurs and curettes. **E** Spinal fixation is accomplished and the spine manually extended and rods placed.

instrumentation. The authors argue that this approach minimizes the risks of vascular injury, pseudoarthrosis of the vertebral surfaces, and nerve root compression. Furthermore, they have obtained correction of 75 degrees, much greater than we would attempt at a single level. We have had no instances of radiculopathy using standard wedge osteotomy, presumably because of aggressive removal of the pedicles.

Complications Complication rates are the same as for other types of correction of deformity. Styblo et al reported minor skin sores from bracing and a high incidence of cerebrospinal fluid fistula requiring repeat surgery.[106] Early series reported aortic injury and a high incidence of paraplegia.[1,11,46,117] However, the complication rate has decreased significantly, because of less ambitious single-level correction and the incorporation of multilevel correction. In our series, complications have been limited to those typically seen with spinal surgery. We have not seen any neurological deficit, vascular complications, or—to date—hardware failure. The occasional posterior osteotomy nonunion requires a retroperitoneal fusion.

REFERENCES

1. Adams JC: Technique, dangers and safeguards in osteotomy of spine. J Bone Joint Surg 34B:226–232, 1952.
2. Altman RD, Brown M, Gargano F; Low back pain in Paget's disease of bone. Clin Orthop 217:152–161, 1987.
3. Apple DF Jr. Anson C: Spinal cord injury occurring in patients with ankylosing spondylitis: A multicenter study. Orthopedics 18:1005–1011, 1995.
4. Baba H. Maezawa Y, Kamitani K, et al: Osteoporotic vertebral collapse with late neurological complications. Paraplegia 33:281–289, 1995.
5. Barrett-Connor E: The economic and human costs of osteoporotic fracture. Am J Med 98:3S–8S, 1995.
6. Bergkvist L, Adami H, Persson I et al: The risk of breast cancer after estrogen and estrogen-progestin replacement. N Engl J Med 321:293–297, 1989.
7. Bernstein J, Lane JM: Metabolic bone disorders of the spine. In the Spine (vol 2), Philadelphia: WB Saunders, pp 1381–1427, 1992.
8. Bradford DS, Schumacher WL, Lonstein JE, et al: Ankylosing spondylitis: Experience in surgical management of 21 patients. Spine 12:238–243, 1987.
9. Brandolini F, Bacchini P, Moscato M, et al: Chondrosarcoma as a complicating factor in Paget's disease of bone. Skeletal Radiol 26:497–500, 1997.
10. Briancon D, Meunier PJ: Treatment of osteoporosis with fluoride, calcium, and vitamin D. Orthop Clin North Am 12:629–648, 1981.
11. Briggs H, Keats S, Schlesinger PT: Wedge osteotomy of the spine with bilateral intervertebral foraminotomy: Correction of flexion deformity in five cases of ankylosing arthritis of the spine. J Bone Joint Surg 29:1075–1082, 1947.
12. Cooper C, Carbone L, Michet CJ, et al: Fracture risk in patients with ankylosing spondylitis: A population based study. J Rheumatol 21:1877–1882, 1994.
13. Cots R, Gelman SM: Cauda equina syndrome caused by osteosarcoma in a patient with Paget's disease of bone: Value of modern imaging. Revue du Rheum (English ed) 62:807–808, 1995.
14. Creemers MC, Franssen MJ, van de Putte LB, et al: Methotrexate in severe ankylosing spondylitis: An open study. J Rheumatol 22:1104–1107, 1995.
15. Cuellar ML, Espinosa LR: Management of spondyloarthropathies. Curr Opin Rheumatol 8:288–295, 1996.
16. Cuenod CA, Laredo JD, Chevret S, et al: Acute vertebral collapse due to osteoporosis or malignancy: Appearance on unenhanced and gadolinium-enhanced MR images. Radiology 199:541–549, 1996.
17. Dalsky GP: The role of exercise in the prevention of osteoporosis. Compr Ther 15:30–37, 1989.
18. Daniell HW: Osteoporosis of the slender smoker: Vertebral compression fracture and loss of metacarpal cortex in relation to postmenopausal cigarette smoking and lack of obesity: Arch Intern Med 136:298–304, 1976.
19. Deal CL: Osteoporosis: Prevention, diagnosis, and management. Am J Med 102:35S–39S, 1997.
20. Delmas PD: Biochemical markers of bone turnover. J Bone Miner Res 8:S549–55, 1993.
21. Devogelear JP, Malghem J, Stasse P, et al: Biological and radiological responses to oral etidronate and tiludronate in Paget's disease of bone. Bone 20:259–261, 1997.
22. Dick HM, Dick WC, Sturrock RD, et al: Inheritance of ankylosing spondylitis and HLA antigen W27. Lancet 2:24–25, 1974.
23. Dinneen SF, Buckley TF: Spinal nerve root compression due to monostotic Paget's disease of a lumbar vertebra. Spine 12:948–950, 1987.
24. Ettinger B, Genant HK, Cann CE: Postmenopausal bone loss is prevented by treatment with low-dosage estrogen with calcium. And Intern Med 106:40–45, 1987.
25. Farley SM, Wergedal JE, Farley JR, et al: Spinal fractures during fluoride therapy for osteoporosis: Rela-

tionship to spinal bone density. Osteoporosis Int 2:213–218, 1992.
26. Fenlon HM, Sant SM, Breatnach E: Plain radiographs and thoracic high-resolution CT in patients with ankylosing spondylitis. AJR 168:1067–1072, 1997.
27. Fleish H: Experimental basis for the use of diphosphonates in Paget's disease of bone. Clin Orthop 217:72–78, 1987.
28. Fow MW, Onofrio BM, Kilgore JE: Neurological complications of ankylosing spondylitis. J Neurosurg 78:871–878, 1993.
29. Gerscovich EO, Greenspan A, Montesano PX: Treatment of kyphotic deformity in ankylosing spondylitis. Orthopedics 17:335–343, 1994.
30. Gilsanz V, Loro ML, Roe TF, et al: Vertebral size in elderly women with osteoporosis: Mechanical implications and relationships to fractures. J Clin Invest 95:2332–2337, 1995.
31. Goel MK: Vertebral osteotomy for correction of fixed flexion deformity of the spine. J Bone Joint Surg 50A:287–294, 1968.
32. Graham B, Van Peteghem PK: Fractures of the spine in ankylosing spondylitis. Diagnosis, treatment, and complications. Spine 14(8):803–807, 1989.
33. Gran JT, Skomsvoll JF: The outcome of ankylosing spondylitis: A study of 100 patients. Br J Rheumatol 36:766–771, 1997.
34. Gruskiewicz J, Doron Y, Borovich B, et al: Spinal cord compression in Paget's disease of bone with reference to sarcomatous degeneration and calcitonin treatment. Surg Neurol 27:117–125, 1987.
35. Hadjipavlou A, Shaffer N, Lander P, et al: Pagetic spinal stenosis with extradural pagetoid ossification. Spine 13:128–130, 1988.
36. Halm H, Metz-Stavenhagen P, Zielke K: Results of surgical correction of kyphotic deformities of the spine in ankylosing spondylitis on the basis of the modified Arthritis Impact Measurement Scales. Spine 20:1612–1619, 1995.
37. Halvorson TL, Kelley LA, Thomas KA, et al: Effects of bone mineral density on pedicle screw fixation. Spine 19:2415–2420, 1994.
38. Hansson T, Roos B: The effect of fluoride and calcium on spinal bone mineral content: A controlled prospective (3 years) study. Calcif Tissue Int 40:315–317, 1987.
39. Hasegawa K, Takahashi HE, UchiyamaS, et al: An experimental study of a combination method using a pedicle screw and laminar hook for the osteoporotic spine. Spine 22:958–962, 1997.
40. Heggeness MH: Spine fracture with neurological deficit in osteoporosis. Osteoporos Int 3:215–221, 1993.
41. Henderson NK, Sambrook PN: Relationship between osteoporosis and arthritis and effect of corticosteroids and other drugs on bone. Curr Opin Rheumatol 8:365–369, 1996.
42. Herzberg L, Bayliss E: Spinal cord syndrome due to non-compressive Paget's disease of bone: A spinal-artery steal phenomenon reversible with calcitonin. Lancet 2:13–15, 1980.
43. Hidding A, van der Linden S, de Witte L: Therapeutic effects of individual physical therapy in ankylosing spondylitis related to duration of disease. Clin Rheumatol 12:334–340, 1993.
44. Huang TL, Cohen NJ, Sahgal S: Osteosarcoma complicating Paget's disease of the spine with neurologic complications. Clin Orthop 141:260–265, 1979.
45. Ito M, Hayashi K, Yamada M, et al: Relationship of osteophytes to bone mineral density and spinal fracture in man. Radiology 189:497–502, 1993.
46. Jackson RP, Simmons EH: Dural compression as a cause of paraplegia during operative correction of cervical kyphosis in ankylosing spondylitis. Spine 7:846–848, 1991.
47. Jaffray D, Becker V, Eisenstein S: Closing wedge osteotomy with transpedicular fixation in ankylosing spondylitis. Clin Orthop 279:122–126, 1992.
48. Jimenez-Balderas FJ, Mintz G: Ankylosing spondylitis: Clinical course in women and men. J Rheumatol 20:2069–2072, 1993.
49. Johansson C, Mellstrom D, Rosengren K, et al: A community-based population study of vertebral fractures in 85 year old men and women. Age Ageing 23:338–392, 1994.
50. Jones G, Nguyen T, Sambrook PN, et al: Osteoarthritis, bone density, postural stability, and osteoporotic fractures: A population-based study. J Rheumatol 22:921–925, 1995.
51. Kabasakal Y, Garrett SL, Calin A: The epidemiology of spondylodiscitis in ankylosing spondylitis: A controlled study. Br J Rheumatol 35:660–663, 1996.
52. Kadir S, Kalisher L, Schiller AL: Extramedullary hematopoiesis in Paget's disease of bone. AJR 129:493–495, 1977.
53. Kanis JA, Gray RES: Long-term follow-up observations on treatment in Paget's disease. Clin Orthop 217:99–125, 1987.
54. Kanis JA, Gertz BJ, Singer F, et al: Rationale for the use of alendronate in osteoporosis. Osteoporos Int 5:1–13, 1995.
55. Karasick D, Schweitzer ME, Abidi NA, et al: Fractures of the vertebrae with spinal cord injuries in patients with ankylosing spondylitis: Imaging findings. AJR 165:1205–1208.
56. Kelsey JF: Osteoporosis: Prevalence and incidence.

In Proc of the NIH Concensus Development Conf on Osteoporosis, Bethesda, MD, 1984, p 25.

57. Koenigsberg RA, Klahr J, Zito JL, et al: Magnetic resonance imaging of cauda equina syndrome in ankylosing spondylitis: A case report. J Neuroimaging 5:46–48, 1995.

58. Korovessis P, Maraziotis T, Piperos G, et al: Spontaneous burst fracture of the thoracolumbar spine in osteoporosis associated with neurological impairment: A report of seven cases and review of the literature. Eur Spine J 3:286–288, 1994.

59. Krane SM: Paget's disease of bone. Clin Orthop 127:24–36, 1977.

60. Kumano K, Hirabayashi S, Ogawa Y: Pedicle screws and mineral bone density. Spine 19:1157–1161, 1994.

60a. Lane JM, Healey JH, Schwartz E, et al: Treatment of osteoporosis with sodium fluoride and calcium: Effects on vertebral fracture incidence and bone histomorphometry. Orthop Clin North Am 15:729–745, 1984.

60b. Lane JM, Vigorita VJ: Osteoporosis. Orthop Clin North Am 15:711–728, 1984.

61. Laredo JD, Lakhdari K, Bellaiche L, et al: Acute vertebral collapse: CT findings in benign and malignant nontraumatic cases. Radiology 194:41–48, 1995.

62. Law WA: Osteotomy of the spine. Clin Orthop 66:70–76, 1969.

63. Lazenncec JY, Saillant G, Saidi K, et al: Surgery of the deformities in ankylosing spondylitis: Our experience in 31 patients. Eur Spine J 6:222–232, 1997.

64. Lee YL, Yip KM: The osteoporotic spine. Clin Orthop 323:91–97, 1996.

65. Lee YS, Sclotzhauer T, Ott SM, et al: Skeletal status of men with early and late ankylosing spondylitis. Am J Med 103:233–241, 1997.

66. Liberman UA, Weiss SR, Broll J, et al: Effect of oral alendronate on bone mineral density and the incidence of fractures in post menopausal osteoporosis. N En J Med 333:1437–1444, 1995.

67. Linssen A, Meenken C: Outcomes of HLA-27 positive and HLA-27 negative acute anterior uveitis. Am J Ophthalmol 120:351–361, 1995.

68. Lips P: Epidemiology and predictors of fractures associated with osteoporosis. Am J Med 103:3S–8S, 1997.

69. Lopez-Larrea C, Gonzalez-Roces S, Alvarez V: HLA-B27 structure, function, and disease association. Curr Opin Rheumatol 8:296–308, 1996.

70. Maiman DJ, Larson SJ: Paget's disease of the spine. Contemp Neurosurg 5:1–6, 1983.

71. Maldague B, Malghem J: Dynamic radiologic patterns of Paget's disease of bone. Clin Orthop 217:26–151, 1987.

72. Marguiles JY, Payzer A, Nyska M, et al: The relationship between degenerative changes and osteoporosis in the lumbar spine. Clin Orthop 324:45–152, 1996.

73. Mazzuoli GF, Passeri M, Gennari C, et al: Effects of salmon calcitonin in postmenopausal osteoporosis: A controlled double-blind clinical study. Calcif Tissue Int 38:3–8, 1986.

74. McMaster MJ: A technique for lumbar spinal osteotomy in ankylosing spondylitis. J Bone Joint Surg 67B:204–210, 1985.

75. Meema S, Bunker ML, Meema HE: Preventive effect of estrogen on postmenopausal bone loss. Arch Int Med 135:1436–1440, 1975.

76. Mii Y, Miyauchi Y, Honoki K, et al: Electron microscopic evidence of a viral nature for osteoclast inclusions in Paget's disease of bone. Virchows Arch 424:99–104, 1994.

77. Mills BG, Singer FR: Critical evaluation of viral antigen data in Paget's disease of bone. Clin Orthop 217:16–25, 1987.

78. Mizrahi J, Silva MJ, Keavenry TM, et al: Finite-element stress analysis of the normal and osteoporotic lumbar vertebral body. Spine 18:2088–2096, 1993.

79. Okuyama K, Sata K, Abe E: Stability of transpedicle screwing for the osteoporotic spine: An in vitro study of the mechanical stability. Spine 18:2240–2245, 1993.

80. Olerud C, Frost A, Bring J; Spinal fractues in patients with ankylosing spondylitis.Eur Spine J 5:51–55, 1996.

81. Osteoporosis. National Institutes of Health Consensus Development Conference Statement (Review). Natl Inst Health Consens Dev Conf Consens Statement 5, 6 pp, 1984.

82. Papapoulous SE: Paget's disease of bone: Clinical, pathogenetic, and therapeutic aspects. Baillieres Clin Endocrinol Metab 11:117–143, 1997.

83. Patel S, Pearson D, Hosking DJ: Quantitative bone scintigraphy in the management of monostotic Paget's disease of bone. Arthritis Rheum 38:1506–1512, 1995.

84. Peh WC, Ho WY, Luk KD: Applications of diagnostic scintigraphy in ankylosing spondylitis. Clin Imaging 21:54–62, 1997.

85. Perlaky G, Szendroi M, Varga PP: Osteoporosis: A modifying factor in surgical treatment. Acta Med Hung 50:245–256, 1994.

86. Patterson T, Laasonen L, Leirisalo-Repo M, et al: Spinal pseudoarthrosis complicating ankylosing spondylitis: A report of two patients. Br J Rheumatol 35:1319–1323, 1996.

87. Rahlfs VW, Stat C: Reevaluation of some double-

blind, randomized studies of dexibuprofen: A state of the art review. J Clin Pharmacol 36S:33–40, 1996.

88. Ravichandran G: Neurologic recovery of paraplegia following use of calcitonin in a patient with Paget's disease of spine. Spine 4:37–40, 1979.

89. Reid IR, Nicholson GC, Weinstein RS, et al: Biochemical and radiologic improvement in Paget's disease of bone treated with aledronate: A randomized, placebo-controlled trial. Am J Med 101:341–348, 1996.

90. Riggs BL, Seeman E, Hodgson SF, et al: Effect of the fluoride/calcium regimen on vertebral fracture occurrence in post-menopausal osteoporosis: Comparison with conventional therapy. N En J Med 306:446–450, 1982.

91. Riggs BL, Wahner HW, Melton JL III, et al: Rates of bone loss in the appendicular and axial skeletons of women: Evidence of substantial bone loss before menopause. J Clin Invest 77:1487–1491, 1986.

92. Riggs BL, Hodgson S, O'Fallon W, et al: Effect of fluoride treatment on the fracture rate in post-menopausal women with osteoporosis. N En J Med 322: 845–846, 1990.

93. Riis B, Thomsen K, Christiansen C: Does calcium supplementation prevent postmenopausal bone loss? A double-blind, controlled clinical study. N En J Med 316:173–177, 1987.

94. Ritzel H, Amling M, Posl M, et al: The thickness of human vertebral cortical bone and its changes in aging and osteoporosis: A histomorphometric analysis of the complete spinal column from thirty-seven autopsy specimens. J Bone Miner Res 12:89–95, 1997.

95. Rupp RE, Ebraheim NA, Coombs RJ: Magnetic resonance imaging differentiation of compression spine fractures or vertebral lesions caused by osteoporosis or tumor. Spine 20:2499–2504, 1995.

96. Ryan MD, Taylor TK: Spinal manifestations of Paget's disease. Aust N Z J Surg 62:33–38, 1992.

97. Ryan PJ, Fogelman I: Osteoporotic vertebral fractures: Diagnosis with radiography and bone scintigraphy. Radiology 190:669–772, 1994.

98. Ryan PJ: Overview of role of BMD measurements in managing osteoporosis. Semin Nucl Med 27:197–209, 1997.

99. Ryan PJ, Fogelman I: Bone scintigraphy in metabolic bone disease. Semin Nucl Med 27:291–305, 1997.

100. Sant SM, O'Connell D: Cauda equina syndrome in ankylosing spondylitis: A case report and review of the literature. Clin Rheumatol 14:224–226, 1995.

101. Simmons EH: Kyphotic deformity of the spine in ankylosing spondylitis. Clin Orthop 128:65–77, 1977.

102. Sinaki M, Wollan PC, Scott RW, et al: Can strong back extensors prevent vertebral fractures in women with osteoporosis? Mayo Clin Proc 71:951–956, 1996.

103. Singer FR, Mills BG: The etiology of Paget's disease of bone. Clin Orthop 127:37–42, 1977.

104. Siris E, Weinstein S, Altman R, et al: Comparative study of alendronate versus etidronate for the treatment of Paget's disease of bone. J Clin Endocrinol Metab 81:961–967, 1996.

105. Smith EL, Raab DM: Osteoporosis and physical activity. Acta Med Scand Suppl 711:149–156, 1986.

106. Styblo K, Bossers GT, Slot GH: Osteotomy for kyphosis in ankylosing spondylitis. Acta Orthop Scand 56:294–297, 1985.

107. Tanaka S, Kubota M, Fujimoto Y, et al: Conus medullaris syndrome secondary to an L1 burst fracture in osteoporosis: A case report. Spine 18:2131–2134, 1993.

108. Thiranont N, Netrawichien P: Transpedicular decancellation closed wedge vertebral osteotomy for treatment of fixed flexion deformity of spine in ankylosing spondylitis. Spine 18:2517–2522, 1993.

109. Thomasen E: Vertebral osteotomy for correction of kyphosis in ankylosing spondylitis. Clin Orthop 194:142–146, 1985.

110. Thorngren KG, Liedberg E, Aspelin P: Fractures of the thoracic and lumbar spine in ankylosing spondylitis. Arch Orthop Trauma Surg 98:101–107, 1981.

111. Tyrrell PN, Davies AM, Evans N: Neurological disturbances in ankylosing sondylitis. Ann rheum Dis 53:714–717, 1994.

112. Viitanen JV, Kokko ML, Lehtien K, et al: Correlation between mobility restrictions and radiologic changes in ankylosing spondylitis. Spine 20:492–496, 1995.

113. Wallace E, Wong J, Reid IR: Pamidronate treatment of the neurologic sequelae of pagetic lumbar stenosis. Arch Intern Med 155:1813–1815, 1995.

114. Wasnich RD: Vertebral fracture epidemiology. Bone 18:179–183, 1996.

115. Watts N: Treatment of osteoporosis with biphosphonates. Rheum Dis Clin North Am 20:717–729, 1994.

116. Weale AE, Marsh CH, Yeoman PM: Secure fixation of lumbar osteotomy: Surgical experience with 50 patients. Clin Orthop 321:216–222, 1995.

117. Weatherly C, Jaffray D, Terry A: Vascular complications associated with osteotomy in ankylosing spondylitis: Report of two cases. Spine 1:43–46, 1988.

118. Yost JH, Spencer-Green G, Krant JD: Vascular steal mimicking compression myelopathy in Paget's disease of bone. J Rheumatol 20:1064–1065, 1993.

CHAPTER 5

Disc Degeneration

Intervertebral Disc Herniation

Discogenic Pain

Raised Intraosseous Pressure

Zygapophyseal ("Facet") Joints

Degenerative Spondylolisthesis

Degenerative Scoliosis

Lumbar Stenosis

Fusion

Outcomes

Disc Degeneration

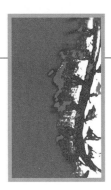

Changes in the structure of the intervertebral disc begin in early childhood and continue throughout life, and this normal process of aging can be accelerated by trauma. The associated alterations in the hydrostatic and biomechanical properties of the disc can lead to a variety of clinical problems, such as disc herniation, zygapophyseal joint degeneration, increased intraosseous pressure, spondylosis with stenosis, degenerative spondylolisthesis, and degenerative scoliosis.

Intervertebral Disc Herniation

Lumbar disc herniations had been recognized at autopsy as a cause of radiculopathy as early as 1911,[114] but the first clinical identification was made by Dandy during surgery for what had been presumed to be a metastatic tumor.[33] Mixter and Barr[117] were the first to make the diagnosis of herniated disc prior to surgery and to design the operation accordingly. They recognized the possibility of postoperative instability and raised the question of fusion as part of the operation. From their observations they concluded that "rupture of the intervertebral disc is not an uncommon cause of symptoms." They used myelography, but because initially 2 ml or less of the Lipiodol was used, it was only possible to identify subarachnoid block. Of the patients operated upon for lumbar lesions, 6 were paraparetic, and a block was demonstrated in each. A myelogram was done in 3 of 4 patients with symptoms and findings of monoradiculopathy, was negative in each, and the diagnosis was made on clinical grounds. When Lipiodol became more readily available, 5 ml was found sufficient to demonstrate a filling defect produced by a protruded disc. Mixter and Ayer[116] found that "in the last 10 cases of the series the demonstration has been so certain that a preoperative diagnosis of herniated disc has been made. In 5 patients who complained solely of unilateral pain who showed no objective sensory, motor or reflex abnormality, a characteristic notching of the Lipiodol shadow correctly indicated a disc hernia."

At first, their conclusions and recommendations were met with skepticism and resistance. Mixter found that the best way to overcome this was to invite the skeptic to scrub in with him and to observe the lesion and its removal at firsthand. For example, Love spent several days with Mixter and by 1940 was able to report a series of 500 consecutive patients operated upon for disc herniation.[106]

Clinical Presentation and Diagnosis

In the early years, considerable variation existed regarding diagnostic criteria. Dandy considered low back pain with radiation down the posterior portion of one or both lower limbs with intensification of the pain by coughing or sneezing to be characteristic, and considered the only important physical finding to be alteration of the Achilles reflex.[35] He did not believe that L4–L5 herniations could be distinguished from those at L5–S1. Mixter considered the pain with straight leg raising to be an important finding in his patients, one-third of whom had bilateral radiation.[115,116] Of Love's patients, 78% had unilateral sciatica and 6% had backache alone. He considered pain with straight leg raising, sciatic tenderness, and alteration of the Achilles' reflex to be the most helpful neurological signs.[106] Spurling and Grantham[154] felt that muscle spasm with a list away from the side of the lesion was important, and placed greater emphasis on alteration of sensory perception. They concluded that the level of herniation could be determined by physical findings, particularly changes in patellar and Achilles' reflexes and location of sensory loss.

Each considered increased pain in association with coughing to be an important symptom, and none believed that muscle weakness was significant, attributing it when present to inhibition of muscle contractions secondary to associated pain. This view gradually changed to the present general reliance on unilateral pain, paresthesias and sensory loss in a radicular distribution, muscle weakness, and pain with straight leg raising, especially with crossed reference, as diagnostic criteria for identification of the level. In most instances, lateral herniation at L5–S1 is associated with pain radiating into the heel and lateral aspect of the foot with paresthesias in the same distribution. Sensory perception is usually diminished over the lateral aspect of the foot, and weakness of the flexor hallucis is usually present. With L4–L5 herniations, the pain radiates down the lower limb into the ankle, the dorsomedial aspect of the foot, and the large toe, with paresthesia and sensory loss in the same distribution. Gluteal and extensor hallucis muscles are usually weak, and the extensor digitorum brevis is frequently atrophic. Patients with L3–L4 herniation experience pain radiating into the thigh and medial portions of the leg, with weakness of the tibialis anterior and extensor hallucis muscles. The quadriceps may also be involved. Large central protrusions can produce bilateral weakness and urinary retention but are uncommon, comprising 3.2% of cases in one series.[65]

Diagnostic Procedures

Methods to determine diagnoses have been controversial from the beginning. Although Mixter and Barr were able to make the diagnosis of disc herniation on clinical grounds, in a later paper Mixter and Ayer state that "both the examination of the spinal fluid and x-ray examination with Lipiodol are of the greatest importance. We can say with equal emphasis that without increase of protein in the spinal fluid and without positive roentgenological evidence, even a tentative diagnosis of rupture of intervertebral disc in the lumbar region should not be made."[116] Others[34,35,146] believed that the diagnosis of herniated disc could be made on the basis of symptoms and physical findings and considered myelography to be unnecessary in most patients. They were also concerned about the possible adverse effects of retained Lipiodol, which was either left in place or incompletely removed through a meningeal incision during the operation. With the advent of Pantopaque, myelography became widely used despite reservations regarding the adverse effect of retained Pantopaque, which frequently was not entirely removed. This problem was resolved by the newer, water-soluble contrast media, which produced myelograms of excellent diagnostic quality without the development of arachnoidal adhesions.[72]

Before the development of computed tomography (CT) and magnetic resonance imaging (MRI), we had stopped doing myelograms in patients with clear-cut radicular symptoms and findings because the myelograms were done for localization after the decision for surgery had already been made. If the symptoms and findings indicated an L5 radiculopathy, the operation was directed at L4–L5, and if a significant lesion was not found, the L5–S1 disc was examined. Conversely, if the clinical features suggested a S1 radiculopathy, the L5–S1 interspace was approached first. Myelography was reserved for patients in whom the clinical diagnosis was less obvious. It could be argued that CT or MRI are also unnecessary in a clear-cut radiculopathy with apparently good clinical localization. However, even apparently good clinical localization is not always reliable. For example, a 32-year-old woman presented with pain radiating down the right lower limb to the ankle, gluteal and extensor hallucis weakness, normal sensory perception, and pain with straight leg raising to 30 degrees. Although the clinical features suggested an L5 radiculopathy, the MRI demonstrated a disc herniation at L5–S1 (Fig. 5–1). Similarly, a 42-year-old man had back pain radiating into the distal portion of the left leg, decreased sensory perception over the medial aspect of the left foot and leg, and weakness of the left gluteal, tibialis anterior, and extensor hallucis muscles. Again, although the clinical features suggested an L5 radiculopathy, the MRI demonstrated disc herniation at L3–L4 (Fig. 5–4).

CT and MRI have virtually eliminated the need for myelography except in patients with metallic fixation devices, which can significantly degrade the image. However, good CT scans can be obtained in the presence of titanium implants (Fig. 5–43). Electromyography is not useful in the evaluation of the patient with characteristic clinical find-

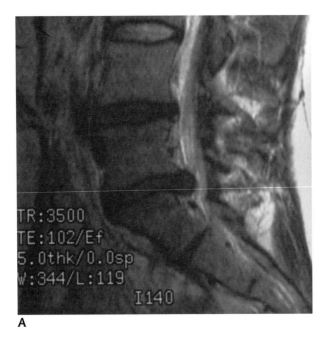
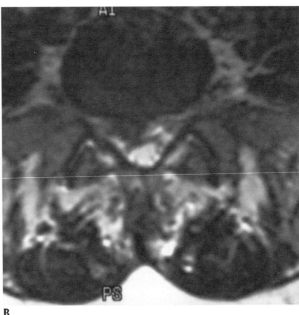

FIGURE 5-1. **A and B** MRI demonstrating extruded disc fragment at L5–S1.

ings of herniated nucleus pulposus. A normal electromyogram (EMG) does not exclude a radiculopathy, and an abnormal examination only confirms the clinical observations at the cost of patient discomfort and increased expense. Although a case can perhaps be made for discography in some situations, radiculopathy is not one of them.[161] Evoked potential recordings may occasionally be useful. For example, a patient had back pain radiating down the right lower limb into the big toe with gluteal and toe extensor weakness and sensory loss in the medial aspect of the foot. Extension of the spine was restricted, but flexion was much better. Myelogram, postmyelogram CT, and MRI had been done without demonstration of a disc herniation. Spine films had demonstrated posterior displacement of L4 on L5 in extension reduced in flexion, and evoked potentials demonstrated reduction in amplitude of the response to right peroneal nerve stimulation during extension. (Fig. 5–2).

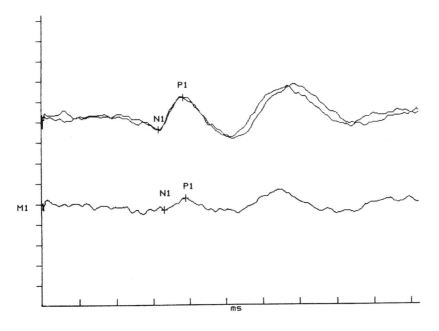

FIGURE 5-2.
Somatosensory evoked potentials recorded from scalp electrodes secondary to stimulation of the right paroneal nerve. Horizontal calibration is 10 msec per vision; vertical is 1.22 μv per division. The upper recording is before, and the lower immediately after extension of the lumbar spine sufficient to produce lower limb pain.

Management

Nonsurgical Treatment

Initial treatment should be *nonsurgical*, a term which is preferable to *conservative*. *Radical*, not *surgical*, is the antonym of *conservative*. The conservative treatment of acute appendicitis is appendectomy. Bedrest should not be used for more than a few days. Once the acute symptoms have subsided, *physical therapy* can be started emphasizing *exercise* to strengthen the paravertebral and abdominal muscles. These will help convert the abdominal cavity into a weight-bearing cylinder, relieving the load on the intervertebral discs. In this regard, Williams' exercises, which were designed to decrease the lumbar lordosis,[174] are not helpful. The efficacy of epidural steroid injections is not clear, and we no longer use them. If steroids are to relieve pain by reducing inflammation, then presumably inflammation must be present. Swollen and inflamed nerve roots have been described,[106] but this is not a common phenomenon. In patients operated upon for the first time we have not been impressed by discoloration of the dura or adherence to the extruded fragment or floor of the spinal canal. Although nerve degeneration was found in 3 of 10 nerve roots biopsied during surgery for herniated disc, inflammation was not identified.[100] Additionally, histological examination of surgical specimens from 100 patients did not identify evidence of acute or chronic inflammation.[122,183]

The size of the disc herniation decreases in some, but not all, patients who improve without surgical treatment. Twenty-one patients in whom repeat CT scans were done after 6 to 27 months (mean 12.9), the herniation disappeared or was substantially smaller in 10, but was not significantly changed in 11.[39] Straight leg raising was painful initially in 29 of 30 patients with herniations demonstrated by CT scan, and subsequent scans were done at 3 and 24 months.[158] Straight leg raising was positive in 10 at 3 months and in 3 at 30 months. There was no correlation between size of the herniation and severity of straight leg raising initially, nor between reduction in size and improvement in straight leg raising. The greatest decrease in size occurred during the first 3 months.

Surgical Treatment

Pain The most common indication for surgery is pain. In most patients, the neurological deficit is not functionally significant, and those with complete foot drop usually do not recover much function. Difference of opinions exists as to whether operations should be done early in at least some patients[113] or only after more prolonged nonsurgical treatment.[77] Those who recover without surgery usually begin to show significant improvement within a week of onset of radicular pain (Fig. 5–3). The patient in Figure 5–3 developed severe right sciatica, and her physician ordered a CT scan. The pain was already subsiding when the scan was done and had almost com-

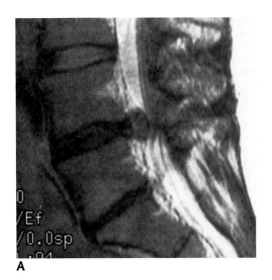
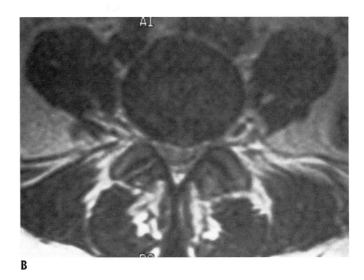

FIGURE 5–3. **A and B** Large central disc herniation at L4–L5, more pronounced on the right side of the canal.

pletely subsided in less than 2 weeks. Disabling symptoms that persist for more than 2 weeks without significant improvement usually will not subside without an operation. The patient's occupation also has an influence. Since the pain is aggravated by physical activity, someone with a sedentary occupation may be able to get by without surgery, in contrast to one whose work is more strenuous. Persistence in nonsurgical treatment in the face of continued disabling pain only delays return to the previous level of activity. In a frequently quoted paper,[167] long-term results in patients treated nonsurgically have been reported to be as good as for those operated upon. However, in this report, patients with definite indications for surgery were excluded, and the comparison made was between those with more equivocal indications who agreed to be selected at random into one group for surgery and another for continued physical therapy. At one year follow-up the patients operated upon had a better result, but at 10 years the difference between the two groups was not statistically significant.

Central Protrusion The other major indication for surgery is cauda equina syndrome secondary to a large central protrusion. Although traditionally this has been considered a surgical emergency, a relationship has not been found to exist between the interval from the onset of symptoms to surgery and the extent of recovery.[38,65,90]

Initially a multilevel laminectomy was done with transdural removal of the herniated disc.[117] Enemas were given on the day prior to surgery and on the third postoperative day. Patients remained at bedrest for 10 days and were discharged 12 days after surgery.[106] Subsequently, the procedure was modified to a unilateral exposure with hemilaminotomy and extradural removal.[106] More recently, microsurgical techniques have been developed.[175,176,178]

The advantages of microdiscectomy include a smaller skin incision and less extensive muscle dissection and therefore less postoperative pain, permitting earlier discharge from the hospital. However, intraoperative radiography is necessary for localization. Even with a microsurgical approach, laminar exposure is required and at least above L5–S1 some bone must be removed. The standard hemilaminotomy approach provides better exposure of the nerve root and related structures and improves the ability to deal with lateral recess and foraminal stenosis. Intraoperative radiography is not required because the appropriate level can be identified by anatomical landmarks. If the extruded fragment is in the axilla of the root, reflection of the root medially at the level of extrusion is difficult and is facilitated by beginning the process more rostrally. This, however, requires more extensive laminotomy than can be readily done through a microsurgical exposure. The microsurgical approach is also not well suited for the removal of the inferiorly migrated sequestered fragment at L4–L5 or L3–L4 where the root lies alongside the pedicle (Fig. 5–4) and retraction is difficult. Again, a more

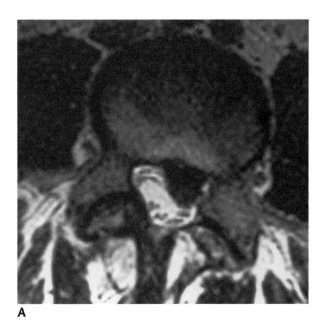
A

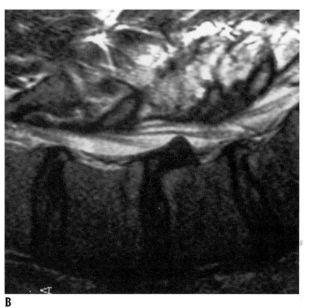
B

FIGURE 5–4. **A and B** Sequestered disc herniation at L3–L4.

extensive laminotomy is required than is feasible with a microsurgical approach.

Reduction in length of hospital stay is not necessarily related to the extent of the operation. In 1981 Wilson and Harbaugh[178] reported an average length of stay of 4.12 days after microdiscectomy as compared with 6.75 days after the standard approach. Same-day surgery for microdiscectomy is now being done, and we discharge most patients who have had standard hemilaminotomy on the following day. Since it is unlikely that postoperative pain is any less severe in 1998 than in 1981, the driving force behind decreased hospital stays appears to be the refusal of the insurance companies to pay for more than abbreviated hospitalization. Patients with substantial pain who would prefer to remain in the hospital accept discharge rather than face a financial penalty. Although hospital stay may be one day longer with the standard approach, the increased operating time associated with microdiscectomy and the necessity for intraoperative radiography tends to equalize the cost. Another disadvantage of microdiscectomy is the greater possibility of operating at the wrong level. Although the incidence is not known and probably never will be, based on our experience in reviewing cases where malpractice has been alleged, operation at the wrong level appears to occur more frequently with microdiscectomy. The clinical results are no better with microdiscectomy, and the amount of scar no less.[159]

Disc Removal A difference of opinions exists regarding the amount of disc that should be removed. Removal of the extruded fragment and whatever additional loose pieces of disc that can be readily identified appears sufficient. Vigorous curettage and attempts at evacuation of the interspace are not associated with lowered incidence of recurrent herniation.[9] Retention of as much disc as possible preserves some of the biomechanical functions of the disc. It has been shown that the biomechanical properties of the lumbar motion segment are more adversely affected by total as opposed to partial discectomy.[66,67] Furthermore, if only the herniated fragment is removed, it is unlikely that vascular, ureteral, or intestinal injury will occur. The annulus is thicker anteriorly, and only vigorous attempts at discectomy are likely to penetrate an intact annulus.[4] It seems likely that the instrument reaches the prevertebral space through an annulus that is already at least partially defective. The integrity of the anterior portion of the annulus can be established by failure of saline solution introduced into the interspace to drain from it.

Other Herniations The diagnosis of far lateral disc herniation has also been facilitated by CT and MRI. When only myelography was available, intraforaminal herniations could be suspected by slight asymmetry of the root sheath and by probing the foramen with a blunt nerve hook. However, extraforaminal herniations could not be identified by myelography, and probably account for some of the patients who failed to improve following hemilaminotomy and discectomy. Most far lateral herniations occur at L3–L4 and L4–L5.[47,48] The physical findings are much the same as those associated with intraspinal herniations except that pain with straight leg raising is less frequent.[1] Intraforaminal herniations are best approached by standard hemilaminotomy and medial facetectomy. For extraforaminal herniations, medial facetectomy can be avoided by the intertransverse approach. This can be readily accomplished at the L3–L4 and L4–L5 levels, where most of these herniations occur (Fig. 5–5). However, the intertransverse approach is much more difficult at L5–S1 because of the configuration and more lateral projection of the sacral articular process and the relatively small space between the transverse process and the sacral ala as compared with the intertransverse distance at more rostral levels. For extraforaminal herniations at L5–S1 we have found it necessary to do a total facetectomy. Although it has been suggested that in this case fusion should be done,[93] this does not appear necessary since instability following unilateral facetectomy is uncommon.[47,48]

However, if instability is already present, then fusion is justifiable. For example, the patient whose films are shown in Figure 5–6 had severe back pain

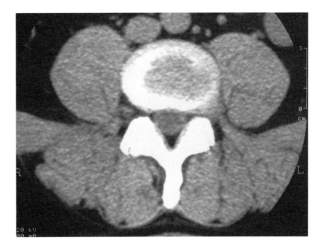

FIGURE 5–5. Far lateral disc herniation on the left at L4–L5.

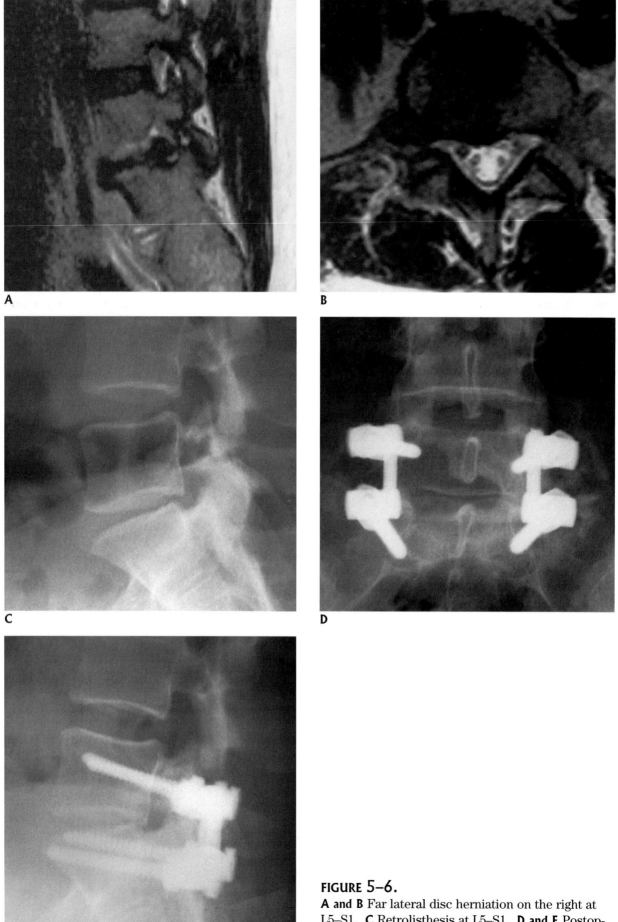

FIGURE 5–6.
A and B Far lateral disc herniation on the right at L5–S1. **C** Retrolisthesis at L5–S1. **D and E** Postoperative films.

radiating down the right lower limb to the medial aspect of the ankle. Motion of the spine was limited in both flexion and extension. The right gluteal muscles were weaker than the left, and extension of the right foot and toes was also weaker than the left. Sensory perception was diminished over the medial aspect of the right foot and leg. Straight leg raising was painful at 45 degrees. A facetectomy was done for removal of the extruded fragment, and fusion was performed because of the retrolisthesis and the severe back pain.

Percutaneous Techniques Percutaneous techniques have been advocated as an alternative to open surgery. *Intradiscal treatment* is attractive because it can be done under local anesthesia and requires little, if any, hospitalization. It is relatively painless and inexpensive. The rationale is reduction of disc volume and therefore intradiscal pressure, whether by chemical action or by actual removal of tissue. A reduction of intradiscal pressure, however, may merely reflect relaxation of the annulus, which is not well suited to withstand vertical loads.

Chymopapain injection was the first method of intradiscal therapy to be introduced, and although a substantial number of patients selected for this treatment were placebo reactors,[58] nevertheless, many patients had significant improvement.[19,109,168,179] The mystery is why, since pain relief was immediate in some and prompt in most, whereas reduction in height of the disc took much longer.[85,109]

Good results have also been reported with *percutaneous discectomy*, a procedure that should be limited to protrusions contained beneath the posterior longitudinal ligament,[136] because it is not effective for the management of sequestered or extruded fragments. We have operated on patients who have had persistent symptoms following the procedure and found extruded fragments beneath the root, although the central portion of the disc had been nicely evacuated.

Despite initial good results in some patients after intradiscal treatment, reservation should be entertained regarding a procedure whose major goal is removal of as much of the disc as possible because of the subsequent adverse effect on the biomechanical properties of the discs.[66,67]

Recurrent Pain Following removal of the disc herniation, most patients experience prompt relief of pain. In others this is more gradual and in some initial relief is followed by recurrent pain several days later which then subsides. This may be related to the increased sensitivity to the root that has been involved with the disc protrusion. In patients operated upon for herniated disc, Smyth and Wright placed a loop of nylon suture around the root at the site of compression and brought the ends of the loop out through the incision.[152] In some patients loops were placed around uninvolved roots as well. Several days after surgery mild tension was applied to the loops, reproducing preoperative symptoms at the level of herniation. The uninvolved roots were less sensitive.

Different opinions have been expressed regarding postoperative resumption of activity with return to work, which varies from 4 to 16 weeks.[71] Carragee et al found that their patients could return to work in less than 2 weeks, including those who did heavy work.[22] It appears reasonable, however, to restrict heavy lifting for several weeks to allow time for the opening in the annulus to close.

Recurrent pain is a difficult problem, particularly if it occurs within 6 months of surgery. Postoperative imaging studies performed in patients whose symptoms had been satisfactorily relieved demonstrated persistent defects at 2 to 3 months[119,159] and at one year in a substantial number of patients.[41,159] Furthermore, the presence and extent of scar could not be correlated with symptoms.[81,159] Consequently, recurrent sciatica within the first year following surgery should not automatically be ascribed to recurrent disc herniation or scar. For example, a 38-year-old lady had back pain radiating down the left lower limb into the calf with paresthesias in the lateral aspect of the foot. The left flexor hallucis longus was weaker than the right, sensory perception was diminished over the lateral aspect of the left foot, and straight leg raising was painful at 20 degrees. Her symptoms and physical findings resolved following removal of an extruded fragment at L5–S1. Four months later she slipped and fell and developed recurrent pain radiating down the left lower limb into the foot. Flexion of the spine was moderately limited and straight leg raising was painful at 45 degrees on the left. Her sensory perception and muscle strength remained normal. CT scan appeared much the same as at the preoperative examination (Fig. 5–7). Because muscle strength and sensory perception remained normal, surgery was not recommended and the symptoms gradually subsided.

Recurrent or persistent radicular pain after surgery for herniated disc is a major problem. If a cause for the radiculopathy can be identified,

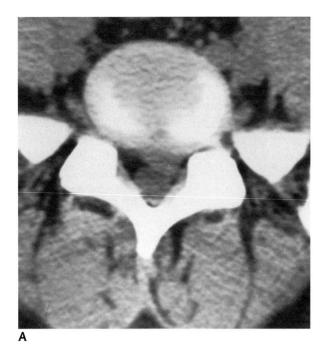 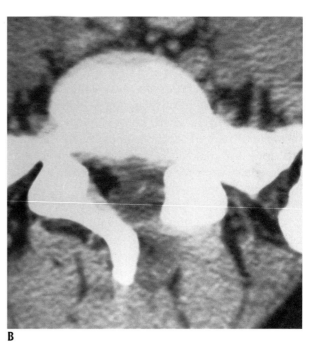

FIGURE 5–7. **A** CT scan prior to removal of an extruded disc fragment at L5–S1. **B** CT scan 5 months following operation.

such as retained or recurrent disc fragment, foraminal stenosis, entrapment in the lateral recess, or instability, then improvement can be anticipated following correction of the abnormality. Symptoms not related to these factors can be difficult to explain. Involvement of the root sheath by scar is frequently used to account for the pain but appears to be an overused whipping boy, and "adhesive arachnoiditis" is much less frequently invoked now that oil-based contrast media are no longer used.

The patient operated upon for vertebral body fracture or osteomyelitis can be expected to have dural adhesions at least as severe as those associated with disc surgery, These patients, however, rarely develop persistent radicular pain. When a cause cannot be identified, treatment is difficult and usually less than successful.

Surgery performed to free up the nerve root can be expected to provide at most only temporary relief, and this is probably secondary to manipulation of the root, producing some loss of function in afferent fibers as in the compression operation for trigeminal neuralgia. Dorsal rhizotomy has been proposed, but the results have been variable. White and Sweet reported good results in 6 of 7 patients with a single-level rhizotomy and good results in 5 patients with L5 and S1 rhizotomy.[171] However, 3 had weakness requiring use of an ankle brace. In another series successful relief of pain was achieved in approximately 50% of patients overall, although results were somewhat better when two roots were divided rather than one.[157] Our experience is similar to that of Onofrio and Campa,[131] who observed successful relief of pain in only 17% of patients who had rhizotomy following previous lumbar disc surgery. They found diagnostic selective root blocks unreliable prognostic indicators of the result of rhizotomy. The overall failure of one level rhizotomy and the somewhat better results with division of two roots suggest that the cause for pain does not lie within the root but rather within the tissues to which it is distributed. This is also supported by the results of diagnostic root blocks.[128]

Because experiments in monkeys suggested that application of current to the nerve root could block afferent conduction,[124] we implanted electrodes on the lumbar roots of patients with persistent and intractable radicular pain. In most instances, the electrodes were placed under local anesthesia in the L5 and S1 root foramina and led out through the skin. Subsequently, currents were applied through the electrodes at 100 rectangular pulses per second. If the pain was successfully relieved, a radio receiver was implanted subcutaneously through a separate incision and connected to the electrodes. The initial results were excellent, but with time nearly all patients experienced progressively decreasing relief of pain, probably for the same reason that rhizotomy was not successful. Dorsal column stimulators have also been used. With successful results defined as 50% reduction in pain 2 years or more after implant, the success rate is approximately 50%.[127]

Patient Selection for Surgery Good patient selection has been identified as a major factor in the prevention of the failed back surgery syndrome.[52] Certainly the patient with severe pain restricted to the distribution of a single root, appropriate sensory loss, muscle weakness, pain with straight leg raising, and demonstration of an extruded fragment by CT or MRI can be expected to have excellent relief of pain. In patients who have radicular symptoms and findings that are less well defined, who have a greater component of back pain, and whose imaging studies demonstrate a diffusely bulging disc more prominent on the side of pain present a greater problem.

Dysfunctional personality is also a major factor in determining the patient's assessment of the outcome, even in those with well-defined radicular syndromes. Although it is gratifying to have the patient acknowledge that symptoms have been relieved, the major goal of treatment is relief of symptoms. Personality disorder is not a guarantee of immortality, and persistent complaints do not necessarily mean that the patient has not been helped. For example, one of our patients who had an obvious personality problem presented with progressive paraparesis secondary to a meningioma at T8. She was unable to walk. Following laminectomy and removal of the tumor, recovery of neurological function was excellent and she could walk without assistance. The patient, however, complained bitterly of severe pain in the region of the incision, and stated that if she could do it over again she would not have had the operation.

Fusion The issue of whether fusion should be done at the time of surgery for herniated disc was raised by Mixter and Barr[117] and has been a continuing controversy ever since.[60] Patients whose symptoms are predominantly radicular and who do not have radiographic evidence of instability do not require a fusion. For example, the patient whose MRI is shown in Figure 5–8A had pain radiating down the right lower limb to the lateral aspect of the foot. Plantar flexion of the right foot and toes was weaker than of the left. Sensory perception was diminished over the lateral aspect of the right foot. Straight leg raising was painful at 20 degrees on the right and 40 degrees on the left with pain referred to the right lower limb. A hemilaminotomy was done at L5–S1 and a large extruded fragment removed. The symptoms were relieved and neurological function returned to normal. The patient was discharged on the second postoperative day and returned to work 2 weeks following surgery. Two years later while dancing at his wedding he developed recurrent pain in the back and right lower limb. These symptoms persisted and he was unable to work. The pain radiated into the lateral aspect of the right foot. MRI (Fig. 5–8B) demonstrated recurrent herniation almost identical to that prior to the operative 2 years previously. He was operated upon and a large extruded fragment was removed. The patient was discharged the day following surgery and returned to work approximately 2 weeks later.

It could be argued that fusion at the time of the first operation would have prevented the recurrence requiring the second. If this had been done, however, the hospital stay would have been substantially longer, postoperative pain would have been greater, and much more time would have been lost from work. In some circumstances, however, a fusion is appropriate.

The patient whose films are shown in Fig. 5–9 was involved in an automobile accident and developed pain in the back radiating down the right lower limb into the heel. She was a physical education major and was unable to continue playing on her university soccer team. The pain was minimal upon getting up in the morning but progressively increased during the day and was also aggravated by sitting. Physical activities were significantly restricted.

Examination 8 months later demonstrated atrophy of the right extensor digitorum brevis and weakness of dorsiflexion and plantar flexion of the right foot. Weakness subsequently developed in the right gluteal muscles. Spine films showed progressive narrowing of the L5–S1 interspace. Although a CT scan did not demonstrate disc herniation, the increased pain associated with sitting and the progression of pain during the day suggested bulging of the disc and constriction of the root foramen as a function of applied load. Fourteen months following injury, posterior lumbar interbody fusion was done with good relief of symptoms and return of neurological function to normal. The patient was able to resume full physical activity and return to the soccer team.

Compared with transverse process fusion, posterior lumbar interbody fusion requires less dissec-

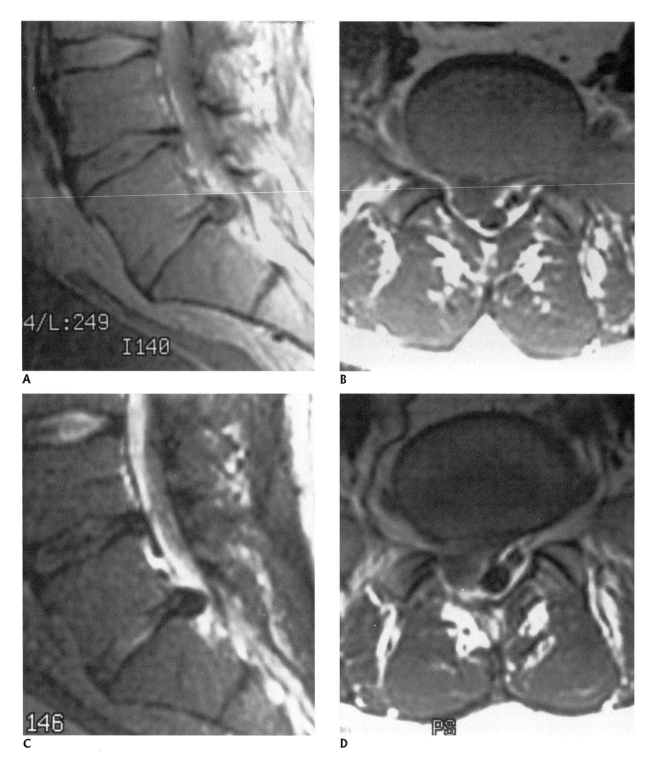

FIGURE 5-8. **A** CT scans prior to removal of an extruded disc fragment at L5–S1. **C** and **D** CT scans 2 years later.

tion, and bony union takes place in the axis of rotation of the motion segment. However, the incidence of postoperative neurological deficits is greater,[99,138] probably related to stretch of the L5 root as it moves around the pedicle secondary to retraction at the L4–L5 level. Root stretch is not as much a problem at L5–S1 because of the more oblique course of the S1 root.

Another patient, a 22-year-old man, sustained a lifting injury at work and developed back pain

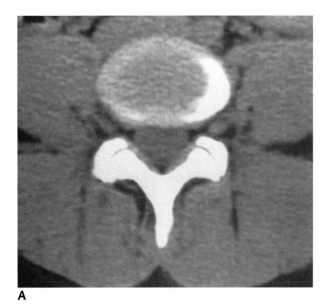 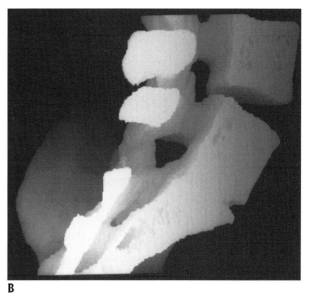

FIGURE 5-9. **A** CT scan demonstrating minimally building disc. **B** 3-D CT scan 1 year following posterior lumbar interbody fusion at L5–S1. The tip of the S1 articular process has been removed.

which radiated down both lower limbs to the distal portion of the leg. The pain was not relieved by lying down. It was worse in connection with cold, damp weather. Extensive nonsurgical treatment did not provide relief of symptoms. Motion of the spine was significantly restricted in extension, which produced pain radiating into both thighs. Flexion was done better. Muscle strength was normal in the lower limbs. MRI demonstrated degenerative change in the disc at L4–L5 and L5–S1 with bulging to the left of midline at L5–S1 (Fig. 5–10). A bivalved Spica orthosis was made, and the patient was fairly comfortable while wearing the orthosis but when out of it had significant pain. However, with restriction of activity, the pain was tolerable. The symptoms became more severe and persistent, and he developed pain radiating down the left lower limb into the lateral aspect of the foot. Dorsiflexion and plantar flexion of the left big toe were weaker than the right, and straight leg raising was painful at 35 degrees on the left. Two years following injury, an extruded disc fragment was removed at L5–S1 on the left. Because back pain was very prominent and was relieved by an orthosis, fusion was done from L4 to the sacrum with pedicle fixation, and relief of preoperative symptoms was satisfactory. Although some back discomfort persisted, analgesics were not required. He was unable to return to his previous occupation as a construction worker but is employed at a job requiring less strenuous physical activity.

Discogenic Pain

Discography

The disc itself can also be a source of back pain.[27] In disc surgery under local anesthesia, palpation of the disc was associated with local back pain.[154,173] Since both disc degeneration and back pain are common, a correlation between anatomical change and symptoms can be difficult, and discography has been used for this purpose. Discography is controversial, and has been considered both useful[151] and useless.[125] The reason for pain production during discography is not clear.[15] End plate deflection[73] and end plate disruption have been proposed.[80] Back pain is the predominant symptom, and injection of even a normal disc can cause pain.[28] MRI has made discography obsolete for diagnostic purposes, although a few patients with normal MRI have abnormal discograms.[13,86] The pain of discography has been considered related to herniated nucleus pulposus by some,[110,118] whereas others consider intradiscal pathology to be the major factor.[161] Discography is mainly used now to determine whether the pain associated with injection of contrast medium is similar or dissimilar to the patient's symptoms. Similar, or concordant, pain was produced in a series of patients in whom pain was considered sufficiently

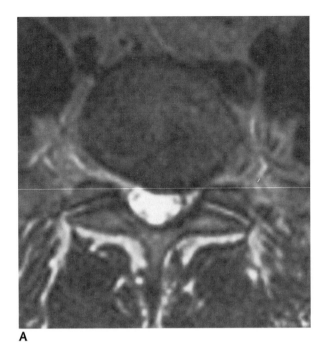 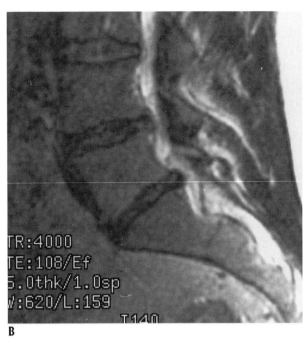

FIGURE 5–10. **A** The L5–S1 disc is bulging mildly into the left side of the canal. **B** The L4–L5 and the L5–S1 discs are degenerated and mildly bulging.

severe to warrant surgery. For those who had concordant pain with only degenerative discs, 50% improved as compared to 75% of those where annular tears were demonstrated.[118] These observations suggest that reproduction of pain by discography alone is not reliable.

Internal Disc Disruption

The syndrome of internal disc disruption has been described in which back pain is considered to be produced by the effect on nerve endings in the annulus by the products of disc metabolism, which are also considered to produce a systemic effect by entry of these materials through the subchondral veins into the general circulation, leading to weight loss.[30,31] However, it does not appear likely that a structure as hypocellular as the intervertebral disc and one without a blood supply and nourished only by diffusion across the end plate can generate enough metabolic products to create a systemic effect. Persistence of pain despite recumbency is one of the factors used in support of the syndrome, but a group of patients has been described in which pain is aggravated during recumbency and is relieved by motion. In these patients, CT scan did not demonstrate changes in the apophyseal joints, but pain was relieved following fusion. Histological examination of the joints removed at surgery demonstrated changes similar to those found in chondromalacia patellae. The authors designated this as chondromalacia facetae.[44] In other patients whose symptoms are precipitated by standing and by applied loads and relieved by lying down, the major factor appears to be mechanical. Loss of the normal biomechanical properties of the disc is followed by greater stress on the annulus. The annulus is not well suited to withstand vertical loads,[126] and an applied stress may excite the nerve endings in the periphery of the annulus with or without the development of fissures.

Raised Intraosseous Pressure

Pathology

Raised intraosseous pressure has been identified as a source of pain in long bones[97] and has been implicated in the development of lumbar pain.[5] Vertebral intraosseous pressure was least when measured with the patient prone, intermediate when standing, and greatest when sitting. In these patients, injection of saline into the vertebral body was promptly followed by pain.[50] Vertebral bodies with abnormal signal on MRI were found to have substantially greater pressure than those with normal signal.[121]

Clinical Presentation and Diagnosis

Two types of signal in homogeneity have been described. In Type I, signal intensity was decreased on T1 images but increased on T2. Type II had increased signal on T1 and no alteration or only slightly increased signal on T2. Most of the patients with Type I changed to Type II over a period of 1 to 3 years. In those who were operated upon, histological examination demonstrated disruption of the end plate in both types. Vascularity and osteoblasts were increased in Type I, with replacement of hemopoietic elements by fat. The bony trabeculae were thickened in both types.[121] Raised intraosseous pressure has been shown to follow end plate disruption in vitro.[181] Clinically, end plate disruption was identified during discography, which produced concordant pain in 13 of 14 patients, compared with concordant pain in 34% where the end plates were normal.[80] Similiarly, end plate disruption with intraosseous disc herniation was found in 8 patients who had sustained an acute compression injury. Each had back pain, and two also had thigh pain. The herniations were identified by discography. The pain was reproduced by injection, and this effect was blocked by introduction of local anesthetic into the disc space.[112] Also, bone scan demonstrated increased uptake in the affected vertebral bodies, reflecting increased osteoblastic activity.[56]

Management

This apparent correlation between raised intraosseous pressure and back pain is illustrated (Fig. 5–11) by one of our patients who had severe and disabling low back pain, relieved by lying down and precipitated by sitting and standing. Spine films demonstrated narrowing at L5–S1, but the apophyseal joints appeared normal. Bone scan with single-photon emission tomography (SPECT) demonstrated increased uptake in the bodies of L5 and S1. Following fusion with pedicle fixation, the pain was relieved and the patient returned to full activity. Four years later pain recurred and was persistent. A bone scan with SPECT done as part of the evaluation now demonstrated substantially reduced uptake at L5–S1 but increased uptake at a more rostral motion segment.

In another patient whose predominant symptom was low back pain relieved by lying down and precipitated by sitting and standing, MRI demonstrated altered signal on either side of a degenerated disc, and bone scan with SPECT showed increased uptake in the L5 and S1 vertebral bodies (Fig. 5–12). Pain was relieved following transverse process fusion with pedicle fixation. In these patients, it is likely that the end plates had become incompetent, allowing transmission of pressure from the disc into the vertebral body by the increased loads associated with sitting and standing. Pedicle fixation provided prompt relief of pain by shielding the presumably defective end plates, and therefore the vertebral bodies, from applied loads.

Zygapophyseal "Facet" Joints

Pathology

The correct term for the posterior intervertebral joints is *zygapophyseal*, but *facet joint* has come into common usage, and being less cumbersome will be employed here. Degenerative changes in these joints, such as cartilage necrosis and defects in subchondral bone, are the same as those observed in other synovial joints.[98] Pressure on the articular surfaces is increased by extension and with narrowing of the disc.[180] Degenerative changes in the joints are closely connected with degenerative changes in the discs of the same motion segment.[79] The "facet syndrome" was first described by Ghormley,[64] who considered the pain to be secondary to degenerative changes in the joints and in some instances to pressure by hypertrophic joints on neural elements. Although the existence of a definite "facet syndrome" has been questioned,[144] the posterior intervertebral joints are recognized as a source of pain.[7,144] This is supported by the excellent relief of back pain which followed facetectomy when back pain was the only or major symptom.[147] Mooney and Robertson found that injection of hypertonic saline into the joints produced pain in the back, the thigh, and sometimes into the leg.[120] The distribution of pain, however, was not joint specific. The injections were associ-

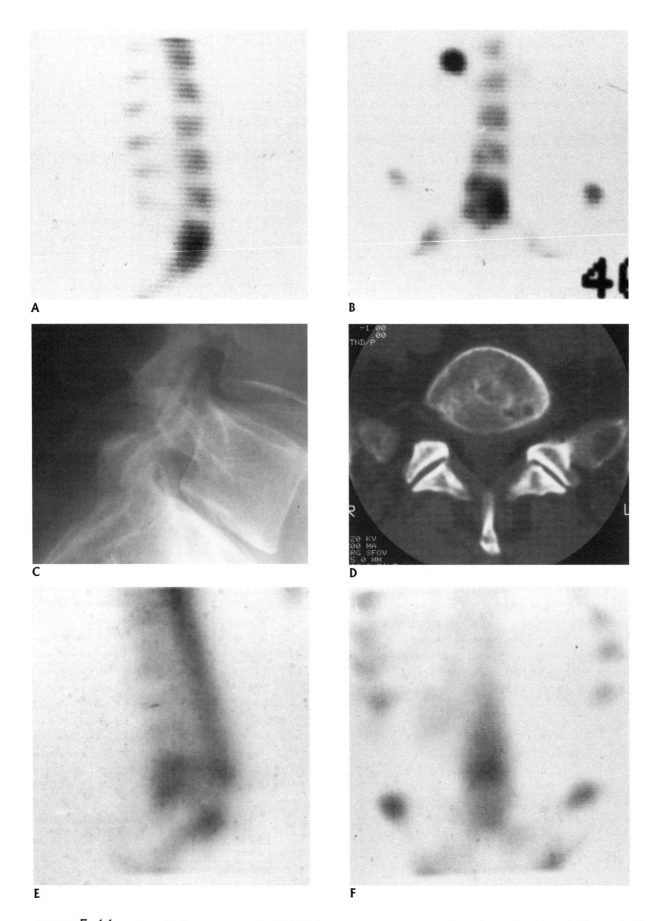

FIGURE 5–11. **A and B** Bone scan with SPECT demonstrating increased uptake in the L5 and S1 vertebral bodies. **C** The disc height at L5–S1 is significantly decreased. **D** CT scans demonstrating relatively normal joints. **E and F** Bone scan with SPECT done 4 years later. The uptake at L5–S1 has decreased considerably, but there is increased uptake at more rostral levels.

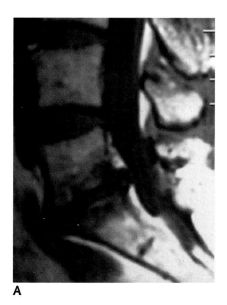 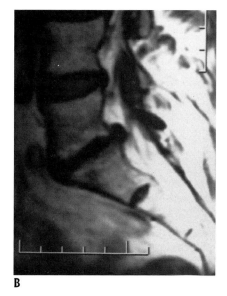 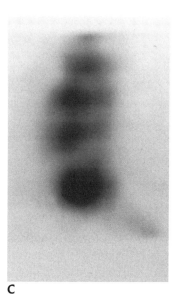

FIGURE 5–12. **A** Signal is decreased on either side of narrowed L5–S1 disc on T1. **B** Signal is increased on T2. **C** Bone scan with SPECT shows increased uptake in the L5–S1 vertebral bodies.

ated with increased myoelectric activity in the hamstring muscles and the development of pain with straight leg raising at 70 degrees, which was considered secondary to hamstring tension. These effects and the production of pain by injection of hypertonic saline could be blocked by the introduction of local anesthetic agents into the joints.

Clinical Presentation and Diagnosis

Facet pain can be restricted to the low back, but it usually radiates. Patients can experience pain in the buttock, inguinal area, thigh, and less frequently the leg. Some describe abdominal pain. It can be either unilateral or bilateral and is increased by extension, which causes increased pressure on the articular surfaces.[104,180] Flexion is usually not painful, and patients tend to stand in a flexed position. Lateral bending can also produce pain but not as consistently as extension. Focal tenderness over the affected joint is frequently present.[74,101] Although symptoms are relieved in most instances by lying down, in some patients pain is more severe during rest and recumbency.[44] Fusion was followed by good relief of symptoms. Although plain films were normal, histological examination of the joints demonstrated abnormalities similar to those found in chondromalacia patellae, including foci of full-thickness cartilage necrosis with ulceration, fibrillation, and exposure of subchondral bone. The authors coined the term *chondromalacia facetae* for this condition.[44]

Management by Injection

Variable results have been reported following injection of the joints with local anesthetic and steroids. In general, the results were better if radiographic or scintigraphic abnormalities of the joints could be demonstrated. In one series of patients with symptoms consistent with facet pain, injection of joints in which CT had demonstrated narrowing or erosion was followed by immediate and complete relief of pain. This did not occur after injection of joints that appeared normal.[23] In another report when bone scan with SPECT was normal, injection of the joints did not provide relief of symptoms, but in 12 patients in whom increased uptake was demonstrated, 8 obtained good relief.[78] Patients with pain in the back, thigh, or groin increased by extension are more likely to respond than those with only back pain.[74] Intra-articular injection has been found to be necessary,[108] and when this was not confirmed radiographically, the results were poor.[51] Patients who responded to facet blocks were reported to have better results with facet denervation than those who did not.[103] Failure of facet denervation to provide good long-term results may be related to the innervation of these joints from the anterior, posterior, and lateral aspects, and from at least three spinal levels.[6] In a prospective study, a correlation was shown between relief of pain after facet injection and after fusion.[107] Although pain relief is only transient in the majority of cases, this at least identifies the joint as the source of pain, and a substantial number of patients experience prolonged relief of 6 months or more.[40,108,120]

For example, a 66-year-old lady had back pain radiating down the left lower limb to the ankle for about 6 months. The pain had become progressively more severe and was increased by walking short distances. Lumbar stenosis had been demonstrated radiographically (Fig. 5–13A), and a laminectomy had been recommended. Extension was limited to the neutral position but flexion was good. The neurological examination was normal. Spine films demonstrated anterior displacement of L4 on L5 increased in flexion (Fig. 5–13B), and uptake was increased bilaterally at L4–L5 on bone scan with SPECT. Injection of the left L4–L5 joint with local anesthetic and steroid was followed by excellent relief of pain. The patient returned 3 years later with recurrent pain. Spine films showed increased translational motion at L4–L5. Again injection of the left L4–L5 joint was followed by good relief of pain. Symptoms recurred after 3 months, and another injection produced prolonged relief of symptoms. Two years later the pain recurred but was tolerable, and the patient did not believe it was sufficiently severe to have another injection.

Although this patient had severe lumbar stenosis, her symptoms are clearly related to the left L4–L5 joint, and while the instability was in flexion, pain was experienced in extension probably because of the increased pressure on the articular surfaces associated with that movement. Although the joints were abnormal bilaterally, only the left side produced pain, demonstrating that radiograhic and scintigraphic abnormalities can be present without associated pain.

Hip/Spine Syndrome

The hip/spine syndrome has been described[129] in patients with degenerative changes in both the hip and the spine. Pain from the abnormal hip can be experienced in the gluteal area, in the groin, and in the anterior aspect of the thigh. A fixed flexion deformity of the hip joint may develop, leading to extension of the spine and pressure on the articular surfaces, resulting in back pain. On the other hand, lumbar scoliosis can produce pelvic tilt, accelerating degenerative changes in the hip. Relief of pain following injection of the hip joint with local anesthetic identifies the hip as the source of pain, and successful selective root block or facet block implicates the spine.[129]

Degenerative Spondylolisthesis

Degenerative spondylolisthesis is usually discussed in connection with spondylolisthesis secondary to congenital or traumatic abnormalities of the pars interarticularis, but since it is a consequence of disc degeneration, it will be considered in this chapter. It is more common in women and does not develop before the fifth decade.[142] Since the translational displacement can be either anterior or posterior, *spondylolisthesis* and *anterolisthesis* should not be considered synonyms.[42] Spondylolisthesis was present in 28.6% of 500 patients with low back pain, and posterior displacement was more common than anterior.[123]

Pathology

Retrolisthesis appears related to laxity of the joint capsules secondary to disc degeneration and decreased disc height (Fig. 5–14). In anterolisthesis, the upper facets of the joint grind through the lower,[55] and this process is facilitated by sagittally oriented articular processes (Fig. 5–15), although it may occur with more coronally oriented joints (Fig. 5–16). The sagittal orientation is significantly more common in patients with degenerative anterolisthesis than in normal individuals or patients with lumbar stenosis.[70] Anterior displacement is usually more pronounced than posterior, but does not exceed 30% of vertebral body height.[142] Anterior displacement is most common at L4–L5, perhaps because L4 is more mobile than L5, which is anchored by the iliolumbar ligament.[55] This hypothesis is supported by the observation that L4–L5 anterolisthesis is more frequent when L5 is sacralized.[142] Osteoarthritis of the hips is present in 17% of patients with anterolisthesis,[55] sometimes causing diagnostic problems.[129]

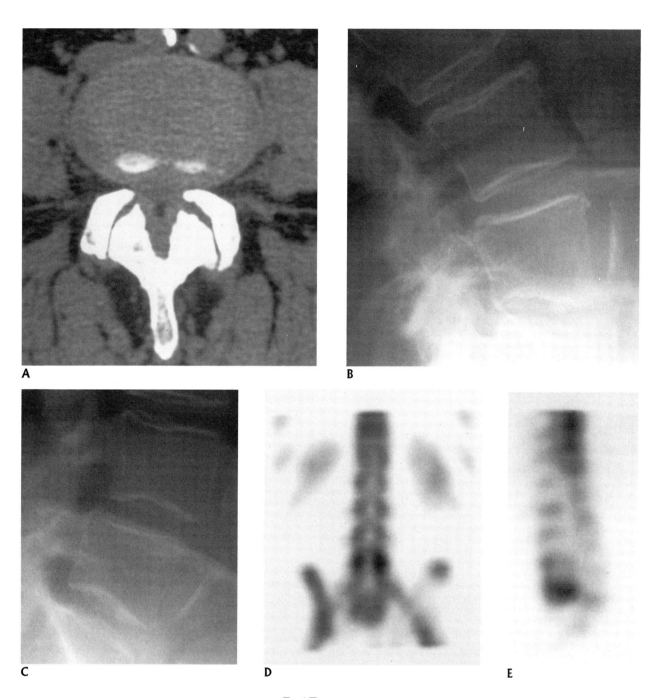

FIGURE 5-13. **A** CT scan demonstrating lumbar stenosis at L4–L5. **B** Mild anterolisthesis at L4–L5. **C** The anterolisthesis is increased in flexion. **D and E** Uptake is increased in the L4–L5 joints bilaterally on bone scan with SPECT.

Clinical Presentation and Diagnosis

The symptoms are much the same as those associated with lumbar stenosis, including back pain, radicular or nonradicular lower limb pain, and neurogenic claudication.[3,46,49] Radiculopathy is common, the L5 being the most frequently involved root.[83,84] Nonradicular lower limb pain usually is relieved by lying down, but radicular pain persists, although it may become less severe.

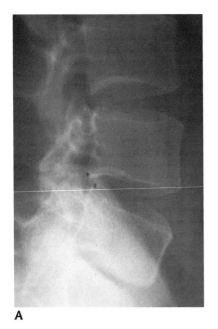 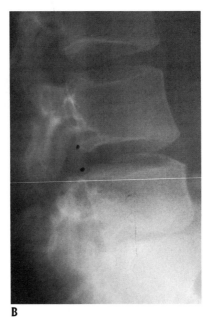 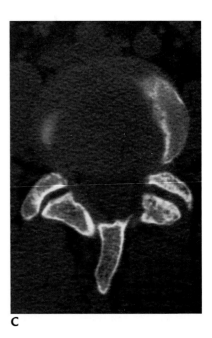

FIGURE 5–14. **A and B** Retrolisthesis at L4–L5 in extension, reduced in flexion. **C** CT scan demonstrating widened left L4–L5 joint consistent with relaxation of the joint capsule.

Management

Surgical Treatment

Surgery is usually performed because of intractable pain, although in a few patients muscle weakness may also be significant. As with lumbar stenosis, considerable disagreement exists with regard to the appropriate operation.[53] Laminectomy with medial facetectomy[46,49,76] and laminectomy and facetectomy[32] have been advocated. Increased displacement following surgery either was not observed,[46,49] or if it did occur did not affect the results.[32,76] In one series results were better with facetectomy,[32] but in others results were poor.[102,139]

Nonsurgical treatment such as physical therapy or epidural steroids is not especially effective.

Fusion Disagreement also exists with regard to fusion. Some consider it unnecessary[46,49,132] or only necessary if preoperative flexion and extension films demonstrated instability,[76] but others consider it to be a factor in achieving better results.[83,84,102,139] In a prospective study comparing the results of laminectomy and medial facetectomy alone or in combination with fusion, significantly better results were found in the fusion group.[75] However, since in this study all patients had translational motion during flexion and extension, it is perhaps not surprising that the results were better in those patients who were fused.

A decision regarding fusion should not be made on an all-or-none basis. A patient with back or back and nonradicular lower limb pain with increased translational movement during flexion and extension and without radiculopathy does not require a laminectomy but needs fusion. A patient with predominantly radicular symptoms and findings but without instability does not need a fusion. If both radiculopathy and instability are present, then decompression and fusion is the best operation.

For example, a laminectomy and facetectomy had been done in and 80-year-old woman (Fig. 5–17) with only transient relief of symptoms. A myelogram demonstrated adequate dimensions of the spinal canal and posterior displacement of L4 on L5. She had severe back and right lower limb pain with a right L5 radiculopathy. The symptoms were relieved by lying down but were precipitated by standing. She spent much of her day lying down. A lateral approach was used for discectomy and interbody fusion. Because the bone was very soft, pedicle fixation was not used. She was kept in a Spica cast until fusion occurred.

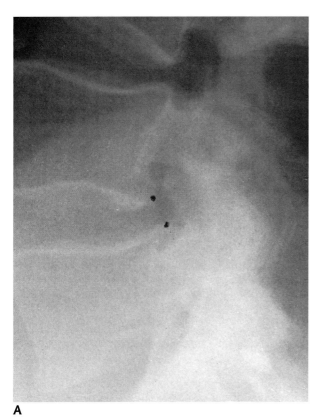
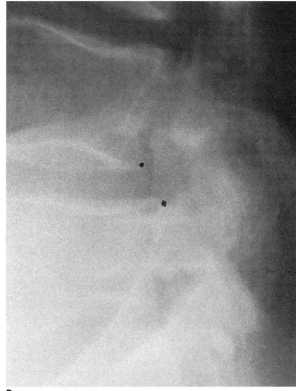
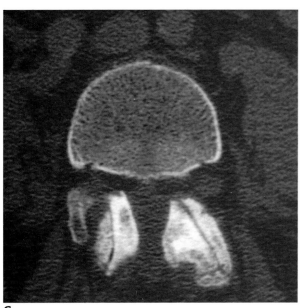

FIGURE 5-15.
A Anterolisthesis at L4–L5. B Displacement is increased during flexion. C The L4–L5 joints are sagitally oriented and degenerated.

Degenerative Scoliosis

As with degenerative spondyolisthesis, symptomatic degenerative scoliosis usually develops after age 50 and is more common in women. Benner and Ehni considered it be a result of asymmetric disc degeneration (Fig. 5–18).[11] Unlike degenerative spondylolisthesis, where the displacement is limited, the deformity in degenerative scoliosis is frequently but slowly progressive, less than 3 degrees per year (Fig. 5–19). A formula has been developed to predict the rate of progression.[87]

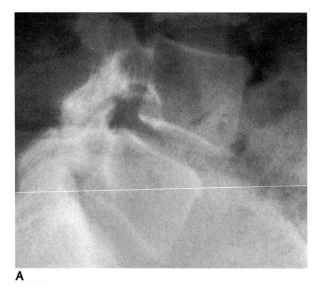
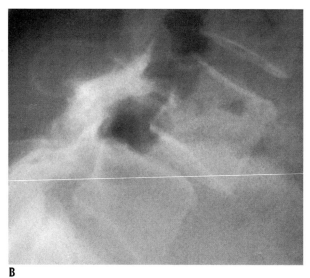
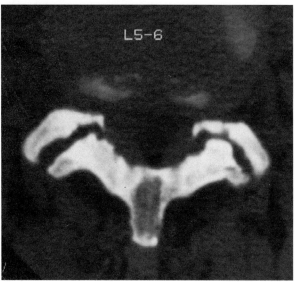

FIGURE 5–16.
A Anterolisthesis at L5–L6. **B** The anterolisthesis is increased during flexion. **C** These more coronally oriented joints have severe degenerative changes.

Clinical Presentation and Diagnosis

The symptoms are much the same as in degenerative spondylolisthesis, including back pain with or without nonradicular or radicular lower limb pain and neurogenic claudication. Radicular symptoms and findings can be related either to stenosis of the canal or to the root foramina (Fig. 5–20). Lateral displacement of the apical vertebrae may also affect the root immediately below by stretching it across the pedicle.[150] Radiculopathy usually occurs on the concave side of the curve.

Surgical Management

Different opinions have been expressed regarding the extent of the surgical procedure. Good results have been reported following laminectomy and foraminotomy, which sometimes requires facetectomy, and adverse effects were not observed following facetectomy, which, although usually unilateral, was sometimes bilateral.[45] However, others observed progression of deformity following laminectomy with significant increase in symptoms requiring fusion.[11] Different opinions also existed among those who considered a fusion necessary. Kostuik achieved good correction of deformity

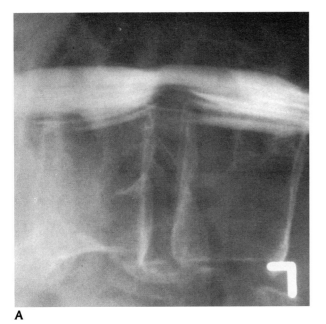
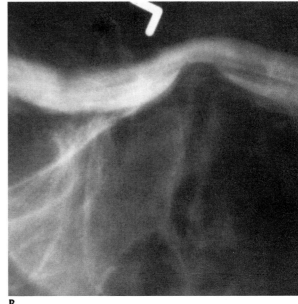
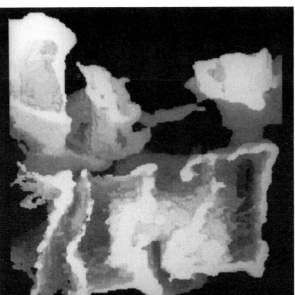

FIGURE 5–17.
A Myelogram done prior to an L4–L5 laminectomy and facetectomy. **B** Postoperative myelogram. L4 is displaced posteriorly on L5. **C** 3-D CT scan following lateral approach for discectomy, resection of the posterior superior portion of L4, and interbody fusion with iliac crest graft. Pedicle fixation was not used because the bone was very soft. The patient was placed in a SPICA cast for postoperative immobilization.

with a two-stage procedure. At the first stage multilevel anterior discectomy and bone grafting were performed, followed by posterior instrumentation at a second operation.[88,89] Substantial but less complete correction was obtained with posterior resection of ligaments and joint capsules with pedicle fixation from L1 to the sacrum.[111] Simmons and Simmons obtained good results following laminectomy and foraminotomy with pedicle fixation no higher than the first vertebra with a level superior surface.[149]

Since degenerative scoliosis is progressive, laminectomy and foraminotomy cannot be expected to arrest this process, and may indeed accelerate it. If the major problem is radiculopathy, the bone removal necessary to decompress the nerve root (Fig. 5–20) can introduce further instability. This may be followed by a relatively rapid increase in curve (Fig. 5–21). Consequently, foraminotomy should be accompanied by fusion (Fig. 5–22). If radiculopathy is not a factor, fusion with instrumentation is all that is required (Fig. 5–19).

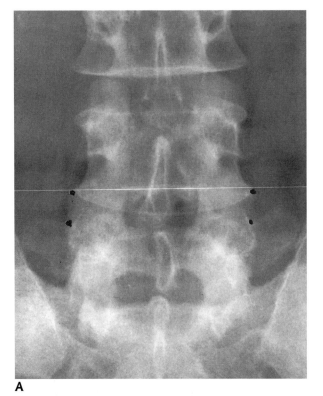
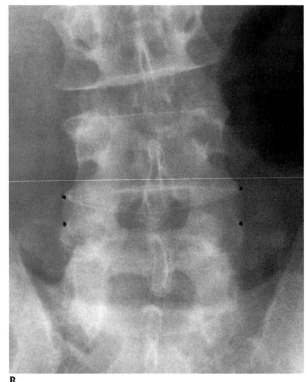
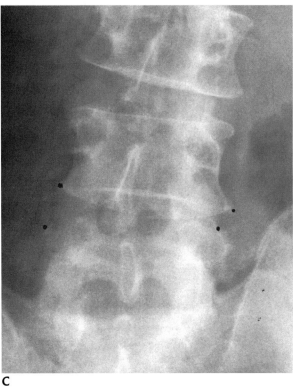

FIGURE 5-18.
A AP film with the patient in neutral position.
B Film during right lateral bending. **C** Displacement is asymmetrical during left lateral bending which is consistent with more pronounced degeneration of the left side of the disc.

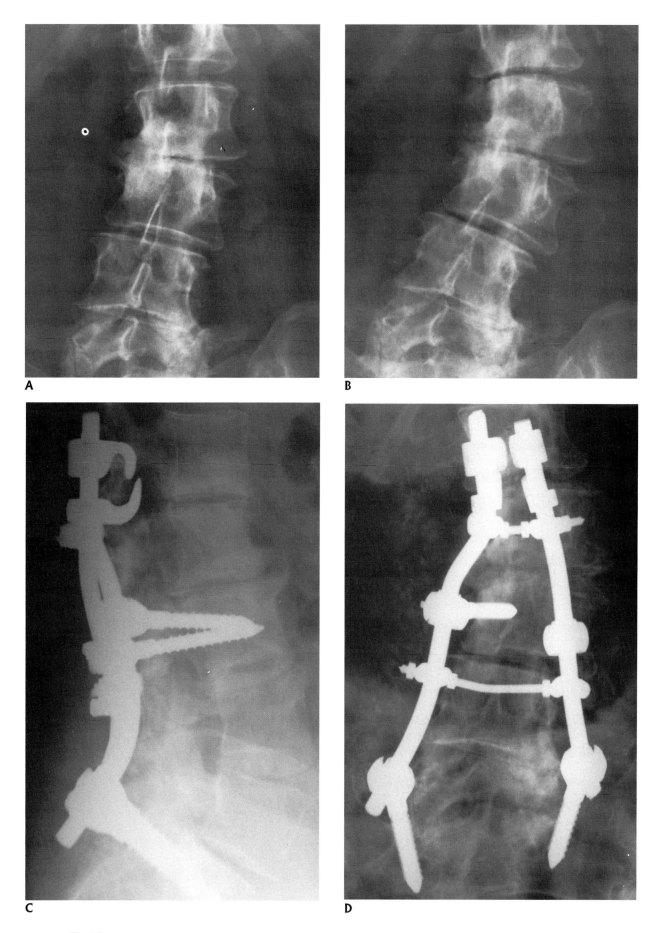

FIGURE 5-19. **A** Film demonstrating early degenerative scoliosis. **B** Same patient 4 years later. There has been slow progression of scoliosis with development of L1–L2 disc degeneration. The pain had become increasingly more severe. **C and D** Postoperative films. The L1 pedicle was too small to accept a screw.

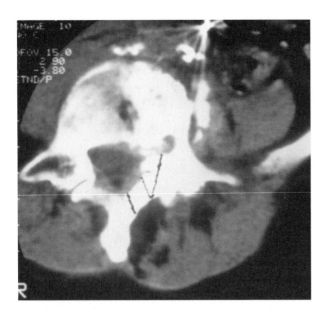

FIGURE 5–20. CT demonstrating a left L5 foraminal stenosis in a patient with degenerative scoliosis and left L5 radiculopathy. Laminectomy (parallel lines) would be ineffective and at least a medial facetectomy is required.

Lumbar Stenosis

Lumbar stenosis can be classified as developmental, idiopathic, and acquired.

Developmental Lumbar Stenosis

In achondroplasia, the most common developmental type, the pedicles are thick and short, resulting in constriction of the spinal canal. Other abnormalities include a dorsal lumbar kyphosis and an exaggerated lumbar lordosis. Neurological deficits can be related to both the kyphosis and the stenosis. Low back pain is common and perhaps related to the lumbar lordosis.[2] The patient whose films are shown in Figure 5–23 is a 55-year-old man with achondroplasia. Laminectomy had been done from T12 through L3 because of pain and weakness in the lower limbs associated with walking

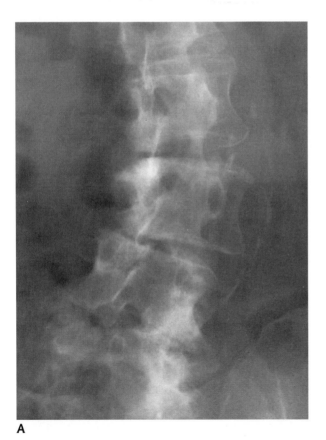
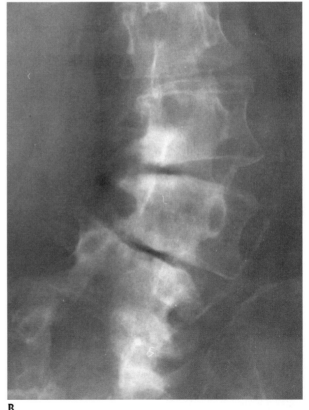

FIGURE 5–21. **A** AP film prior to laminectomy for lumbar stenosis. **B** Two years later the deformity has increased and a left L5 radiculopathy has developed.

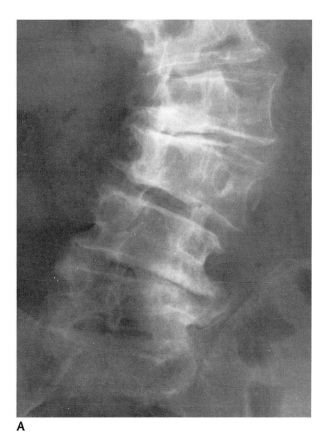
A

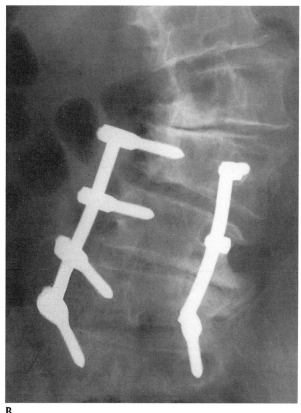
B

FIGURE 5–22. Preoperative films in a patient with left L5 radiculopathy. **A** The L5–S1 interpedicular space is less on the left, consistent with foraminal stenosis. **B** Postoperative film. A screw could not be placed in the left L5 pedicle because of the proximity to that of S1.

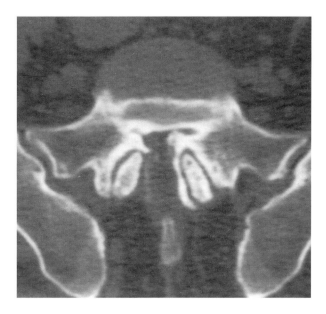

FIGURE 5–23. CT scan in a patient with achondroplasia and bilateral L5 and S1 radiculopathy. The radiculopathy was more severe on the right, although the radiographic abnormality is more pronounced on the left.

short distances. Following the operation he improved and did well for 17 years, when the symptoms recurred. The pain and weakness became progressively worse, and he was unable to walk more than 50 feet. Dorsiflexion and plantar flexion of the feet and toes were weak bilaterally, worse on the right. Perception of joint rotation was diminished in the toes of the right foot, and perception of pain and touch was decreased bilaterally in the feet and legs, more pronounced over the lateral aspect than the medial. Following laminectomy at L4 and L5, strength was recovered fully in the dorsiflexors and plantar flexors of the feet. Sensory perception improved but remained mildly impaired in the right foot. Walking also improved but was limited to approximately one block by back pain, presumably secondary to pressure on the lumbar articular surfaces related to the hyperlordosis. The patient was unwilling to consider a fusion, and therefore further evaluation was not pursued.

Idiopathic Lumbar Stenosis

Idiopathic lumbar stenosis occurs most frequently between L3 and L5. The pedicles are short and the lamina and articular processes are thick. It is most common at L3, L4, and L5. Symptoms develop during adult life secondary to stenosis that is related to only slight spondylotic changes.[162-164]

Acquired Lumbar Stenosis

Acquired stenosis is produced by hypertrophy of the posterior joints, thickening of the ligamentum flavum, and by osteophytic ridges. The stenosis can be central (Fig. 5–24) or limited to the lateral recess (Fig. 5–25) or root foramen (Fig. 5–26).

Clinical Presentation and Diagnosis

Back pain may be the only or principal symptom in patients with lumbar stenosis. It is unrelated to the stenosis, but rather is related to the abnormal posterior joints that contribute to the stenosis. The stenosis itself can cause radicular symptoms and findings, more often unilateral than bilateral. Even with unilateral radiculopathy, radiographic examination may show bilateral abnormalities (Fig. 5–27). In most patients, the symptoms are increased by extension of the lumbar spine and by walking. The dimensions of the spinal canal have been shown to decrease during extension,[133] and the pain associated with walking is probably related to the extension that occurs with each step. The constriction of the canal that occurs during extension can, under some circumstances, cause significant neurological deficit. Paraparesis during application of an extension cast with partial recovery following laminectomy was reported by Goldthwait, who attributed it to transient spondylolisthesis.[69] However, the relationship between lumbar stenosis and development of severe neurological deficit associated with sustained extension during general anesthesia was recognized by Ehni.[43]

Although the increased radicular pain experienced by patients with lumbar stenosis associated with walking can be broadly considered neurogenic claudication, it is monoradicular in most instances and is at most only partially relieved by lying down. Neurogenic claudication is usually defined as lower limb discomfort that is absent at rest and appears after extension of the spine and walking. Some are able to walk without limitation if they maintain a flexed position, as in pushing a shopping cart. One of our patients could play tennis without difficulty, but developed pain in the right buttock and lower limb after walking less than half a city block. He stood in flexion, and was unable to extend to the neutral position. The neurological examination was normal. After a hemilaminectomy and foraminotomy, walking was unrestricted. The pain of neurogenic claudication usually does not follow a radicular distribution suggesting involvement of more than one root. Some patients described a sensation of numbness or weakness after walking. In most, the symptoms subside after a few minutes, and they are able to resume walking.

Pathology

Although a vascular etiology has been proposed for neurogenic claudication,[134] mechanical factors appear more likely. The symptoms are almost simultaneous with extension and appear within at most a few minutes of walking. In contrast, median nerve conduction was not found to decrease until 20 minutes after inflation of a pneumatic cuff to above systolic pressure and was 50 to 70% of control after 30 minutes. Although response amplitude reduction occurred earlier in patients with carpal tunnel syndrome, nevertheless, it developed after 5 minutes in only 1 of 14 patients, and only after 10 minutes in the others.[61] However, in neurogenic claudication, reduction of somatosensory evoked potential amplitude develops immediately after extension of the spine (Fig. 5–28) and after walking for less than 5 minutes (Fig. 5–29). In some patients, extension was followed by a greater reduction in amplitude of the response than after walking (Fig. 5–30). This reduction of response amplitude in lumbar stenosis suggests involvement of L4, L5, and S1 in most cases, since if only one root is affected, the amplitude of the response to peroneal nerve stimulation is not significantly reduced (Fig. 5–31).

Surgical Treatment

The objective of surgical treatment is to enlarge the spinal canal. Because hypertrophic joints encroach

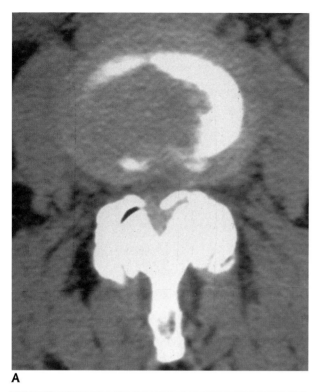
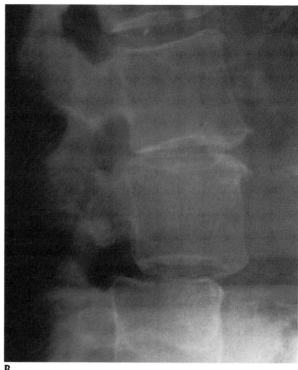
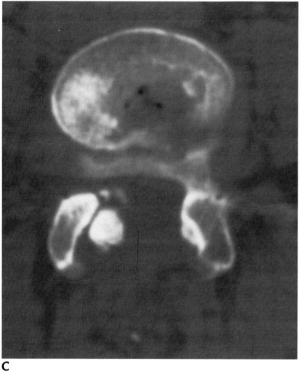

FIGURE 5-24.
A Lumbar stenosis in a patient with left L5 radiculopathy. A laminectomy, left facetectomy, and medial right facetectomy were done. **B** Film taken 1 year later. Anterolisthesis has developed with annoying but tolerable low back discomfort. **C** Postoperative CT scans showing a left facetectomy and partial right facetectomy.

medially, resection limited to the lamina can result in only a narrow midsagittal removal of bone. This has two potential disadvantages. In one, enlargement of the canal will be limited with the possibility of persistent symptoms. In the other, the dura will tend to protrude through the opening, increasing the possibility of a dural tear. If this occurs, the roots erupt from their confined quarters, cerebrospinal fluid drains, and epidural bleeding begins. Under these conditions, bone removal sufficient to return the roots to their normal location and to repair the dura is difficult and trying. To prevent this,

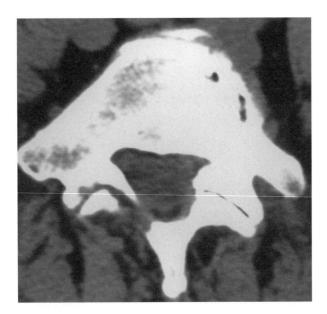

FIGURE 5-25. Left lateral recess stenosis. A left L5 radiculopathy was relieved by a medial facetectomy.

the laminectomy should be advanced on as broad a front as possible. Resection of hypertrophic joints and hypertrophic laminae can be facilitated by thinning them with a brace and bit, such as the D'Errico. Residual bone can be removed with curettes and punches with narrow foot plates. The resection can be extended laterally with a narrow osteotome. This provides a wider laminectomy than can easily be done with bone-biting instruments, and mini-

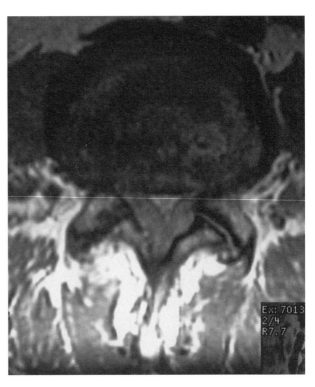

FIGURE 5-27. MRI showing symmetrical stenosis in a patient with unilateral radiculopathy.

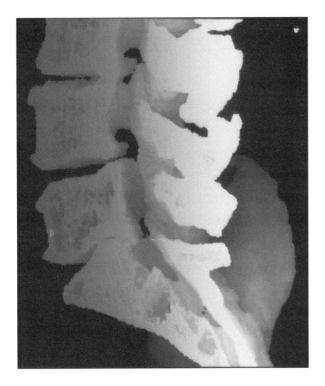

FIGURE 5-26. 3-D CT scan demonstrating stenosis of the right L5 foramen.

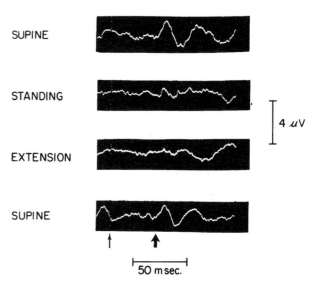

FIGURE 5-28. Potentials evoked by stimulation of the controlateral peroneal nerve after standing and after extension. The responses were allowed to return to control values after standing and after extension.

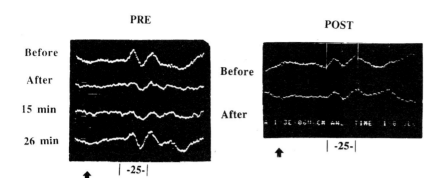

FIGURE 5-29.
Potentials evoked by peroneal nerve stimulation before and after walking. The responses on the left were recorded prior to surgery and on the right after laminectomy.

mizes the possibility of dural laceration and root injury. Delay in removing the ligamentum flavum until bone resection has been completed further decreases the chance of a dural tear.

The importance of an intact dura is illustrated by the patient whose MRI scans are shown in Figure 5-32. He gave a history of developing headaches, swelling in the area of the incision, and severe pain in the left lower limb radiating into the lateral aspect of the foot 10 days after a laminectomy at L2, L3, and L4. He was admitted to a hospital, where a drain was placed in the cystic swelling. The headaches subsided, but the area of swelling persisted. It was approximately 3 cm in diameter and was tender. Palpation of the swollen area produced pain radiating down the left lower limb. Plantar flexion of the left big toe was weak, and straight leg raising was painful at 30 degrees. He was operated upon, and when the meningocele was opened a nerve root hernia was seen protruding through a small opening in the dura. It was replaced and the opening was closed with a fascial plug, reinforced by imbrication of the inferior portion of the meningocele capsule.

Laminectomy and Facetectomy

Disagreement exists regarding the extent of the surgical procedure. Laminectomy alone, laminectomy and medial facetectomy, and laminectomy with facetectomy have been advocated. In many patients, the size of the joints makes it virtually impossible to do a laminectomy without at least a medial facetectomy. Even though an attempt may be made to limit the resection of the medial portion of the joints, the pars may fracture, resulting in a complete facetectomy. In vitro studies have demonstrated that instability did not follow medial facetectomy, but was observed after total facetectomy even when unilateral.[130] Clinically, Shenkin and Hash[148] observed anterolisthesis in 6 of 59 patients with bilateral facetectomy, two of whom required fusion. Others reported postoperative slip in 20%[82] and 31%.[20] However, this occurred in only 1 of 27 patients who had facetectomy at two levels on one side and medial facetectomy at corresponding levels on the other.[95] The variable incidence of displacement could be related to a variable extent of stabilization secondary to development of osteophytes and joint ossification.

Postfacetectomy Instability Although postfacetectomy instability is variable, it does occur (Fig. 5-24). Surgical treatment is usually not necessary, but occasionally symptoms may be severe enough to require an operation (Fig. 5-33). This patient had back pain that was precipitated by standing and

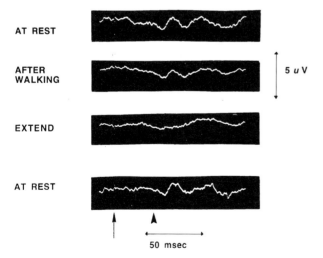

FIGURE 5-30. Recordings evoked by peroneal nerve stimulation with return to control values before the next recording. Extension produces a greater decrease in evoked response amplitude than does walking.

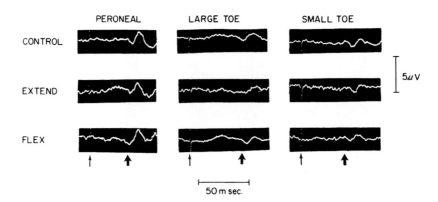

FIGURE 5-31. Somatosensory evoked potentials secondary to stimulation of the peroneal nerve (left), digital nerves of the large toe (center), and digital nerves of the small toe (right). Only the response to stimulation of the large toe digital nerves was reduced during extension sufficient to cause pain.

relieved by fusion. Occasionally in osteopenic patients, the postfacetectomy deformity may become severe, causing significant neurological deficit. The patient whose films are shown in Fig. 5-34 had a laminectomy with facetectomy because of back pain. He developed difficulty walking and required a walker. The right hip flexors, hamstrings, quadriceps, and foot extensors were weak. A lateral approach was done for resection of the pedicle and posterior portion of L3 with fusion to the iliac bone. Recovery of function was good, and he was able to walk without assistance. Another patient gave a history of laminectomy from T11 to L3 because of back pain and lower limb paresthesias. Progressive deformity developed (Fig. 5-35A-C). A myelogram demonstrated stenosis at L2 (Fig. 5-35D). When evaluated in our clinic, major symptoms were back and right lower limb pain and inability to detect bladder filling. The patient was incontinent of urine, and it was necessary for her to void hourly during the day and four times during the night. Gluteal and lower limb muscles were weak bilaterally. Six years after the original procedure a lateral approach was used for reconstruction of the spinal canal by L2 resection and interbody fusion from L1 to L3 with iliac crest graft (Fig. 5-35E, F). Recovery of strength in the affected muscles was good, and bladder function returned to normal. The back pain was not relieved. In this patient, the deformity was such that metallic instrumentation was not feasible. However, the bone grafts that were fitted as a modified mortise and tenon joint served as an instrument.

Laminectomy Overall, laminectomy has provided good relief of sciatica and claudication.[20,82,163] Recurrent symptoms were related to postoperative anterolisthesis[20,82] or to recurrent stenosis or development of stenosis at new levels.[20] Persistent low back pain accounted for poor results in 18 of 92 patients with less extensive bone removal.[164] Perhaps some of the patients with poor results following laminectomy may not have had neurogenic claudication, but rather symptoms related to abnormalities of the facets. In 45 patients with good results following laminectomy, evoked potentials recorded after walking and extension of the spine were abnormal in 42, whereas in 16 patients with poor results, evoked potentials were normal in 12.[94] The abnormal responses in 4 of the patients with poor results can be explained by compression sufficient to affect large fibers but not the smaller fibers, which are less sensitive to pressure; consequently, the pain was probably not neurogenic. Perhaps the good results in the 3 patients with normal responses were related to partial or total facetectomy incidental to efforts at enlarging the spinal canal. The 12 patients with poor results and normal evoked potentials probably had arthrogenic pain.

Fusion

Decisions regarding fusion should not be all or none. If the major problem is radiculopathy or

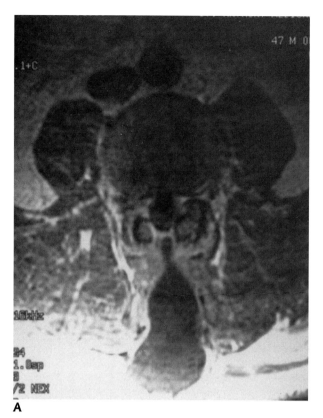
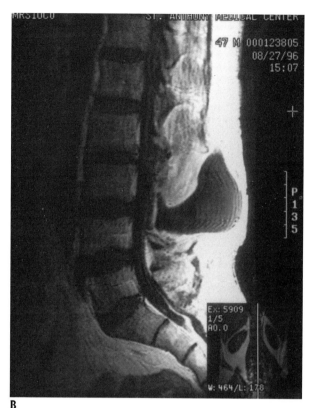
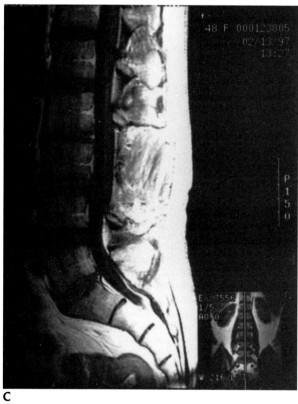

FIGURE 5-32.
A and B MRI scan demonstrating a postoperative meningocele. **C** MRI after repair of the meningocele.

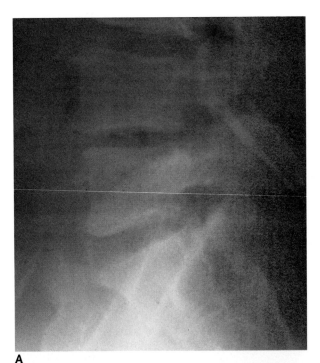

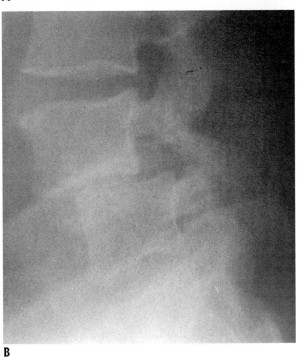
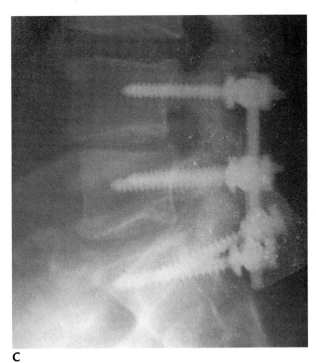

FIGURE 5–33.
A Lateral film with the patient supine. **B** Film taken with patient standing. **C** Film following transverse process fusion with pedicle fixation.

neurogenic claudication, then fusion is not necessary because of the relatively low incidence of symptomatic anterolisthesis. However, if back pain is a major component, particularly if function films demonstrate instability or if bone scan with SPECT demonstrates increased uptake in the joints, then fusion is appropriate.

Fusion

Regardless of the indications, once fusion has been decided upon, the next question is the method to be employed. Because in the publications concerned with fusion the indications are widely variable, the

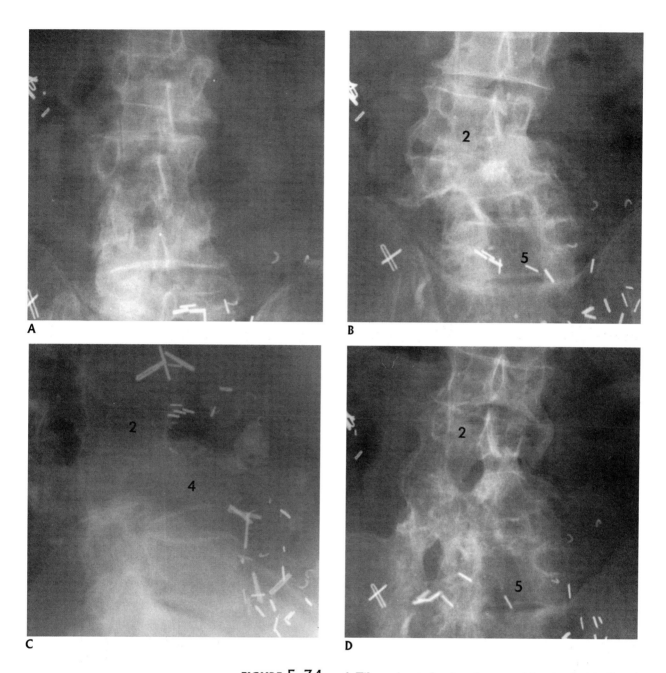

FIGURE 5–34. **A** Film prior to laminectomy and facetectomy. **B and C** AP and lateral films 2 years following surgery. **D** One year after lateral approach for reconstruction of the spinal canal and fusion to the ilium with iliac crest graft.

methods for fusion should not be evaluated by the associated relief of symptoms, but by the efficiency with which fusion is achieved. For each method, the reported rates of fusion vary considerably. Reliance only upon the appearance of an anteroposterior (AP) film can be expected to give a higher fusion rate than when supplemented by bending films. Even with bony continuity and no motion on films taken in flexion and extension, the apparent fusion rate will be less than the actual.[25] Direct inspection at surgery provides the only assurance that fusion has occurred. In a series of 175 patients in whom reoperation was done, a substantial lack of correlation was found between the assessment of fusion on plain films, polytomograms, bending films, and CT scans and the surgical findings.[17] In

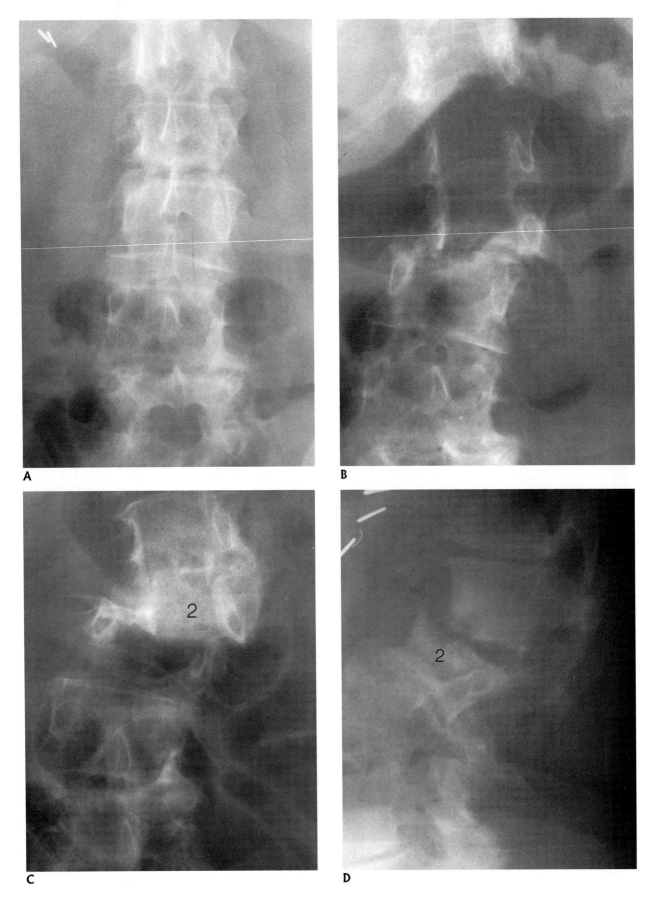

FIGURE 5-35. **A** AP film prior to laminectomy from T11 to L3 with L2–L3 facetectomy. **B** Film taken 2 years later. **C and D** Seven years following surgery.

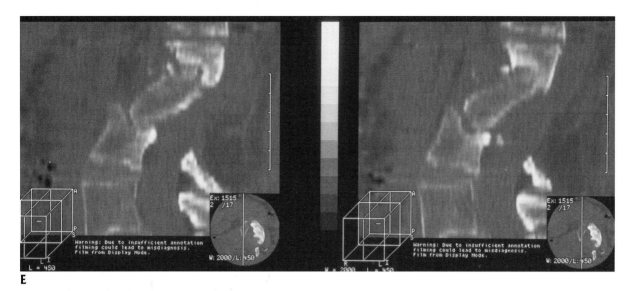

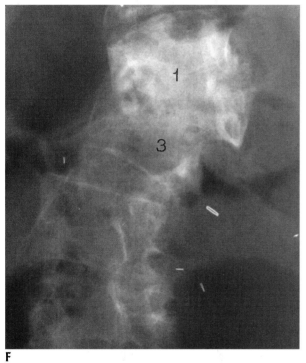

FIGURE 5-35.
E CT scan demonstrating area of resection and graft with beginning union. F One year postoperative.

some patients, bending may be inhibited by pain and will be reflected by lack of motion in the unfused segments as well. Smoking appears to have an adverse effect.[18]

Midline Fusion

Midline fusion, the original technique, has disadvantages. Since it is posterior to the axis of rotation, elasticity of bone allows some motion,[140] which can lead to hypertrophy and neural compression or permit disc herniation beneath the fusion. (Fig. 5–36).

Posterior Lumbar Interbody Fusion

Posterior lumbar interbody fusion (PLIF), which was introduced by Cloward,[26] is in the axis of rotation. Back bone can be used successfully, although

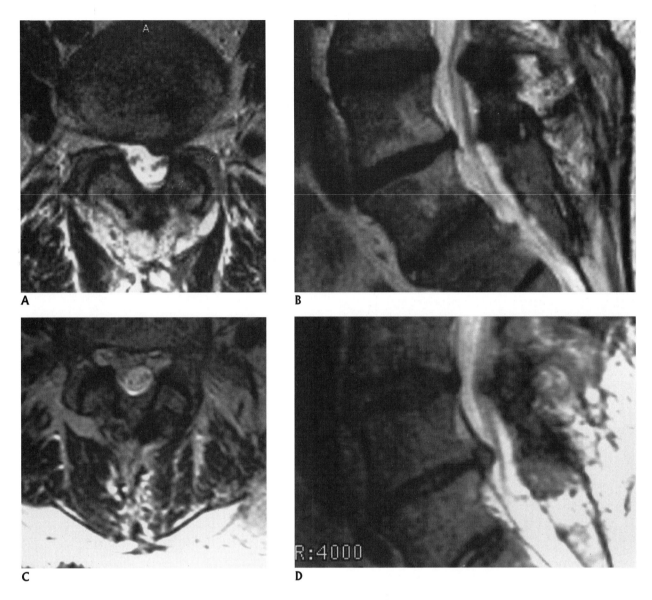

FIGURE 5-36. **A and B** MRI done because of back pain. A posterior midline fusion had been done 15 years earlier. The increased signal on either side of the interspace suggests that the midline fusion is not shielding the motion segment from applied loads. **C and D** MRI 4 months later. A right L5 radiculopathy had developed during the interim. The fusion was solid, and it was necessary to drill through it to remove an extruded fragment.

autologous graft provides earlier union. Tricortical iliac crest grafts should be countersunk beneath the cortical margin of the vertebral body to minimize the possibility of graft dislocation. Because these grafts will penetrate into the cancellous bone, disc space narrowing can be expected. This can lead to nerve root compression, which can be prevented by removing the tip of the articular process (Fig. 5-9). Fusion rates of 88%[28] and 84%[99] have been reported. The incidence of root injury is higher than that associated with standard discectomy,[99,138] probably because of the more extensive root retraction required. Metallic cages containing bone (Fig. 5-37) provide more immediate immobilization, and a fusion rate of 96% has been reported despite the relatively small amount of bone graft that can be introduced.[138] This is perhaps related to the tendency for titanium to be incorporated by bone.[12] Since locally resected bone is available, iliac crest graft is unnecessary. The disadvantages

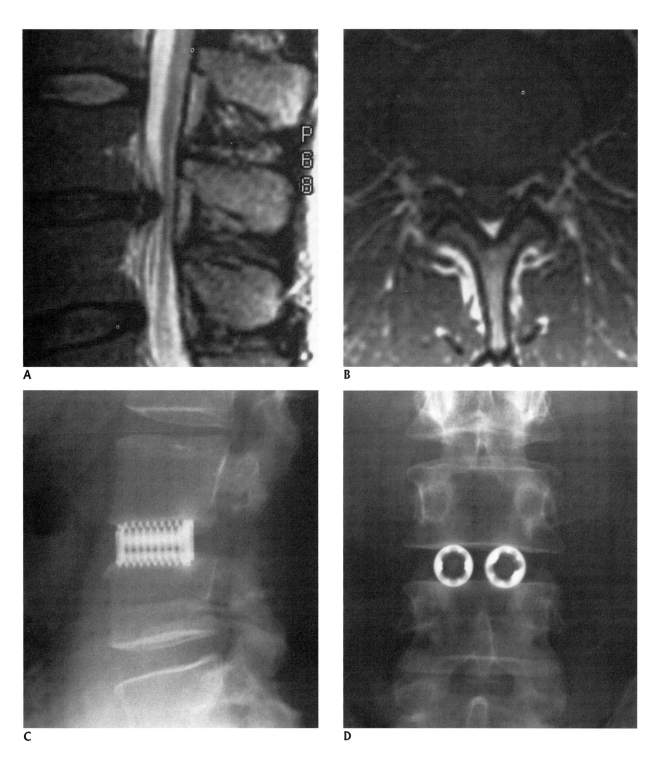

FIGURE 5–37. **A and B** MRI demonstrating large central disc herniation at L3–L4 in a patient with cauda equina syndrome. **C and D** Films following removal of the herniated disc and fixation with titanium cages.

of cages are the necessity for more extensive resection of the joints, especially at levels above L5–S1, and the more vigorous retraction compared with PLIF where the bone grafts can be moved from lateral to medial.

Anterior Fusion

Anterior fusion has been used principally for treatment of low back pain, but also for failed posterior fusion. Reported fusion rates for a single-level procedure are 79%,[14] 85%,[24] and 91%[68]; at two levels they are 48%[24] and 72%[68]; at three levels the rate is 62%.[68] Fusion may also depend upon the level, with 90% for anterior fusion at L5–S1 and 60% at L4–L5.[145] For a single-level fusion a retroperitoneal approach can be used, but laparotomy is necessary if two or more motion segments are to be fused.[145] The development of endoscopic techniques has decreased the morbidity associated with anterior fusion. Because the potential for complications is greater, we have used anterior fusion only as an alternative to the posterior approach for the management of a failed transverse process fusion.

Circumferential Fusion

Circumferential or 360-degree fusion was developed because of dissatisfaction with results of anterior fusion.[145] Kozak and O'Brien summarized the observations from a number of publications regarding uninstrumented fusions and found that rates at one level for anterior or posterior fusion, respectively, were 82.5 and 81.5%, at two levels 69.5 and 67.4%, and at three levels 51.2 and 53.5%.[92] Their results with anterior interbody and posterior transverse process fusion with Knodt rod fixation were 91.5% fusion at one level, 91.5% at two levels, and 77.8% at three levels. Proposed indications for circumferential fusion are major degenerative instability, combined anterior and posterior degenerative changes, and poor results from a previous operation.[145] The development of pedicle fixation and metal cages has made circumferential fusion obsolete as a primary procedure.

Transverse Process Fusion

Transverse process fusion is probably the most widely used method. It has the advantage of being close to the axis of rotation and does not require root retraction. A disadvantage is the necessity for autologous graft with associated donor site discomfort, which was found to be persistent in 37% of patients.[59] We have found that donor site symptoms are substantially diminished if only the iliac crest is exposed. After cortical bone is removed from the crest, cancellous bone is taken from between the inner and outer tables, thus avoiding the necessity to dissect the gluteal muscles. For uninstrumented fusions, the reported rates are variable. Based on appearance of the AP film alone, a rate of 100% was reported[37] for a single-level fusion and 94% for two motion segments. When lack of movement on bending films with good motion at adjacent segments is added as a criterion, then fusion rates are lower. Stauffer and Coventry reported a fusion rate of 80%, but three-fourths of these procedures were done at one level.[155] Grubb and Lipscomb found a 70% fusion rate at one level and 50% at two levels.[71]

Instrumentation

Immobilization promotes bony union. This was recognized thousands of years ago by the Egyptians, who splinted fractures with linen stiffened by starch, clay, or egg albumin.[166] Consequently, it is not surprising that fusion rates are better if instrumentation is employed for fixation. The rigidity of fixation appears to influence the results. Because bone remodels under pressure, metal to metal to bone devices using laminar fixation with hooks or wires will tend to loosen more readily than metal to metal to bone configurations. With Knodt rod fixation from L4 to the sacrum, the fusion rate was 82%[170] and 86% with Luque lamina fixation.[91] With more rigid devices, fusion rates were 100% at one level and 92% at two levels,[71] and 93% at one level, 92% at two levels, and 92% at three levels.[156] The historical cohort study also demonstrated significantly better fusion rates with pedicle fixation as compared to uninstrumented fusion.[62,184] Pseudoarthrosis is most frequently detected by bending films demonstrating motion. However, if pain limits bending, failure of fusion can be implied by bone resorption adjacent to the screws, or by increased uptake on bone scan with SPECT (Fig. 5–42).

Of the devices available, *Knodt rods* are relatively easy to install, but unless distraction is continued to full flexion, immobilization may be incomplete and rod dislocation may occur. Also, if

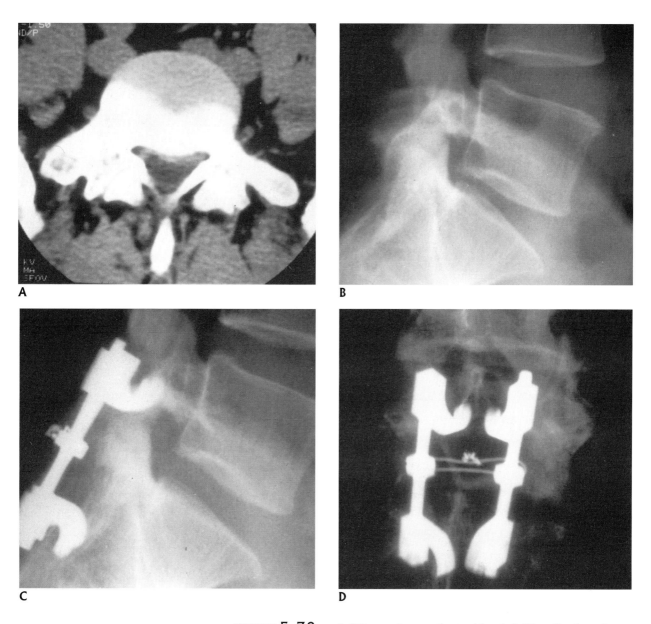

FIGURE 5-38. **A** CT scan in a patient with a left S1 radiculopathy. **B** Lateral film demonstrating slight retrolisthesis at L5–S1. **C and D** Postoperative films demonstrating correction of retrolisthesis and enlargement of the root foramina. The wire is placed to prevent rotation of the threaded rods and subsequent loosening of the hooks.

placed over more than one or two motion segments, lumbar lordosis will be substantially decreased. The major advantage of distraction rods is the capacity to increase the dimension of the root foramina[95] and rapidity of installation. Although Knodt rods can be useful in some situations (Fig. 5–38), they have been almost entirely supplanted by pedicle fixation and metal cages.

Laminar fixation with Luque rods (Fig. 5–39) has been successfully employed,[91] but, like Knodt rods, they have largely been replaced by cages and pedicle screws. Laminar clamping with hooks, although useful in fractures, is not suited to degenerative problems because most lumbar fusions involve the sacrum and usually only one or two motion segments. Laminar hooks can be combined with sacral screws if the pedicles are too small to accept the screw or if this combination offers a mechanical advantage (Fig. 5–40). In this patient, arrest of progressive displacement is theoretically

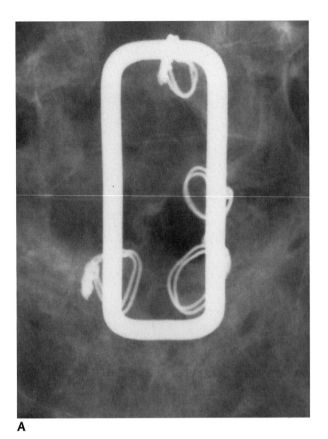
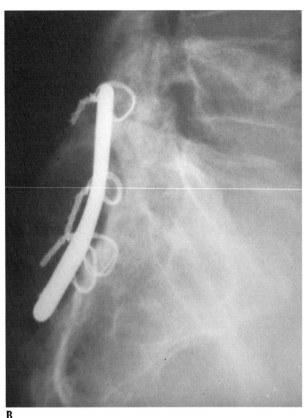

FIGURE 5-39. **A and B** AP, lateral films after transverse process fusion with Luque rectangle fixation. A right L4 and L5 hemilaminectomy had been done previously. The operation was done before pedicle fixation was available.

more effective than pedicle fixation alone. Bone resorbs under pressure, and screws may pull out (Fig. 5-41), although this is unusual.

Pedicle screw devices can be classified into categories. One is metal-to-bone (Fig. 5-41), and the other is metal-to-bone with two subsets, screw plate and screw rod.

In personal (SJL) series of 720 consecutive fusions (Table 5-1), overall fusion rates were better when more rigid devices were used (Table 5-2). With the Cotrel-Dubousset and Artifex devices, the fusion rate at L5-S1 was 100% and at L4-S1 94.9%. In this series, the deep infection rate was 0.7% and superficial rate 1.2%. Two patients had neurological complications, both after pedicle fixation. One developed a significant L5 radiculopathy after she began walking. The medial wall of the pedicle had fractured into the spinal canal, probably because the screw had been placed too obliquely. Full recovery followed removal of the screw and displaced bone. The other patient (Fig. 5-43) had radicular pain without neurological deficit, and symptoms subsided after removal of the screw. Both went on to fusion.

Complications

Infection Infection rates from other series have varied from 2.6%, of which 0.6% were deep,[36] to a deep infection rate of 5%.[185] Nerve root injury associated with pedicle fixation occurred in 5%[172] and 1.6%[169] of cases with recovery following screw removal. Although postoperative CT demonstrated that the screws were lateral to the pedicle in 4% and encroached on the canal in 6%,[63] in only one patient were symptoms suggestive of radiculopathy, and these were transient. Arterial injury is a potential complication if the screw penetrates the anterior cortex of a lumbar vertebra, but none were re-

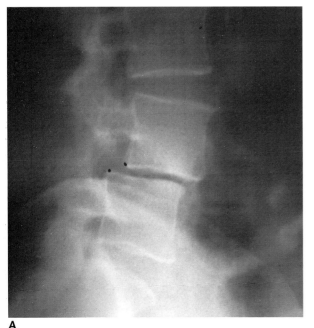

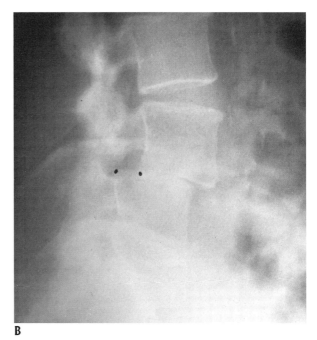

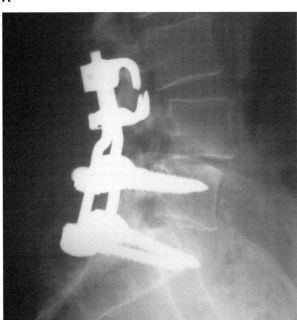

FIGURE 5-40.
A Film prior to laminectomy and facetectomy at L4–L5. **B** Two months following surgery. Back pain had become severe and disabling. **C** Postoperative film. Although the anterolisthesis was largely corrected and the fusion appeared to be successful, pain was only partially relieved and continued to be significant.

ported in any of the papers reviewed for this book.[36,63,105,111,143,156,172,185]

Increased Stress on Motion Segments

Increased stress on motion segments adjacent to a fusion has been demostrated and may cause clinical problems.[137] Acquired spondylolysis was observed in 2.5% of patients.[59] Symptomatic degeneration adjacent to the fusion is uncommon and is late in development but occasionally requires treatment (Fig. 5–44).[96] In this patient, the radiologic appearance suggested infection, but ESR and Gallium scan were normal. Although the incidence of problems below the so-called floating fusion is low,[16] it nevertheless appears prudent to include a subjacent vertebra in the fusion if the disc appears abnormal on MRI. The addition of L5–S1 to an L4–5 fusion does not greatly increase operating time or morbidity and may preclude the necessity of reoperation.

Metal Allergies
The increased use of metallic implants in surgery has led to concern regarding the development of allergic reactions or an ad-

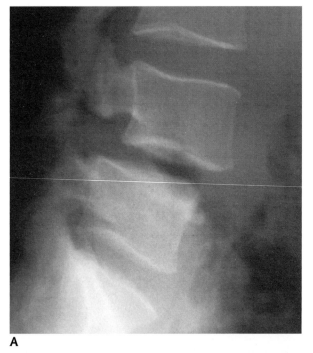

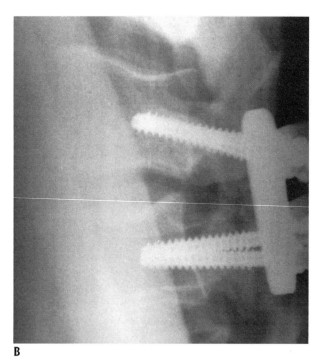

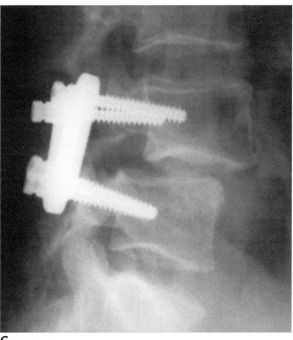

FIGURE 5–41.
A Spondylolisthesis at L4–L5. **B** Intraoperative film. The spondylolisthesis has been reduced. **C** Film taken 5 days following surgery.

verse effect related to a pre-existing metal allergy. Metal concentrations were increased in blood, urine, and adjacent tissue with metal-to-metal hip prostheses, but in patients with metal-to-plastic devices, blood and urine levels were normal and tissue levels only slightly elevated.[54] Sensitivity did not develop following surgery.[141] Metal allergy following spinal instrumentation has not been reported as a complication in any of the publications reviewed for this book, but has been observed in association with subcutaneous screws [10] or screw plates.[29] This is not surprising, since contact dermatitis is mediated by epidermal Langerhans cells.[8] These cells can be reached by metallic ion either through the skin or from immediately beneath it but not in sufficient concentration from more distant locations. Although skin testing has been recommended for patients scheduled to have spinal instrumentation,[12] this does not appear necessary. Patients with known metal allergies are

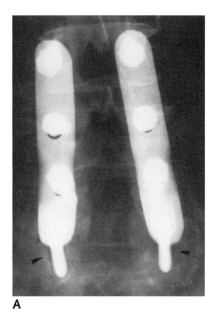 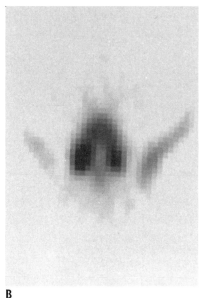

FIGURE 5–42.
A This patient had severe and persistent back and nonradicular lower limb pain following fusion. Motion was not evident on bending films, but radiolucency developed around the S1 screws (*arrows*). This can be seen most clearly on the right side. **B** Locally increased uptake on a bone scan with SPECT 1 year after surgery.

usually apprehensive regarding spinal instrumentation but can be reassured that evidence to support this apprehension does not exist. Metal allergy is more common in women.[54] However, of the 720 patients previously referred to, none developed cutaneous problems related to the implants, and the deep infection rate was 0.7% in men and 0.7% in women. The presence of metal allergy is not a contraindication even to subcutaneous, implants which can be removed if necessary after bone union has occurred,[21] and certainly not to spinal instrumentation.

TABLE 5–1

Device	
Knodt rods	62
Luque rods	83
Steffee	34
Luque plate	75
Cotrel-Dubousset	265
Artifex	201

TABLE 5–2

Device	
Knodt	71
Luque loop	82
Luque plate	80
Steffee	91
Cotrel-Dubousset	94
Artifex	97

Outcomes

Although a sure thing does not exist in spinal surgery, the closest to it is the treatment of radiculopathy secondary to an extruded disc fragment. However, even though radiculopathy may be completely relieved, some patients have persistent back pain. For example, a 34-year-old woman had excellent relief of sciatica after removal of an L5–S1 extruded fragment, but had persistent back pain that was relieved by lying down, partially relieved by wearing a bivalved plastic orthosis, and aggravated by sitting for more than short periods of time. Consequently, she was unable to return to work as a secretary. Bone scan with SPECT and bending films were normal. MRI demostrated degenerative changes at L4–5 and L5–S1 (Fig. 5–45). It is likely that her pain is discogenic, but since the symptoms were tolerable with restriction of activity, a fusion was not done.

Reasonably good results can also be anticipated for the treatment of neurogenic claudication,[177] radiculopathy secondary to lumbar

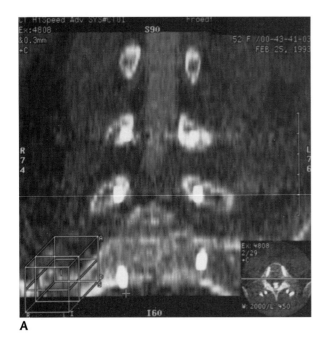

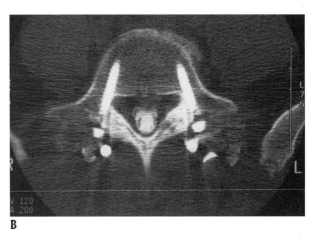

FIGURE 5–43.
A and **B** Postmyelogram CT. The right L4 screw is partly outside the pedicle.

stenosis,[164] or degenerative spondylolisthesis,[46,49] but persistent or developing postoperative back pain can be a problem.[164] It is not surprising that the results of surgery done principally for back pain with or without nonradicular lower limb pain are not as good as surgery done for radiculopathy.[132]

Back pain is much more likely to be produced by multiple factors (see Fig. 1–3, Chapter 1). For example, persistent and disabling back pain is experienced by a substantial number of patients with healed lumbar vertebral fractures and has been attributed to soft tissue injury.[153] A major problem in deciding whether surgical treatment is indicated in patients whose major problem is back pain is the lack of correlation between radiological abnormality and clinical presentation. The patient whose films are shown in Figure 5–46 had back pain following an accident. Physical therapy and facet injection were recommended. Instead he decided to try a dietary supplement from a health emporium. The pain went away. In contrast, another patient with less radiological abnormality (Fig. 5–47) had severe

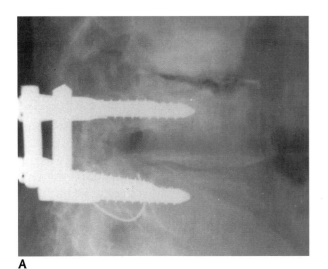

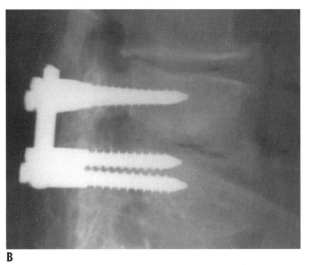

FIGURE 5–44. **A** Bone destruction at L3–L4 suggesting infection, but ESR and gallium scan were normal. **B** Union is taking place after L3–L4 pedicle fixation and transverse process fusion, but retrolisthesis has developed at L2–L3.

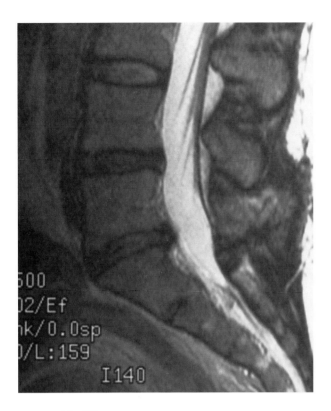

FIGURE 5-45. Disc degeneration at L4–L5 and L5–S1 without changes in bone signal intensity.

back and nonradicular lower limb that was refractory to nonsurgical treatment and that subsided after transverse process fusion. The same lack of correlation exists with intracranial meningioma, where large tumors can be an incidental finding on CT or MRI done for trauma, or at autopsy, whereas small tumors can cause significant problems. However, once problems do develop, they can be reliably connected to the tumor. This is, unfortunately, not always the case with degenerative spinal disorders, which probably accounts for some of the poor results associated with spinal fusion.

An evaluation of the results of fusion from a survey of publications is compromised by the variable indications for surgery and by the criteria used for evaluation of the results. If return to a previous occupation is a measure of a good result, then the results will be poor if the preoperative job requires substantial physical activity and if the patient has been off work for more than a few months.[57,132] The probability of return to work had been reported to be 50% for someone who has been off work for 6 months and 25% at 1 year.[165] Age and previous back surgery are also factors that diminish the likelihood of return to work.[57] Consequently, it is unrealistic to expect that a middle-to late-middle-aged foundary worker who has severe pain despite having been off work will return to the same job following a fusion. However,

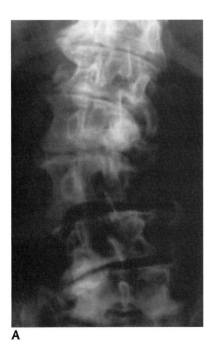

A

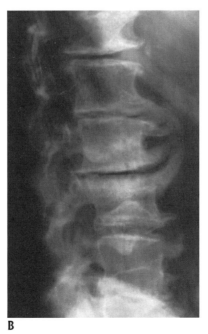

B

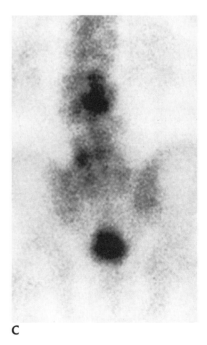

C

FIGURE 5-46. **A and B** AP, lateral films in a patient with back pain. **C** Bone scan from the same patient.

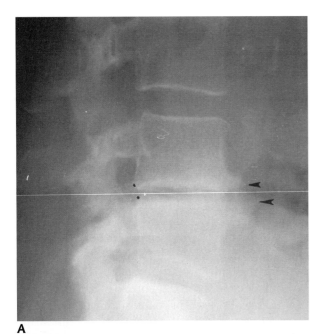
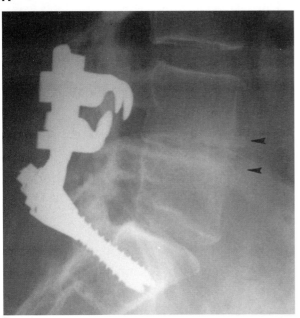
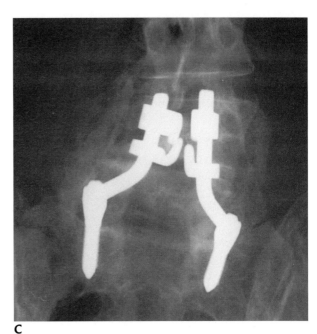

FIGURE 5–47.
A Slight retrolisthesis at L4–L5 and traction spurs on L4 and L5 (*arrows*). **B** The traction spurs have become smaller following fusion. The L4 pedicles were too small for the screws available when the operation was done. **C** The transverse process fusion appears satisfactory, and motion was not apparent from L4 to the sacrum on bending films.

if the indication for surgery is pain that is intolerable even with restriction of activity and a satisfactory result is considered to have intolerable pain become tolerable, then the results of an operation will be considerably better. This may account for the finding from a survey of 47 articles that the average satisfactory outcome after a fusion was 68%,[160] whereas 68% of patients with industrial injury remained disabled 2 years after fusion.[57] In this connection it may be significant that when good results were equated with return to work, 85% of patients with fair or poor results considered themselves completely limited for work or recreational activity, but approximately half of them were satisfied with the overall results.[132]

Patients who have symptoms that are related to their job or other necessary activity and that are considered tolerable are, in most circumstances, not candidates for surgery. If the symptoms become severe enough to preclude working but are tolerable with restricted activity, then less strenuous employment is the preferable alternative. However, if the symptoms have become intolerable even with restrictions, then surgical treatment is appropriate, with the proviso that return to the premorbid level of activity is unlikely.

Poor results have been ascribed to poor patient selection.[52] In that paper, the indications for surgery in those with poor results were clearly inappropriate. The major problem, however, is not poor results with poor indications, but rather poor results with good indications (Fig. 5–40).

REFERENCES

1. Abdullah AF, Wolber PGH, Warfield JR, et al: Surgical management of extreme lateral lumbar disc herniations: Review of 138 cases. Neurosurgery 22(4):648–653, 1988.

2. Alexander E: Significance of the small lumbar spinal canal: Cauda equina compression syndromes due to spondylosis. Part 5: Achondroplasia. J Neurosurg 31(November):513–519, 1969.

3. Alexander E Jr, Kelly DL Jr, Davis CJ Jr, et al: Intact arch spondylolisthesis: A review of 50 cases and description of surgical treatment. J Neurosurg 63:840–844, 1985.

4. Anda S, Aakhus S, Skaanes KO, et al: Anterior perforations in lumbar discectomies: A report of four cases of vascular complications and a CT study of the prevertebral lumbar anatomy. Spine 16(1):54–60, 1991.

5. Arnoldi C: Intraosseous hypertension. A possible cause of low back pain. Clin Orthop 115:30–34, 1976.

6. Auteroche P: Innervation of the zygapophyseal joints of the lumbar spine. Anatomia Clinica 5:17–28, 1983.

7. Badgley CE: The articular facets in relation to low-back pain and sciatic radiation. J Bone Joint Surg 23(2):481–496, 1941.

8. Baer RL: The mechanism of allergic contact hypersensitivity. In Contact Dermatitis, ed. A.A. Fisher, Lea & Febiger, Philadelphia, pp. 1–8, 1986.

9. Balderston RA, Gilyard GG, Jones AAM, et al: The treatment of lumbar disc herniation: Simple fragment excision versus disc space curettage. J Spinal Disord 4(1):22–25, 1991.

10. Barranco VP, Solomon H; Eczematous dermatitis caused by internal exposure to nickel. South Med J 66(4):447–448, 1973.

11. Benner B, Ehni G: Degenerative lumbar scoliosis. Spine 4(6):548–551, 1979.

12. Bennett GJ: Materials and material testing. In Spinal Instrumentation, ed. E.C. Benzel, American Association of Neurological Surgeons, Park Ridge, pp. 31–43, 1994.

13. Bernard TN Jr: Lumbard discography followed by computed tomography: Refining the diagnosis of low-back pain. Spine 15(7):690–707, 1990.

14. Blumenthal SL, Baker J, Dossett A, et al: The role of anterior lumbar fusion for internal disc disruption. Spine 13(5):566–569, 1988.

15. Brodsky AE, Binder WF: Lumbar discography: Its value in diagnosis and treatment of lumbar disc lesions. Spine 4(2):110–120, 1979.

16. Brodsky AE, Hendricks RL, Khalil MA, et al: Segmental ("floating") lumbar spine fusions. Spine 14(4):447–450, 1989.

17. Brodsky, AE, Kovalsky ES, Khalil MA: Correlation of radiologic assessment of lumbar spine fusions with surgical exploration. Spine 16(6):261–265, 1991.

18. Brown CW, Orme TJ, Richardson HD: The rate of pseudarthrosis (surgical nonunion) in patients who are smokers and patients who are nonsmokers: A comparison study. Spine 11(10):942–943, 1986.

19. Brown MD: Chemonucleolysis with disease: Technique, results, case reports. Spine 1(2):115–120, 1976.

20. Caputy AJ, Luessenhop AJ: Long-term evaluation of decompressive surgery for degenerative lumbar stenosis. J Neurosurg 77:669–676, 1992.

21. Carlsson A, Moller H: Implantation of orthopaedic devices in patients with metal allergy. Acta Derm Venereol (Stockh) 69:62–66, 1989.

22. Carragee EJ, Helms E, O'Sullivan, GS: Are postoperative activity restrictions necessary after posterior lumbar discectomy? A prospective study of outcomes in 50 consecutive cases. Spine 21(16):1893–1897, 1996.

23. Carrer GF: Lumbar facet joint injection in low back pain and sciatica. Neuroradiology 137:665–667, 1980.

24. Chow SP, Leong JCY, Ma A, et al: Anterior spinal fusion for deranged lumbar intervertebral disc: A review of 97 cases. Spine 5(5):452–458, 1980.

25. Cleveland M, Bosworth DM, Thompson FR: Pseudoarthrosis in the lumbosacral spine. J Bone Joint Surg 30A(2):302–312, 1948.

26. Cloward RB: The treatment of ruptured lumbar intervertebral discs by vertebral body fusion. I. Indications, operative technique, after care. J Neurosurg 10:154–168, 1953.

27. Cloward RB: Lesions of the intervertebral disks and their treatment of interbody fusion methods: The painful disk. Clin Orthop 27:51–77, 1963.

28. Collis JS, Gardner WJ: Lumbar discography: An analysis of one thousand cases. J Neurosurg 19:452–461, 1962.

29. Cramers M, and Lucht U: Metal sensitivity in patients treated for tribial fractures with plates of stainless steel. Acta Orthop Scand 48:248–249, 1977.

30. Crock HV: Internal disc disruption: A challenge to disc prolapse fifty years on. Spine 11(6):650–653, 1986.
31. Crock HV: Internal disc disruption. In The Adult Spine, ed. J.W. Frymoyer, Raven Press, New York, pp. 2015–2025, 1991.
32. Dall BE, Rowe, DE: Degenerative spondylolisthesis: Its surgical management. Spine 10(7):668–672, 1985.
33. Dandy WE: Loose cartilage from intervertebral disk stimulating tumor of the spinal cord. Arch Surg 19:660–672, 1929.
34. Dandy WE: Concealed ruptured intervertebral disks: A plea for the elimination of contrast mediums in diagnosis. JAMA 117(10):821–823, 1941.
35. Dandy WE: Recent advances in the diagnosis and treatment of ruptured intervertebral disks. Ann Surg 115(4):514–520, 1942.
36. Davne SH, and Myers DL: Complications of lumbar spinal fusion with transpedicular instrumentation. Spine 17(6S):S184–S189, 1992.
37. Dawson EG, Lotysch M III, Urist MR: Intertransverse process lumbar arthrodesis with autogenous bone graft. Clin Orthop 154(Jan–Feb):90–96, 1981.
38. Delamarter RB, Sherman JE, Carr JB: Cauda equina syndrome: Neurologic recovery following immediate, early, or late decompression. Spine 16(9):1022–1029, 1991.
39. Delauche-Cavallier M-C, Budet C, Laredol J-D, et al: Lumbar disc herniation: Computed tomography scan changes after conservative treatment of nerve root compression. Spine 17(8):927–933, 1992.
40. Destouet JM, Gilula LA, Murphy WA, et al: Lumbar facet joint injection: Indication, technique, clinical correlation and preliminary results. Radiology 145:321–325, 1982.
41. Deutsch AL, Howard M, Dawson EG, et al: Lumbar spine following successful surgical discectomy: Magnetic resonance imaging features and implications. Spine 18(8):1054–1060, 1993.
42. Dupuis PR, Yong-Hing K, Cassidy JD, et al: Radiologic diagnosis of degerative lumbar spinal instability. Spine 10(3):262–276, 1985.
43. Ehni G: Significance of the small lumbar spinal canal: Cauda equina compression syndromes due to spondylosis. Part 4: Acute compression artificially-induced during operation. J Neurosurg 31(November):507–512, 1969.
44. Eisenstein SM, Parry CR: The lumbar facet arthrosis syndrome: Clinical presentation and articular surface changes. J Bone Joint Surg 69-B(1):3–7, 1987.
45. Epstein JA, Epstein BS, Jones MD: Symptomatic lumbar scoliosis with degenerative changes in the elderly. Spine 4(6):542–547, 1979.
46. Epstein NE, Epstein JA, Carras R, et al: Degenerative spondylolisthesis with an intact neural arch: A review of 60 cases with an analysis of clinical findings and the development of surgical management. Neurosurgery 13(5):555–561, 1983.
47. Epstein NE, Epstein JA, Carras R, et al: Far lateral lumbar disc herniations and associated structural abnormalities: An evaluation in 60 patients of the comparative value of CT, MRI, and Myelo-CT in diagnosis and management. Spine 15(6):534–539, 1990.
48. Epstein NE: Evaluation of varied surgical approaches used in the management of 170 far-lateral lumbar disc herniations: Indications and results. J Neurosurg 83:648–656, 1995.
49. Epstein JA, Epstein BS, Lavine LS, et al: Degenerative lumbar spondylolisthesis with an intact neural arch (psuedospondylolisthesis). J. Neurosurg 44(Feb):139–147, 1976.
50. Esses SL, Moro JK: Intraosseous vertebral body pressures. Spine 16(6 Supplement):S155–S159, 1992.
51. Esses SL, Moro JK: The value of facet joint blocks in patient selection for lumbar fusion. Spine 18(2):185–190, 1993.
52. Fager CA, Freidberg SR: Analysis of failures and poor results of lumbar spine surgery. Spine 5(1):87–93, 1980.
53. Feffer HL, Wiesel SW, Cuckler JM, et al.: Degenerative spondylolisthesis: To fuse or not to fuse. Spine 10(3):287–289. 1985.
54. Fisher AA: Dermatitis due to medical mechanical devices. In Contact Dermatitis, Lea & Febiger, Philadelphia, pp. 338–341, 1986.
55. Fitzgerald J, Newman P: Degenerative spondylolisthesis. J Bone Joint Surg 56B:184–192, 1976.
56. Foley RK, Kirkaldy-Willis WH: Chronic venous hypertension in the tail of the Wistar rat. Spine 4(3):251–257, 1979.
57. Franklin GM, Haug J, Heyer NJ, et al: Outcome of lumbar fusion in Washington state workers' compensation. Spine 19(17):1897–1904, 1994.
58. Fraser RD: Chymopapain for the treatment of intervertebral disc herniation: A preliminary report of a double-blind study. Spine 7(6):608–612, 1982.
59. Frymoyer JW, Hanley E, Howe J, et al: Disc excision and spine fusion in the management of lumbar disc disease: A minimum ten-year followup. Spine 3(1):1–6, 1978.
60. Frymoyer JW, Matteri RE, Hanley EN, et al: Failed lumbar disc surgery requiring second operation: A long-term follow-up study. Spine 3(1):7–11, 1978.
61. Fullerton PM: The effect of ischaemia on nerve conduction in the carpal tunnel syndrome. J Neurol Neurosurg Psychiatry 26:385–397, 1963.
62. Garfin SR: Summation. Spine 19(20 Suppl):2300S–2305S, 1994.

63. Gertzbein SD, Robbins SEI: Accuracy of pedicular screw placement *in vivo*. Spine 15(1):11–14, 1990.
64. Ghormley RK: Low back pain with special reference to the articular facets, with presentation of an operative procedure. JAMA 101(23):1773–1777, 1933.
65. Gleave JRW, MacFarlane R: Prognosis for recovery of bladder function following lumbar central disc prolapse. Br J Neurosurg 4:205–210, 1990.
66. Goel VK, Goyal S, Clark C, et al: Kinematics of the whole lumbar spine: Effect of discetomy. Spine 10(6):543–554, 1985.
67. Goel VI, Fromknecht SJ, Nishiyama K, et al: The role of lumbar spinal elements in flexion. Spine 10(6):516–523, 1985.
68. Goldner JL, Urbaniak JR, McCollum DE: Anterior disc excision and interbody spinal fusion for chronic low back pain. Orthop Clin North Am 2(2):543–568, 1971.
69. Goldthwait JE: The lumbo-sacral articulation: An explanation of many cases of "lumbago," "sciatica" and paraplegia. Boston Medical and Surgical Journal 164:365–372, 1911.
70. Grobler LJ, Robertson PA, Novotny JE, et al: Etiology of spondyloisthesis: Assessment of the role by lumbar facet joint morphology. Spine 18(1):80–91, 1993.
71. Grubb SA, Lipscomb HJ: Results of lumbosacral fusion for degenerative disc disease with or without instrumentation: Two-to five-year follow up. Spine 17(3):349–355, 1992
72. Haughton VM, Eldevik OP, Khang-Cheng H, et al: Arachnoiditis from experimental myelography with aqueous contrast media. Spine 3(1):65–69, 1978.
73. Heggeness MH, Doherty BJ: Discography causes end plate deflection. Spine 18(8):1050–1053, 1993.
74. Helbig T, Lee CK: The lumbar facet syndrome. Spine 13(1):61–64, 1988.
75. Herkowitz HH, Kurz LT: Degenerative lumbar spondylolisthesis with spinal stenosis: A prospective study comparing decompression with decompression and intertransverse process arthrodesis. J Bone Joint Surg 73-A(6):802–808, 1991.
76. Herron LD, Trippi AC: L4-5 degenerative spondylolisthesis: The results of treatment by decompressive laminectomy without fusion. Spine 14(5):534–538, 1989.
77. Hitchon PW, Mouw LJ: Management of lumbar herniated discs. In Principles of Spinal Surgery, eds. A.H. Meneses and V.K.H. Sonntag, McGraw-Hill Health Professions Division, pp. 603–605, 1996.
78. Holder LE, Machin JL, Asdourian PL: Planar and high-resolution SPECT bone imaging in the diagnosis of facet syndrome. J. Nucl Med 36(1):37–44, 1995.
79. Hoyland JA, Freemont AJ, Jayson MIV: Age-related changes in the structures within and bordering the intervertebral foramina: Associations with low back pain. In The Aging Spine, eds. D.W.L. Hukins and M.A. Nelson, Manchester University Press, New York, pp. 94–110, 1987.
80. Hsu KY, Zucherman JF, Derby R, et al: Painful lumbar end-plate disruptions: A significant discographic finding. Spine 13(1):76–78, 1988.
81. Jensen TT, Overgaard S, Thomsen NOB, et al: Postoperative computed tomography three months after lumbar disc surgery: A prospective single-blind study. Spine 16(6):620–622, 1991.
82. Johnsson K-E, Willner S, Johnsson K: Postoperative instability after decompression for lumbar spinal stenosis. Spine 11(2):107–110, 1986.
83. Kaneda K, Satoh S, Nohara Y, et al: Distraction rod instrumentation with posterolateral fusion in isthmic spondylolisthesis: 53 cases followed for 18–89 months. Spine 10(4):383–389. 1985.
84. Kaneda K, Kazama H, Satoh S, et al: Follow-up study of medial facetectomies and posterolateral fusion with instrumentation in unstable degenerative spondylolisthesis. Clin Orthop 2203(February):159–167, 1986.
85. Kato F, Mimatsu K, Kawakami N, et al: Serial changes observed by magnetic resonance imaging in the intervertebral disc after chemonucleolysis: A consideration of the mechanism of chemonucleolysis. Spine 17(8):934–939, 1992.
86. Kornberg M: Discography and magnetic resonance imaging in the diagnosis of lumbar disc disruption. Spine 14(12):1368–1372, 1989.
87. Korovessis P, Piperos G, Sidiropoulos P, et al: Adult idiopathic lumbar scoliosis: A formula for prediction of progression and review of the literature. Spine 19(17):1926–1932, 1994.
88. Kostuik J: Adult scoliosis. In The Textbook of Spinal Surgery, ed. K. Bridwell and R. Dewald, Lippincott, Philadelphia, pp. 249–277. 1991.
89. Kostuik J: Adult scoliosis, assessment and treatment. In The Lumbar Spine, eds. S.W. Wiesel et al., W. B. Saunders, Philadelphia, pp. 1130–1176. 1996.
90. Kostuik J, Harrington I, Alexander D, et al: Cauda equina syndrome and lumbar disc herniation. J Bone Joint Surg 68-A(3):386–391, 1986.
91. Kostuik JC, Errico TJ, Gleason TF: Luque instrumentation in degenerative conditions of the lumbar spine. Spine 15(4):318–321, 1990.
92. Kozak JA, O'Brien JP: Simultaneous combined anterior and posterior fusion: An independent analysis of a treatment for the disabled low-back pain patient. Spine 15(4):322–328. 1990.
93. Kunogi, J-I, Hasue M: Diagnosis and operative treatment of intraforaminal and extraforaminal nerve root compression. Spine 16(11):1312–1320. 1991.

94. Larson SJ: Somatosensory evoked potentials in lumbar stenosis. Surg Synecol Obstet 157(August):191–196, 1983.
95. Lee CK, deBari A: Lumbosacral spinal fusion with Knodt distraction rods. Spine 11(4):373–375, 1986.
96. Lee CK: Accelerated degeneration of the segment adjacent to a lumbar fusion. Spine 13(3):375–377, 1988.
97. Lemperg RK, Arnoldi CC: The significance of intraosseous pressure in normal and diseased states with special reference to the intraosseous engorgement-pain syndrome. Clin Orthop 136(October):143–156, 1976.
98. Lewin T: Osteoarthritis in lumbar synovial joints: A morphologic study. Acta Orthop Scand 73S:2–112, 1964.
99. Lin PM, Cautilli RA, Joyce MF: Posterior lumbar interbody fusion. Clin Orthop 180(November):154–168, 1983.
100. Lindahl O, Rexed B: Histologic changes in spinal nerve roots of operated cases of sciatica. Acta Orthop Scand 20:215–225, 1951.
101. Lippitt AB: The facet joint and its role in spine pain: Management with facet joint injections. Spine 9(7):746–750, 1984.
102. Lombardi JS, Wiltse LL, Reynolds J, et al: Treatment of degenerative spondylolisthesis. Spine 10(9):821–827, 1985.
103. Lora J, Long D: So-called facet denervation in the management of intractable back pain. Spine 1(2):121–126, 1976.
104. Lorenz M, Patwardhan A, Vanderby R Jr: Load-bearing characteristics of lumbar facets in normal and surgical altered spinal segments. Spine 8(2):122–130, 1983.
105. Louis R: Fusion of the lumbar and sacral spine by internal fixation with screw plates. Clin Orthop 203(February):18–33, 1986.
106. Love JG, Walsh MN: Intraspinal protrusion of intervertebral disks. Arch Surg 40(March):454–484, 1940.
107. Lovely T, Rastogi P: The value of provocative facet blocking as a predictor of success in lumbar spine fusion. J of Spinal Disorders 10(6):512–517, 1997.
108. Lynch MC, Taylor JF: Facet joint injection for low back pain: A clinical study. J Bone Joint Surg Am 68-B(1):138–141, 1986.
109. Macnab I, McCulloch JA, Weiner DS, et al: Chemonucleolysis. Can J Surg 14(July):280–289, 1971.
110. Maezawa S, Muro T: Pain provocation at lumbar discography as analyzed by computed tomography/discography. Spine 17(11):1309–1315, 1992.
111. Marchesi DG, Aebi M: Pedicle fixation devices in the treatment of adult lumbar scoliosis. Spine 17(8S):S304–S309, 1992.
112. McCall IW, Park WM, O'Brien JP, et al: Acute traumatic intraosseous disc herniation. Spine 10(2):134–137, 1985.
113. McCulloch JA, Inoue S-i, Moriya H, et al: Surgical indications and techniques. In The Lumbar Spine, eds. J.N. Weinstein and S.W. Wiesel, W. B. Saunders, Philadelphia, pp. 393–421, 1990.
114. Middleton GS, Teacher JH: Injury of the spinal cord due to rupture of an intervertebral disc during muscular effort. In Classics of Orthopaedics, ed. E.M. Bick, J. B. Lippincott, Philadelphia, pp. 139–142, 1976.
115. Mixter WJ: Rupture of the intervertebral disc: A short history of its evolution as a syndrome of importance to the surgeon. JAMA 140:278–282, 1949.
116. Mixter WJ, Ayer JB: Herniation or rupture of the intervertebral disc into the spinal canal: Report of thirty-four cases. N Engl J Med 213:385–393, 1935.
117. Mixter WJ, Barr JS: Rupture of the intervertebral disc with involvement of the spinal canal: N Engl J Med 211:210–215, 1934.
118. Moneta GB, Videman T, Kaivanto K, et al: Reported pain during lumbar discography as a function of annular ruptures and disc degeneration: A re-analysis of 833 discograms. Spine 19(17):1968–1974, 1994.
119. Montaldi S, Fankhauser H, Schnyder P, et al: Computed tomography of the postoperative intervertebral disc and lumbar spinal canal: Investigation of twenty-five patients after successful operation for lumbar disc herniation. Neurosurgery 22(6):1014–1022, 1988.
120. Mooney V, Robertson J: The facet syndrome. Orthopedics Rel Res 115:149–157, 1976.
121. Moore MR, Brown CW, Brugman JL, et al: Relationship between vertebral intraosseous pressure, pH, PO_2, pCO_2, and magnetic resonance imaging signal inhomogeneity in patients with back pain: An in vivo study. Spine 16(6 Suppl):S239–S242, 1991.
122. Moore RJ, Vernon-Roberts B, Fraser RD, et al: The origin and fate of herniated lumbar intervertebral disc tissue. Spine 21(18):2149–2155, 1996.
123. Morgan F, King T: Primary instability of lumbar vertebrae as a common cause of low back pain. J Bone Joint Surg 39B(1):6–22, 1957.
124. Myklebust J, Maiman D, Larson S, et al: Eletrocphysiological effects of lumbar dorsal root stimulation. Neurosurgery 14(6):682–687, 1984.
125. Nachemson A: Lumbar discography: Where are we today? Spine 14(6):555–557, 1989.
126. Nachemson AL, Schultz AB, Berkson MH: Mechanical properties of human lumbar spine motion seg-

ments: Influences of age, sex, disc level, and degeneration. Spine 4(1):1–8, 1979.
127. North RB, Ewend MG, Lawton MT, et al: Failed back surgery syndrome: 5- year follow-up after spinal cord stimulator implantation. Neurosurgery 28(5):692–699, 1991.
128. North RB, Kidd DH, Zahurak M, et al: Specificity of diagnostic nerve blocks: A prospective, randomized study of sciatica due to lumbosacral spine disease. Pain 65:77–85, 1996.
129. Offierski CM, MacNab I: Hip-spine syndrome. Spine 8(3):316–321, 1983.
130. Okawa A, Shinomiya K, Takakuda K, et al: A cadaveric study on the stability of lumbar segment after partial laminotomy and facetectomy with intact posterior ligaments. Spinal Dis 9(6):518–526, 1996.
131. Onorio BM, Campa HK: Evaluation of rhizotomy: Review of 12 years' experience. Neurosurg 36(June):751–755, 1972.
132. Parker LM, Murrel SE, Boden SD, et al: The outcome of posterolateral fusion in highly selected patients with discogenic low back pain. Spine 21(116):1909–1917, 1996.
133. Penning L, Wilmink JT: Posture-dependent bilateral compression of L4 or L5 nerve roots in facet hypertrophy: A dynamic CT-myelographic study. Spine 12(5):488–500, 1987.
134. Porter RWE: Spinal stenosis and neurogenic claudication. Spine 21(17):2046–2052, 1996.
135. Putti V: New conceptions in the pathogenesis of sciatic pain. Lancet July 9:53–60, 1927.
136. Quigley, MR and Maroon, JC: Percutaneous approaches to the lumbar disk. In Principles of Spinal Surgery, eds. AH Menezes and Sonntag, McGraw-Hill, pp. 609–619, 1996.
137. Quinnell RC, Stockdale, HR: Some experimental observations of the influence of a single lumbar floating fusion on the remaining lumbar spine. Spine 6(3):273–267, 1981.
138. Ray CD: Threaded titanium cages for lumbar interbody fusions. Spine 22(6):667–680, 1997.
139. Reynolds JB, Wiltse LL: Surgical treatment of degenerative spondylolisthesis. Spine 4(2):1148–149, 1979.
140. Rolander SD: Motion of the lumbar spine with special reference to the stabilizing effect of posterior fusion: An experimental study on autopsy specimens.
141. Rooker GD, Wilkinson JD: Metal sensitivity in patients undergoing hip replacement. J Bone Joint Surg 62B(4):502–505, 1980.
142. Rosenberg NJ: Degenerative spondylolisthesis: Predisposing factors. J Bone Joint Surg 57-A(4):467–474, 1975.

143. Roy-Camille R, Saillant G, Mazel C: Internal fixation of the lumbar spine with pedicle screw plating. Clin Orthop 203(February):7–17, 1986.
144. Schwarzer AC, April CN, Derby R, et al: Clinical features of patients with pain stemming from the lumbar zygapophysial joings: Is the lumbar facet syndrome a clinical entity? Spine 19(10):1132–1137, 1994.
145. Selby DK, Henderson RJ: Circumferential (360 degree) spinal fusion. In the Adult Spine: Principles and Practice, ed. J.W. Frymoyer, Raven Press, Ltd., New York, pp. 1989–2006, 1991.
146. Semmes RE: Diagnosis of ruptured intervertebral disc without contrast myelography and comment upon recent experience with modified hemilaminectomy for their removal. Yale J Biol Med 11:433–435, 1939.
147. Shenkin HA, Hash CJ: A new approach to the surgical treatment of lumbar spondylosis. J Neurosurg 44(Feb):148–155, 1976.
148. Shenkin HA, Hash, CJ: Spondylolisthesis after multiple bilateral laminectomies and facetectomies for lumbar spondylosis: Follow up review. J Neurosurg 50(Jan):45–47, 1979.
149. Simmons ED, Simmons EHMS: Spinal stenosis with scoliosis. Spine 17(6 Suppl):S117–120, 1992.
150. Simmons ED, Jackson RP: The management of nerve root entrapment syndromes associated with the collapsing scoliosis of idiopathic lumbar and thoracolumbar curves. Spine 4(6):533–541, 1979.
151. Simmons JW, Emeryl SF, McMillin JN, et al: Awake discography: A comparison study with magnetic resonance imaging. Spine 16(6 Suppl):S216–S221, 1991.
152. Smyth MJ, Wright V: Sciatica and the intervertebral disc. J Bone Joint Surg 40-A(6):1401–1418, 1958.
153. Soreff J: Assessment of the late results of traumatic compression fractures of the thoracolumbar vertebral bodies. Trycker and Balder, Stockholm, 1977.
154. Spurling RG, Grantham EG: Neurologic picture of herniations of the nucleus pulposus in the lower part of the lumbar region. Arch Surg 40(3):375–388, 1940.
155. Stauffer RN, Coventry MB: Posterolateral lumbar-spine fusion. J Bone Joint Surg 54A(6):1195–1204, 1972.
156. Steffee AD, Brantigan JW: The variable screw placement spinal fixation system: Report of a prospective study of 250 patients enrolled in food and drug administration clinical trials. Spine 18(9):1160–1172, 1993.
157. Strait TA, Hunter SE: Intraspinal extradural sensory rhizotomy in patients with failure of lumbar disc surgery. J Neurosurg 54(February):193–196, 1981.

158. Thelander U, Fagerlund M, Friberg S, et al: Straight leg raising test versus radiologic size, shape, and position of lumbar disc hernias. Spine 17(4):395–399, 1992.

159. Tullberg T, Rydberg J, Isacsson J: Radiographic changes after lumbar discectomy: Sequential enhanced computed tomography in relation to clinical observations. Spine 18(7):843–850, 1993.

160. Turner JA, Ersek M, Herron L, et al: Patient outcomes after lumbar spinal fusions. JAMA 268(7):907–911, 1992.

161. Vanharanta H, Guyer RD, Ohnmeiss DD, et al: Disc deterioration in low-back syndromes: A prospective, multi-center CT/discography study. Spine 13(12):1349–1351. 1988.

162. Verbiest H: A radicular syndrome from developmental narrowing of the lumbar vertebral canal. J Bone Joint Surg 36B(2):230–237, 1954.

163. Verbiest H: Further experiences on the pathological influence of a developmental narrowness of the bony lumbar vertebral canal. J Bone Joint Surg Am 37-B(4):576–583, 1955.

164. Verbiest H: Results of surgical treatment of idiopathic developmental stenosis of the lumbar vertebral canal: A review of twenty-seven years' experience. J Bone Joint Surg Am 59-B(2):181–188, 1977.

165. Waddell G: A new clinical model for the treatment of low-back pain. Spine 12(7):632–643, 1987.

166. Watson-Jones R: Fractures and Joint Injuries, L E & S Livingston, Edinburgh and London, p. 168, 1955.

167. Weber H: Lumbar disc herniation: A controlled, prospective study with ten years of observation. Spine 8(2):131–140, 1983.

168. Weinstein J, Spratt KF, Lehmann T, et al: Lumbar disc herniation: A comparison of the results of chemonucleolysis and open discectomy after ten years. J Bone Joint Surg 68A(1):43–54, 1986.

169. West JL III, Ogilvie JW, Bradford DS: Complications of the variable screw plate pedicle screw fixation. Spine 16(5):576–579, 1991.

170. White AH, Wynne G, Taylor LW: Knodt rod distraction lumbar fusion. Spine 3(4):434–437, 1983.

171. White JC, Sweet WH: Pain of spinal origin. VI: Limited radicular pain following fracture-dislocation or disc surgery. In Pain and the Neurosurgeon: A Forty-Year Experience, ed. Charles C. Thomas, Springfield, Il, pp. 549–466, 1969.

172. Whitecloud TS III, Butler JC, Cohen JL, et al: Complications with the variable spinal plating system. Spine 14(4):472–476, 1989.

173. Wiberg G: Back pain in relation to the nerve supply of the intervertebral disc. Acta Orthop Scanda 19(2):211–221, 1950.

174. Williams PC: Lesions of the lumbosacral spine: Part II. Chronic traumatic (postural) destruction of the lumbosacral intervertebral disc. J Bone Joint Surg 19:690–703, 1937.

175. Williams RW: Microlumbar discectomy: A conservative surgical approach to the virgin herniated lumbar disc. Spine 3(3):173–182, 1978.

176. Williams RW: Microlumbar discectomy: A 12-year statistical review. Spine 11(8):851–852, 1986.

177. Wilson CB: Significance of the small lumbar spinal canal: Cauda equina compression syndromes due to spondylosis. Part 3: Intermittent claudication. J Neurosurg 31(November):499–506, 1969.

178. Wilson Dh, Harbaugh R: Microsurgical and standard removal of the protruded lumbar disc: A comparative study. Neurosurgery 8(4):422–427, 1981.

179. Wiltse LL, Widell EH, Yuan HA: Chymopapain chemonucleolysis in lumbar disk disease. JAMA 231(5):474–479, 1975.

180. Yang KH, King AI: Mechanism of facet load transmission as a hypothesis for low-back pain. Spine 9(6):557–564,1984.

181. Yoganandan N, Larson SJ, Pintar FA, et al: Intravertebral pressure changes caused by spinal microtrauma. Neurosurgery 35(3):415–421, 1994.

182. Yong-Hing K, Kirkaldy-Willis WH: The three-joint complex. In The Lumbar Spine, eds. J.N. Weinstein and S.W. Weisel, W. B. Saunders, Philadelphia, pp. 80–87, 1990.

183. Yoshizawa H, O'Brien JP, Smith WT, et al: The neuropathology of intervertebral discs removed for low-back pain. J Pathol 132:95–104, 1980.

184. Yuan HA, Garfin SR, Dickman Ca, et al: A historical cohort study of pedicle screw fixation in thoracic, lumbar, and sacral spinal fusions. Spine 19(205):2279S–2296S, 1994.

185. Zucherman J, Hsu K, White A, et al: Early results of spinal fusion using variable spine plating system. Spine 13(5):570–579, 1988.

CHAPTER 6

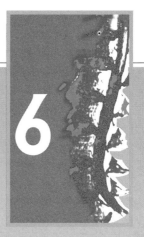

Isthmic Spondylolisthesis

Congenital Isthmic Spondylolisthesis

Isthmic Spondylolysis Secondary to Fracture
of the Pars Interarticularis

Isthmic Spondylolisthesis

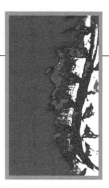

Isthmic spondylolisthesis can be divided into two major categories: the congenital and that secondary to fracture of the pars interarticularis.

Congenital Isthmic Spondylolisthesis

Congenital spondylolisthesis is characterized by an enlongated pars interarticularis and a sacral laminar defect.[21] It has been proposed that the enlogation of the pars is the result of repeated fractures with healing.[30] This appears unlikely, since in the congenital variety progression of displacement is common and can become severe,[4] whereas in children with spondylolisthesis secondary to pars fracture progression is uncommon and mild.[1,7] In addition, in congenital spondylolisthesis the anterior edge of the sacrum does not keep pace with L5, whereas it does with the pars fracture in children (Fig. 6–1).

Clinical Presentation and Diagnosis

Symptoms are back pain with or without nonradicular or radicular lower limb pain with corresponding neurological abnormalities. Progression of displacement with increased symptoms occurs and is most common during the adolescent growth spurt.[3]

Management

Good results have been reported with fusion without reductions.[3,14,17,23] When displacement is severe and progressive, a two-stage procedure for reduction and fusion has been advocated.[4,8,20] However, this involves prolonged hospitalization. It appears that in most instances in situ fusion is adequate.[32] Most operations are done on children and adolescents; only the occasional adult patient with congenital spondylolishtesis requires surgical treatment (Fig. 6–2).

The 20-year-old woman in Figure 6–2 had bilateral S1 radiculopathy, and severe pain not relieved by non surgical treatment. Films had shown progression of displacement during the preceding year. The sacral lamina was removed flush with the sides of the canal. The S1 root on one side was retracted medially and with a diamond burr the posterior edge of the sacrum was drilled out laterally and undercut medially. A similar procedure was done on the other side. The thin layer of bone remaining in the midportion of the floor of the canal was pushed down into the defect that had been created. Transverse process fusion was done with iliac fixation to prevent further displacement, and the radiculopathy was relieved.

Isthmic Spondylolysis Secondary to Fracture of the Pars Interarticularis

Spondylolysis with or without spondylolisthesis is not present at birth, and the youngest reported patient with a pars defect was 4 months old.[31,32] It is present in about 5% of the population at 6 or 7 years of age, increasing to 6% by adulthood.[1,7] Although it is not congenital, there is a strong hereditary component.[1,7] In Alaskan Eskimos admitted for other medical problems, 28% had spondylolysis with associated spondylolisthesis in 15%. The incidence became greater with increasing age and was 17.6% from 6 to 17 years, 26% from 18 to 24 years, and 40.6% in patients 35 to 70 years old.[15] Simper found

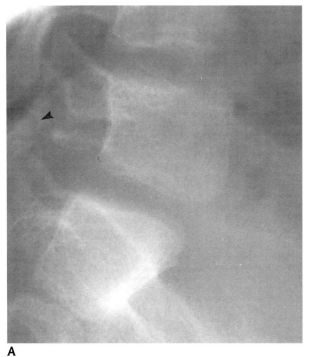

A

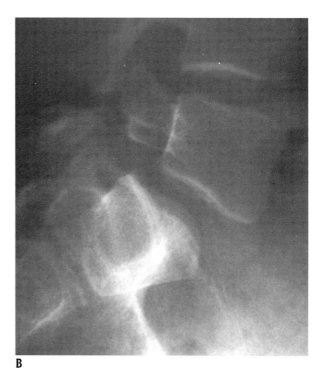

B

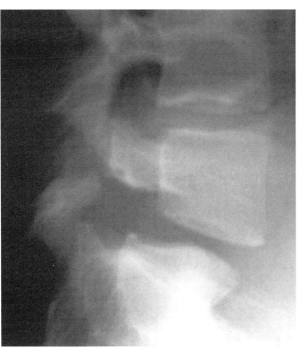

C

FIGURE 6–1
A Pars defect and anterolisthesis at L5–S1 in a 7-year-old boy. L5 and S1 are equal in height. **B** Film taken at age 11. The configuration is normal anteriorly, but L5 height is 90% of S1. **C** Film taken at age 13. S1 has kept pace anteriorly with L5.

spondylolysis in 25 of 46 skeletons from Greenland: 2 of 15 children, and 23 of 31 adults.[25]

Clinical Presentation and Diagnosis

Patients with spondylolysis on the original examination did not develop spondylolisthesis, and of those with spondylolisthesis, progression of displacement was neither common nor severe, it did not occur after age 16, and significant symptoms did not develop until adulthood.[7] For example, bone surveys were done periodically in a child with histiocytosis. The films were normal at 7, 11, and 14 months but demonstrated a pars defect and Grade I spondylolisthesis at 18 months increasing to Grade II at 2 years. The displacement was un-

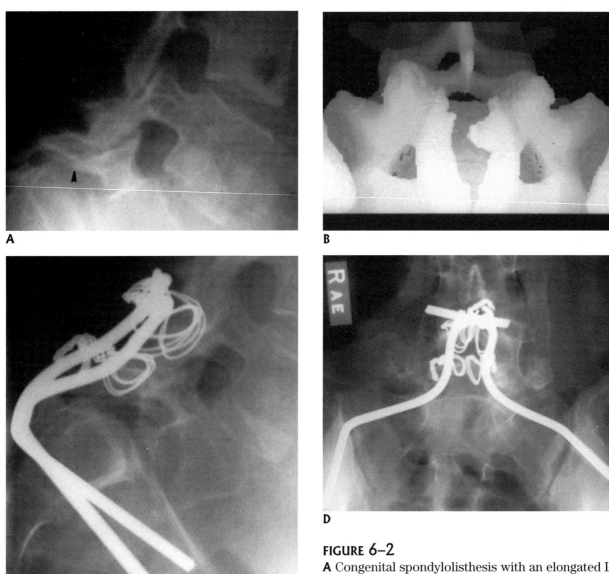

FIGURE 6-2
A Congenital spondylolisthesis with an elongated L5 pars interarticularis (*arrow*). **B** Three-dimensional CT scan. The sacral lamina is defective. **C and D** The posterior edge of the sacrum has been resected and transverse process fusion has been done with iliac fixation.

changed at age 4, and the patient remained asymptomatic.[29] When displacement occurs, the anterior edge of the lower vertebra keeps pace with the anterior inferior edge of the slipping vertebra (Fig. 6–1). The patient in Figure 6–1 was injured when his sled hit a tree. He was 7 years old at the time. The spine films were done because of back pain, which subsequently went away. He continued to be fully active, playing football and soccer. Transient back pain occurred on two occasions, one associated with football and the other with working out on a trampoline. Otherwise, he remained free of symptoms.

The majority of cases occur at L5–S1 and are considered to be fatigue fractures.[30–32] Some patients, most often engaged in gymnastics or ballet, may have unilateral pars defects with hypertrophy of the contralateral lamina (Fig. 6–3). Acute fractures may occur in adolescent athletes engaged in sports that require frequent flexion and extension such as gymnastics. Most were unilateral and associated with increased uptake on bone scans.[18] Low back pain was the presenting symptom and subsided after immobilization in an orthosis, which allowed return to full activity.[18]

Spondylolisthesis can develop in adults and

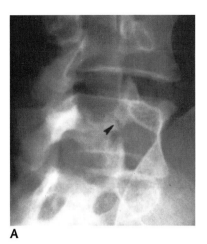
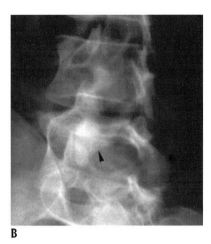

FIGURE 6-3
A and **B** Oblique views demonstrating a unilateral pars defect with hypertrophy of the contralateral lamina.

sometimes can be due to an acute traumatic event,[16] as in the case of the acrobatic dancer who "went onto the stage without the usual 15 or 20 minutes of loosening and limbering. In the course of her dance when, with her spine fully hyperextended and her head between her legs, there was an ominous crack; she suffered agonizing pain, having sustained a fracture of the neural arch of the first lumbar vertebra."[28] The adult onset pars fracture with displacement can be distinguished radiographically from childhood spondylolisthesis by the anterior asymmetry (Fig. 6-4). The patient in Figure 6-4 felt and heard a snap while he was supporting a heavy object with his lumbar spine

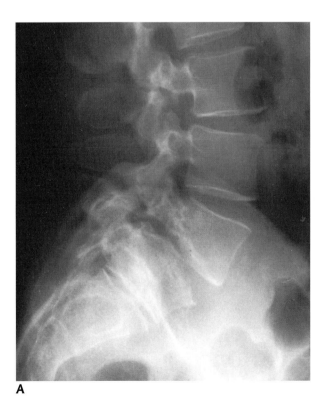
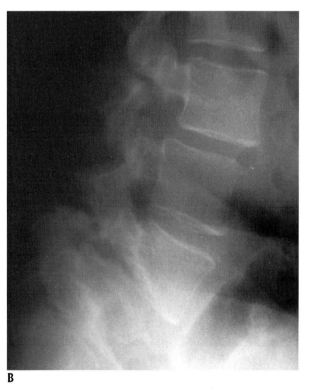

FIGURE 6-4 **A** Childhood onset spondylolisthesis at L5–S1, with a posttraumatic adult onset spondylolisthesis at L2–L3. Height of L5 is 85% that of S1. **B** The displacement at L2–3 is increased during flexion.

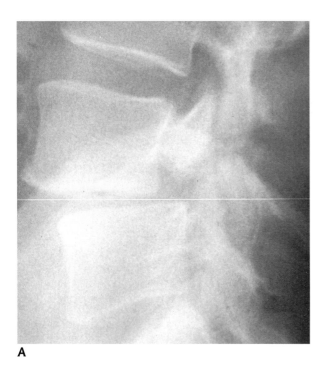 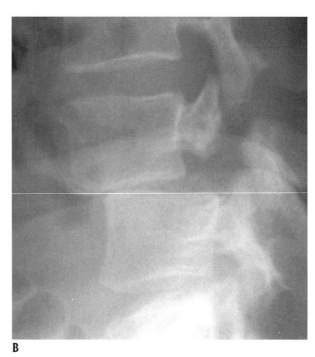

FIGURE 6-5 **A** Adult onset spondylolisthesis at L4–L5 with a right L5 radiculopathy. This patient did not recall an acute traumatic event. **B** The displacement is increased during flexion.

in extension. Instability is also more pronounced in adult onset spondylolisthesis (Fig. 6-5). In addition, progressive displacement can occur (Fig. 6-6).

Management

Treatment is principally determined by pain. The activities of patients with spondylolysis or spondylolisthesis who are not having pain should not be restricted.[7] Patients with unhealed bilateral pars defects have returned to gymnastics and hockey,[18] and 1.5% of players in the National Football League have spondylolisthesis.[24] However, if pain develops and becomes intolerable, then surgical treatment is appropriate.

Foraminotomy

The type of operation is determined by the character of the symptoms. If radiculopathy is the only or highly predominant symptom, then decompression by foraminotomy without fusion is sufficient.[10] Laminectomy, however, need not be done. The radiculopathy is almost always unilateral, and unroofing of the affected root is sufficient. To accomplish this, removal of the loose lamina is inadequate and unnecessary. It is essential that the pars defect be widened and that the remnant of the pars attached to the pedicle be resected.[10] This can be done most efficiently with a narrow and somewhat blunt osteotome that will break the bone rather than slice through it. After the pars remnant has been removed, the root will usually move posteriorly. As with lumbar spondylosis, the best results can be anticipated with a pure radiculopathy. The problem becomes more difficult if back pain with or without nonradicular lower limb pain is the major or only symptom. These symptoms may be unrelated to the spondylolisthesis (Fig. 6-7). The patient in Figure 6-7 had persistent pain despite successful fusion at L5–S1 and was related to L4–5 instability and relieved by fusion at that level. Bone scan with SPECT may show increased uptake, indicating an active process.[9,18,19] As with lumbar spondylosis, back pain may persist despite an apparently successful fusion (Fig. 6-8). The patient in Figure 6-8 was a skilled worker at a job that re-

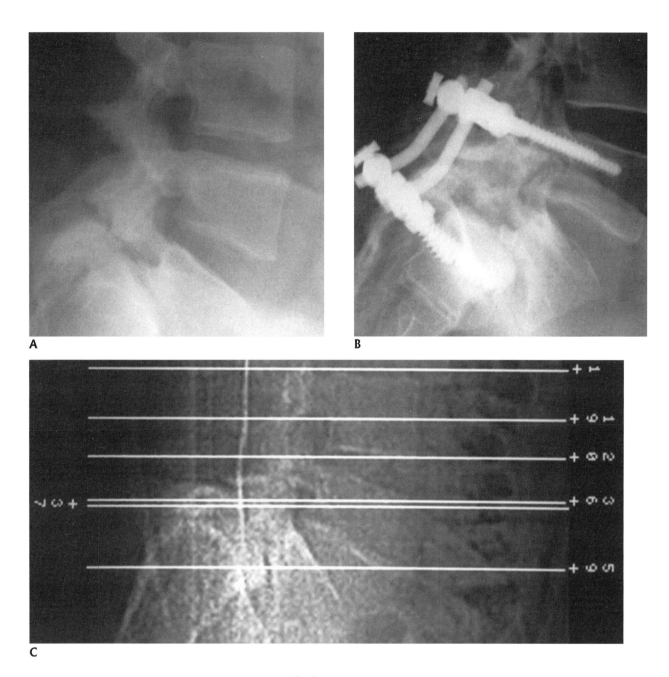

FIGURE 6–6 **A** Adult onset spondylolisthesis at L5–S1. The symptoms have been present for several years without a history of acute trauma. **B** Two years later. This film was taken 2 days following foraminotomy and fusion. Displacement has increased, and the anterior edge of S1 and the inferior surface of L5 appear to have been ground away. This was also seen on the intraoperative radiograph and on the preoperative pedicle CT scout film **C.**

quired substantial physical activity, and workmen's compensation was not a factor. He has returned to a different type of work at significantly lower pay and is not happy.

Although good relief of pain without fusion has been reported, problems can occur after laminectomy (Fig. 6–9). The patient in Figure 6–9 had developed urinary retention. Spine films were reported to show a Grade III spondylolisthesis. A laminectomy was done, but the patient continued to require straight catheterization. Four years later, back pain and significant left L5 radicu-

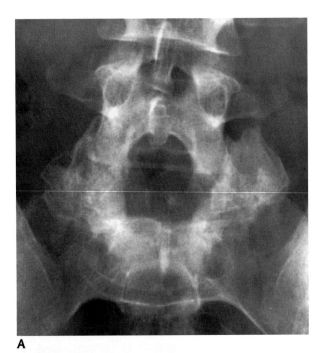

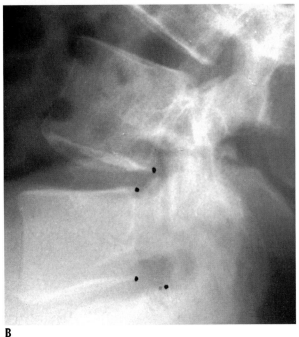
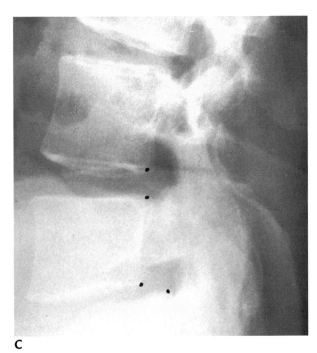

FIGURE 6–7
A The fusion at L5–S1 appears satisfactory. **B** Retrolisthesis at L4–L5 in extension. **C** The retrolisthesis is reduced in flexion.

lopathy developed after a lifting injury. The symptoms became worse, and 12 years after the initial operation a left L5 foraminotomy was done. The posterior superior edge of the sacrum was resected, and transverse process fusion with pedicle fixation was done from L4 to the sacrum. The radiculopathy was relieved and bladder function was recovered, although the patient continued to have some back pain.

Fusion

Foraminotomy alone is adequate for pure radiculopathy, but if back pain is a significant factor, then fusion should probably be done. Methods have been developed to preserve the motion segment. In one, after the pars defect has been cleared of soft tissue and the bone edges freshened, the defect is packed with cancellous bone

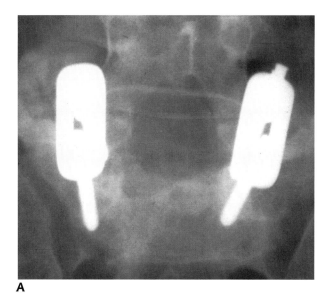
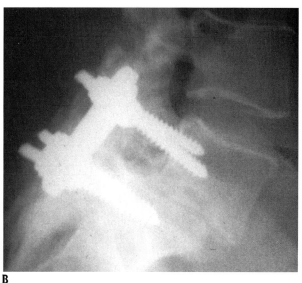

FIGURE 6–8 **A and B** Fusion appears satisfactory, and bending films did not demonstrate motion or instability at more rostral segments. However, the back pain persisted without change.

and a screw placed across the defect from the lamina into the superior articular process. This is done bilaterally.[6] Another method has used wiring from the transverse processes to the spinous process with the bone graft placed in the defect.[5,11,22] These techniques are most successful in patients with little or no slip (Fig. 6–10) and who are less than 30 years of age.[5]

For example, the patient whose films are shown in Figure 6–11 was 53 years old and developed back pain and a left L5 radiculopathy after an extension injury. Pedicle fixation was not available at that time, and Luque rectangle fixation would have required fusion from L4 to the sacrum. Consequently, transverse process wiring with bone grafting of the pars defect was done in conjunction with

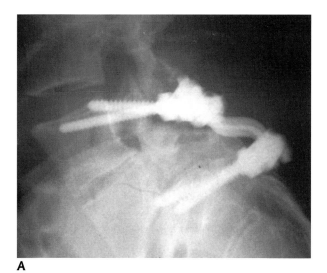
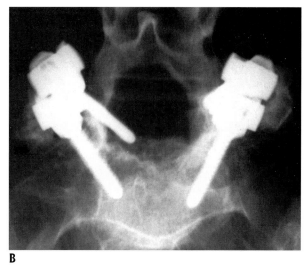

FIGURE 6–9 **A and B** Films after a foraminotomy, resection of the superior edge of the sacrum, and transverse process fusion from L4 to the sacrum.

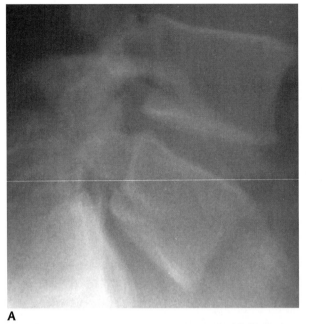
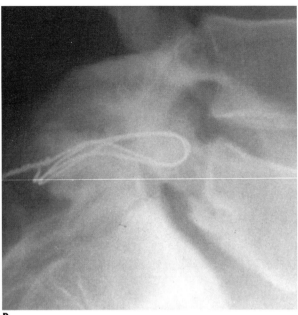
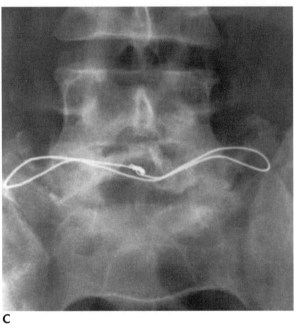

FIGURE 6–10 **A** Spondylolisthesis at L5–S1. **B and C** Films, 1 year after transverse process to spinous process wiring and pars grafting. The increased displacement occurred during the first 2 months following the operation.

foraminotomy. The radiculopathy was relieved, but back pain recurred in association with failure of fusion and increased displacement.

Good results have been reported with anterior interbody fusion,[27] but this method is applicable only to patients with back pain with or without nonradicular lower limb pain. Transverse process fusion with posterior lumbar interbody fusion and pedicle fixation was found to be only slightly more successful than transverse process fusion with instrumentation alone.[26] Since most patients require fixation at only one level, transverse process fusion with pedicle fixation is adequate and the addition of interbody fusion is not necessary. Pedicle fixation has the advantage of providing immediate immobilization and more certain fusion.

Because isthmic spondylolysis and spondylolisthesis are relatively common, considerable caution must be exercised in making the decision for surgery in patients who do not have radicular signs and symptoms. (see Figs. 6–7 and 6–8).

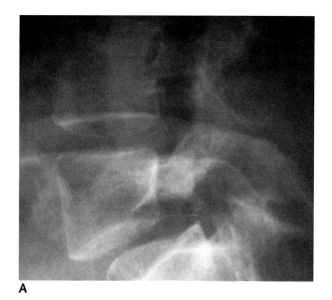 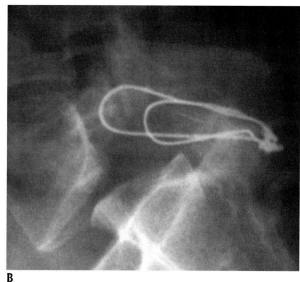

FIGURE 6–11 **A** Adult onset spondylolisthesis at L5–S1. The patient was 52 years old, and symptoms began after an extension injury. **B** The displacement has increased substantially.

REFERENCES

1. Baker DR, McHolick W: Spondylolysis and spondylolisthesis in children. J Bone Joint Surg 38-A(4):933–944, 1956.

2. Blackburne JS, Velikas EP: Spondylolisthesis in children and adolescents. J Bone Joint Surg 59-B(4): 490–494, 1977.

3. Boxall D, Bradford DS, Winter RB, et al: Management of severe spondylolisthesis in children and adolescents. J Bone Joint Surg 61A(4):479–495, 1979.

4. Bradford DS: Treatment of severe spondylolisthesis: A combined approach for reduction and stabilization. Spine 4(5):423–429, 1979.

5. Bradford DS, Iza J: Repair of the defect in spondylolysis or minimal degrees of spondylolisthesis by segmental wire fixation and bone grafting. Spine 10(7):673–679, 1985.

6. Buck JE: Direct repair of the defect in spondylolisthesis: Preliminary report. J Bone Joint Surg 52-B(3):432–437, 1970.

7. Fredrickson BE, Baker D, McHolick WJ, et al: The natural history of spondylolysis and spondylolisthesis. J Bone Joint Surg 66A(5):699–713, 1984.

8. Gaines RW, Nichols WK: Treatment of spondyloptosis by two stage L5 vertebrectomy and reduction of L4 onto S1. Spine 10(7):680–686, 1985.

9. Gainor BJ, Hagen RJ, Allen WC: Biomechanics of the spine in the polevaulter as related to spondylolysis. Am J Sports Med 11(2):53–57, 1983.

10. Gill GG, Manning JG, White HL: Surgical treatment of spondylolisthesis without spine fusion. J Bone Joint Surg 37-A(3):493–520, 1955.

11. Hambly M, Lee CK, Gutteling E, et al: Tension band wiring-bone grafting for spondylolysis and spondylolisthesis: A clinical and biomechanical study. Spine 14(4):455–460, 1989.

12. Hutton WC, Cyron BM: Spondylolysis: The role of the posterior elements in resisting the intervertebral compressive force. Acta Orthop Scand 49:604–609, 1978.

13. Ishikawa S, Kumar SJ, Torres BC: Surgical treatment of dysplastic spondylolisthesis: Results after *in situ* fusion. Spine 19(15):1691–1696, 1994.

14. Johnson JR, Kirwan EOG: The long-term results of fusion in situ for severe spondylolisthesis. J Bone Joint Surg 65B(1):43–46, 1983.

15. Kettelkamp DB, Wright DG: Spondylolysis in the Alaskan Eskimo. J Bone Joint Surg 53-A(3):563–566, 1971.

16. Larson SJ: Hyperextension, hyperflexion, and torsion injuries of the spine. In Neurological Surgery: A Comprehensive Reference Guide to the Diagnosis and Management of Neurosurgical Problems, ed. J.R. Youmans, W.B. Saunders, Philadelphia pp. 2392–2402, 1990.

17. Lenke LG, Bridwell KH, Bullis D, et al: Results of in situ fusion for isthmic spondylolisthesis. J Spinal Disord 5(4):433–442, 1992.

18. Letts M, Smallman T, Afanasiev R, et al: Fracture of the pars interarticularis in adolescent athletes: A

clinical-biomechanical analysis. J Pediatr Orthop 6(1):40–46, 1986.
19. Lowe J, Libson E, Ziv I, et al: Spondylolysis in the upper lumbar spine: A study of 32 patients. J Bone Joint Surg 69-B(4):582–586, 1987.
20. McPhee IB, O'Brien JP: Reduction of severe spondylolisthesis: A preliminary report. Spine 4(5):430–434, 1979.
21. Newman PH, Stone KH: The etiology of spondylolisthesis. J Bone Joint Surg 45-B(1):39–59, 1963.
22. Nichol RO, Scott JHS: Lytic spondylolysis: Repair by wiring. Spine 11(10):1027–1030, 1986.
23. Poussa M, Schlenzka D, Seitsalo S, et al: Surgical treatment of severe isthmic spondylolisthesis in adolescents: Reduction or fusion *in situ*. Spine 18(7):894–901, 1993.
24. Shaffer B, Wiesel S, Lauerman W: Spondylolisthesis in the elite football player: An epidemiologic study in the NCAA and NFL. J Spinal Disorders 10(5):365–370 1997.
25. Simper LB: Spondylolysis in Eskimo skeletons. Acta Orthop Scand 57:78–80, 1986.
26. Suk S, Lee C-K, Kim W-J, et al: Adding posterior lumbar interbody fusion to pedicle screw fixation and posterolateral fusion after decompression in spondylolytic spondylolisthesis. Spine 22(2):210–220, 1997.
27. vanRens TJG, vanHorn JR: Long-term results in lumbosacral interbody fusion for spondylolisthesis. Acta Orthop Scand 53:383–392, 1982.
28. Watson-Jones R: In Fractures and Joint Injuries, E & S Livingstone, Edinburgh and London, p. 967, 1955.
29. Wertzberger KL, Peterson HA: Acquired spondylolysis and spondylolisthesis in the young child. Spine 5(5):437–442, 1980.
30. Wiltse LL: The etiology of spondylolisthesis. J Bone Joint Surg 44-A(3):539–560, 1962.
31. Wiltse LL, Newman PH, Macnab I: Classification of spondylolysis and spondylolisthesis. Clin Orthop 117:23–29, 1976.
32. Wiltse LL, Rothman SLG: Lumbar and lumbosacral spondylolisthesis: Classification, diagnosis, and natural history. In Lumbar Spine, ed. SW Wiesel, et al, W.B. Saunders, Philadelphia, pp. 621–624, 1996.

CHAPTER 7

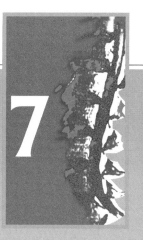

Infection

Pyogenic Hematogenous Osteomyelitis

Disc Space Infection

Epidural Abscess

Tuberculous Vertebral Osteomyelitis

Summary

Infection

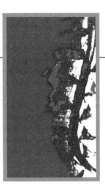

Antibiotics have altered the management or vertebral infections. Nevertheless, a significant number of patients require surgical treatment.

Pyogenic Hematogenous Osteomyelitis

Pyogenic hematogenous osteomyelitis is the most commonly encountered form of vertebral infection. Although it may occur in previously healthy individuals, most patients have predisposing conditions such as diabetes mellitus, immune suppression, intravenous drug abuse, or debilitating disease.[1]

Clinical Presentation and Diagnosis

Back pain is the presenting symptom in virtually all patients. Initially, pain is out of proportion to physical findings, which are usually limited to local tenderness and restricted motion of the vertebral column. Systemic symptoms and findings such as fever, leukocytosis, and weight loss are not prominent in most patients, and if they develop they do so at a considerable interval from the onset of pain. Local pain may progress to radicular pain over periods ranging from several weeks to several months. Neurological complications are not uncommon.[1]

Abnormalities on plain roentgenograms, such as disc space narrowing and bone destruction, do not appear for at least several weeks (Fig. 7–1), but elevation of the erythrocyte sedimentation rate (ESR) and abnormalities on technetium and gallium bone scans develop earlier.[4] Although computed tomography (CT) scans can demonstrate epidural paravertebral granulations, they are most useful for assessing the extent of bone destruction. Magnetic resonance imaging (MRI) more effectively demonstrates epidural granulations and deformity of the neural elements and also has a typical appearance in osteomyelitis: decreased signal intensity on T1-weighted images and increased signal intensity in the same area on T2-weighted images (Fig. 7–2). Occasionally, a degenerative process may mimic infection (Fig. 5–44), but the ESR and gallium scan will be normal.

Management

Drug Therapy

Treatment depends upon several factors and should be medical if the patient is neurologically normal and if bone destruction is minimal. Blood culture and needle biopsies are positive in less than half of the patients.[1] If an organism can be identified, the appropriate antibiotic is given intravenously for 6 weeks, and if cultures are negative, an antibiotic can be selected empirically.

For example, a 78-year-old woman had been operated upon previously with transverse process fusion from L3 to the sacrum and had good relief of symptoms. About 18 months after surgery she abruptly developed severe low back pain and was admitted to a hospital in her community. Spine films demonstrated fusion but were otherwise unremarkable (Fig. 7–3A), as were the myelogram

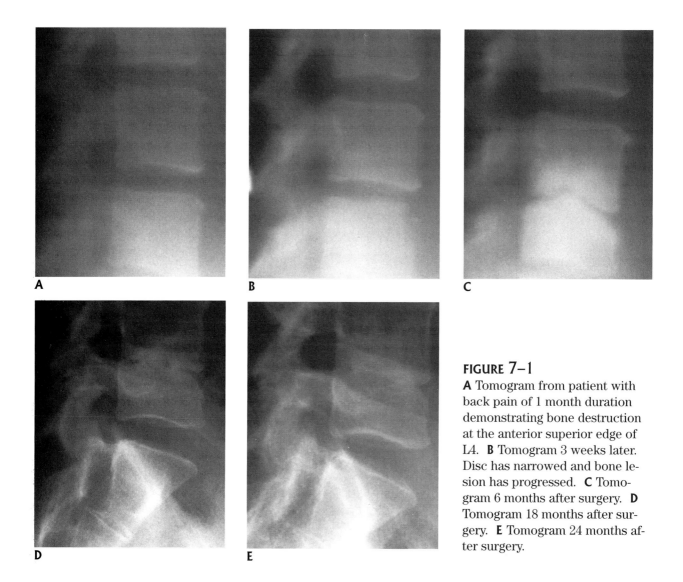

FIGURE 7-1
A Tomogram from patient with back pain of 1 month duration demonstrating bone destruction at the anterior superior edge of L4. **B** Tomogram 3 weeks later. Disc has narrowed and bone lesion has progressed. **C** Tomogram 6 months after surgery. **D** Tomogram 18 months after surgery. **E** Tomogram 24 months after surgery.

and postmyelogram CT scans. The pain progressively increased in severity, and 10 weeks later she was unable to be out of bed because of intolerable pain associated with sitting and standing. Spine films (Fig. 7–3B and C), gallium scan, and MRI were consistent with osteomyelitis at L2–L3, the ESR was 121, and the white blood count (WBC) was 10,500. Needle biopsy and blood cultures did not recover an organism, and consequently she was started on intravenous vancomycin and transferred to an intermediate care unit. The pain subsided and she became able to be out of bed in a bivalved body jacket. The ESR progressively diminished and was 21 at the time of discharge 8 weeks after admission. Films taken 6 months after onset demonstrated beginning union at L2–L3 (Fig. 7–3D), and bone scan with gallium was normal.

Surgical Treatment

If the patient does not improve or if neurological deficit develops, surgical treatment is indicated. Because the pathological process is anterior to the dura, laminectomy is ineffective and also disrupts the posterior ligamentous complex. The subsequent reduction in resistance to flexion is usually followed by more rapid progression of infection and the development or progression of neurological deficit.[1,2] Instead, approaches such as the lateral extracavitary or retroperitoneal sympathectomy should be used. These permit resection of infected tissue without introducing instability.

The patient whose x-ray films are shown in Figure 7–1 was placed on intravenous (IV) antibiotics, but pain persisted, bone destruction and disc narrowing progressed, and the ESR remained ele-

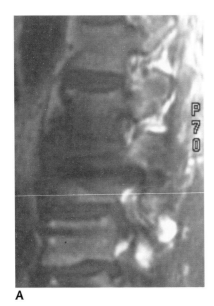 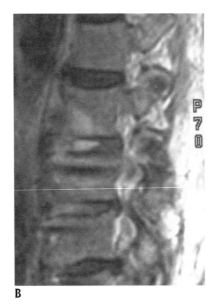

FIGURE 7-2
A T_1-weighted image in a patient with an L2–L3 osteomyelitis.
B T_2-weighted image from the same patient.

vated. A lateral approach was used to remove granulation tissue and infected bone. At the time of treatment appropriate instrumentation was not available and therefore the patient was kept at bedrest for 6 weeks before being allowed up in a bivalved orthosis. Clinical recovery was prompt, although union of the vertebral bodies took place more slowly (see Fig. 7–1C, D, E).

Immobilization and Instrumentation Immobilization has always been important in the management of osteomyelitis and in the preantibiotic era was virtually the only treatment. Consequently, the development of appropriate posterior instrumentation has been a substantial advance, and permits early mobilization and rapid fusion. The importance of immobilization cannot be overemphasized. The patient in Figure 7–4 had bacterial endocarditis, valvular disease with vegetations, congestive failure, and L1–L2 osteomyelitis (Fig. 7–4A). Despite IV antibiotics, pain increased and bone destruction progressed. Because her medical condition was poor and she was neurologically normal, posterior instrumentation was chosen as the primary procedure, laminar fixation was used from T11 to L4 (Fig. 7–4B). Pain was relieved and bone union occurred (Fig. 7–4C).

Before the advent of pedicle screws, distraction rods and rods fixed to the laminae were the only devices available. Multisegment laminar fixation is not desirable in the lumbar area, and because apposition of the vertebral bodies is necessary, distraction rods are inappropriate. However, short-segment laminar fixation may not provide sufficient stiffness. For example, a patient was admitted to the hospital with *Aspergillus* osteomyelitis at L3–L4 (Fig. 7–5A) and was treated with amphotericin. He improved, but renal toxicity developed and the antifungal treatment had to be stopped. This sequence was repeated several times. The infection progressed, and he was operated upon through the lateral approach to remove infected tissue (Fig. 7–5B). About 10 days later L3–L4 laminar fixation was done using a Luque rectangle to allow telescoping to facilitate apposition of the vertebral bodies. Amphotericin treatment resumed, and again renal toxicity developed. The infection continued to progress (Fig. 7–5C), evidently because the Luque rectangle did not provide adequate immobilization. Consequently, through a lumbar sympathectomy approach an iliac crest graft was placed from L3 to L4 (Fig. 7–5D). Full recovery and bony union followed (Fig. 7–5E). In retrospect, primary bone grafting or a more extensive laminar fixation should have been done initially.

More extensive laminar fixation provides greater stiffness, although immobilization of unfused segments can create problems. The patient whose films are shown in Figure 7–6 was a 67-year-old woman with a past history of L4–S1 fusion in whom laminectomy and facetectomy had been done at L2–L3 (Fig. 7–6A). A wound infection developed with profuse purulent drainage and L2–L3 osteomyelitis (Fig. 7–6B). On admission she was febrile and disoriented. The WBC was 10,900, the ESR was 100, and spine films demonstrated progression of the osteomyelitis (Fig. 7–6C). A lat-

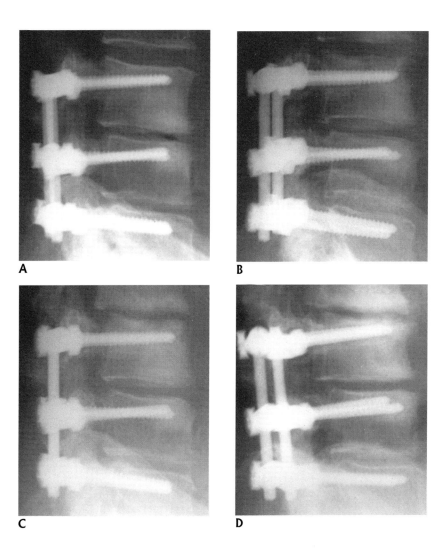

FIGURE 7–3
A Pedicle fixation from L3 to L5. A L5–S1 fusion had been done earlier. **B** Film 10 weeks later demonstrating destructive change at L2–L3. **C** Four months after onset of symptoms. **D** Six months after onset. Bone union is beginning anteriorly.

eral approach was done to evacuate the pus that had reached the dura and to remove granulation tissue and infected bone at L2–L3. Because the patient was diabetic and the infection extensive, the wound was packed open. Staphylococcus grew on cultures, and appropriate antibiotics were administered through a Hickman catheter. The patient's general condition improved, and her mental state cleared. Spine films demonstrated continued instability, and the ESR remained elevated. The wound granulated, and secondary closure was performed followed after 2 weeks by segmental fixation (Fig. 7–6D). Because a pedicle CT scan demonstrated that the pedicular diameter was too small to accept the screws then available, Luque rods were used and fixed to the spinous processes of T11, 12, and L1 to avoid the possibility of spinal cord injury from the extraction of sublaminar wires in the event it would become necessary to remove the device. The caudal ends of the rods were wired to the L4 laminae and to sacral screws. One month later pain had resolved and the WBC and ESR had become normal. The patient returned 3 years later with lumbar pain increased by extension. Spine films demonstrated a broken rod and instability at L3–L4 (Fig. 7–6E), and bone scan with SPECT showed increased uptake in the apophyseal joints at L3–L4. An L3–L4 transverse process fusion was performed. Because fusion and healing had occurred at L2–L3, pedicle screws of an appropriate diameter were placed in L2 for an L2–S1 fixation (Fig. 7–6G). Pain was relieved and fusion occurred.

Pedicle screws and laminar hooks provide the means for rigid, short-segment fixation, and if bone destruction is extensive and a large dead space remains after debridement, primary bone grafting should be done. The patient whose films are shown in Figure 7–7 developed paraparesis and urinary retention secondary to osteomyelitis at L4–L5. A hemilaminotomy was done, but she continued to deteriorate. Admission spine films, CT scans, and

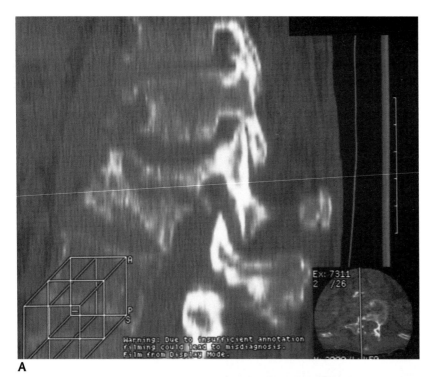

FIGURE 7-4
A CT scan demonstrating osteomyelitis at L1–L2 with extensive bone destruction. **B** Shortly after laminar fixation from T11 to L4. **C** Film taken 6 months after surgery shows that union has occurred.

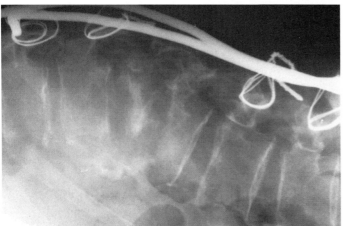

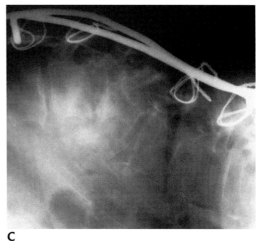

MRI showed infection at L4–L5 with granulation tissue anterior to the dura (Fig. 7-7A). A lateral approach was used for resection of infected tissue, and iliac crest bone grafts were placed from L4 to L5 (Fig. 7-7B). Posterior instrumentation was done 10 days later. The left L4 pedicle had been resected during removal of epidural granulations, precluding pedicle fixation at that level. Even if both pedicles had been available, screws should probably not be placed in the vicinity of infected bone. Consequently, because of osteopenia and the L4 hemilaminectomy, laminar hooks were placed on L3 and connected to sacral screws (Fig. 7-7C). The screws penetrated the anterior sacral cortex to decrease the possibility of screw migration. The patient regained bladder control and became able to walk with a cane. Films done 4 months later demonstrated solid, bony union (Fig. 7-7D).

It is sometimes necessary to use the S2 pedicle. The patient whose films are shown in Figure 7-8 was admitted with a staphylococcal L5–S1 infection that had progressed despite 8 weeks of treatment with intravenous vancomycin. Spine films demonstrated bone destruction at L5–S1 (Fig. 7-8A), the WBC was 6100, and the ESR was 82. CT and MRI demonstrated osteomyelitis at L5–S1. A left lateral extracavitary approach was used for debridement and for placement of an iliac crest bone

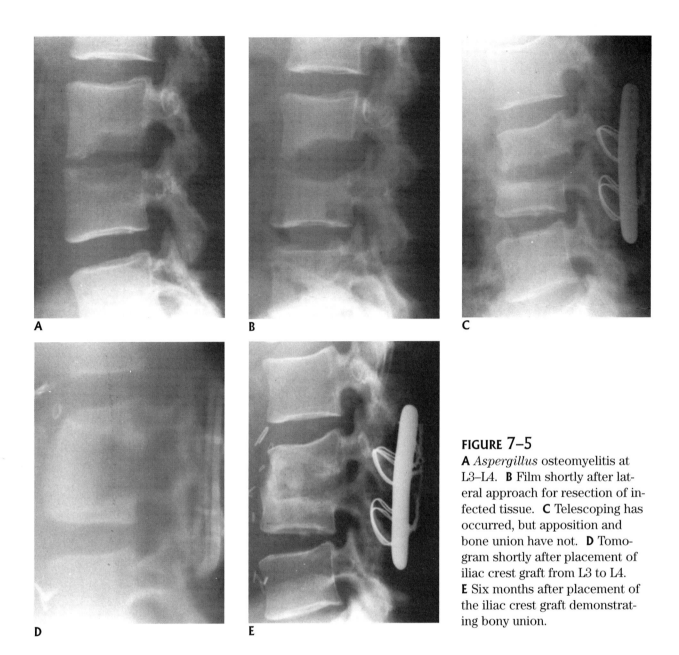

FIGURE 7–5
A *Aspergillus* osteomyelitis at L3–L4. **B** Film shortly after lateral approach for resection of infected tissue. **C** Telescoping has occurred, but apposition and bone union have not. **D** Tomogram shortly after placement of iliac crest graft from L3 to L4. **E** Six months after placement of the iliac crest graft demonstrating bony union.

graft. Posterior instrumentation was done 2 weeks later. Because of S1 involvement, screws were placed in the S2 pedicles and connected to laminar hooks on L4 (Fig. 7–8B). Pedicle screws could have been used, but hooks were selected because of osteopenia. The patient did well following surgery, and films taken 6 months later demonstrated good bony union from L5 to the sacrum. Instrumentation was applied at a second procedure because of reluctance to place foreign material into an infected area. However, single-stage debridement and instrumentation without adverse effects have been reported.[6]

Disc Space Infection

Clinical Presentation and Diagnosis

Disc space infection is an uncommon complication of surgical treatment[8] and chemonucleolysis for herniated vertebral discs.[3] Characteristically the back pain persists and increases in severity following the operation. In most patients the pain is disabling and out of proportion to the physical find-

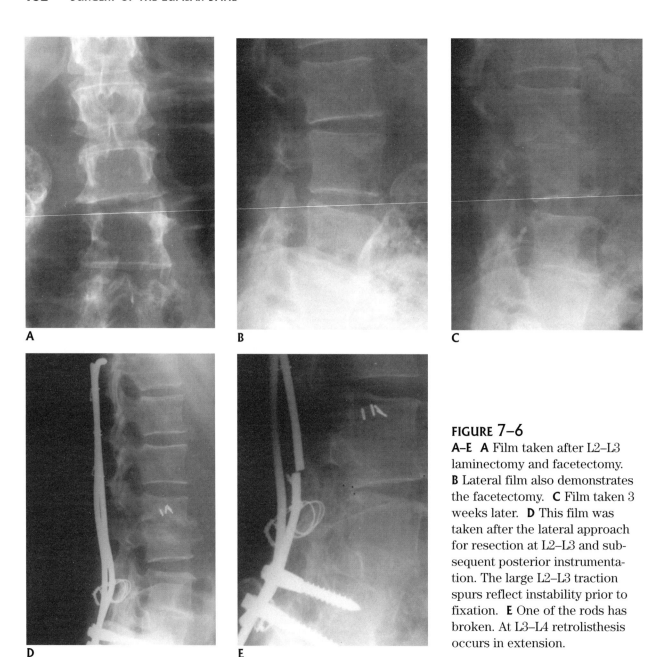

FIGURE 7–6
A–E A Film taken after L2–L3 laminectomy and facetectomy. **B** Lateral film also demonstrates the facetectomy. **C** Film taken 3 weeks later. **D** This film was taken after the lateral approach for resection at L2–L3 and subsequent posterior instrumentation. The large L2–L3 traction spurs reflect instability prior to fixation. **E** One of the rods has broken. At L3–L4 retrolisthesis occurs in extension.

ings. Spine films demonstrate progressive narrowing of the interspace.

Management

Initially, treatment should be *medical*, using antibiotics and immobilization by bedrest. This is continued until the pain subsides sufficiently to permit mobilization in an orthosis. With successful medical management, fusion of the adjacent vertebral bodies occurs in a majority of patients.[8] However, those patients who do not respond to medical management require *surgical treatment*. If bone destruction is minimal and neurological function is normal, approaching the disc to resect infected tissue may not be necessary and posterior instrumentation and fusion can be the primary procedure.

For example, the patient whose films are shown in Figure 7–9 developed disc space infection after hemilaminotomy for L3–L4 discectomy. She had persistent back pain, and despite an adequate course of IV antibiotics the infection persisted (Fig. 7–9A). The pain was increased by extension, and her films also demonstrated posterior displacement of L4 on L5 in extension. Consequently, she

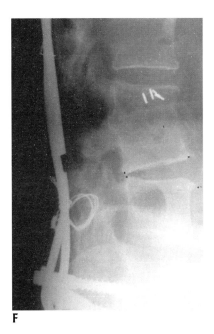
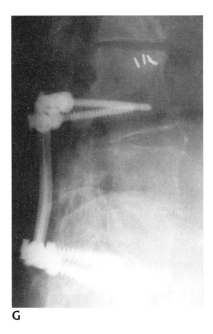

FIGURE 7–6
F and G **F** Alignment is normal in flexion. **G** One year after transverse process fusion and pedicle fixation.

had a transverse process fusion with pedicle fixation from L3 to the sacrum. The symptoms were relieved, interbody fusion took place at L3–L4 (Fig. 7–9B), and the transverse process fusion also appeared satisfactory. An aseptic form has been described with similar symptoms and findings but a much lower ESR and was identified by percutaneous biopsy of the disc.[5]

oped to an extent permitting secondary closure. More recent experiences, however, have shown that extensive laminectomy is unnecessary and that hemilaminotomy of one or more levels can be sufficient to drain an abscess that is usually located posterior to the dura. The wound is closed primarily with drainage.[7]

Epidural Abscess

Clinical Presentation and Diagnosis

Acute epidural abscess is rare. Pain is the presenting symptom and may be followed by neurological deficit, which can be rapidly progressive. MRI is usually diagnostic (Fig. 7–10). However, if myelography is done, the contrast medium should be introduced by lateral cervical puncture to avoid contaminating the cerebrospinal fluid.

Management

In the past, the recommended treatment has been laminectomy over the extent of the abscess with the wound left open until granulations have devel-

Tuberculous Vertebral Osteomyelitis

Tuberculous vertebral osteomyelitis has become an uncommon disorder, and we have not operated on a patient with active infection for more than 15 years. However, this may change because of the increasing number of patients with compromised immune systems.

Clinical Presentation and Diagnosis

Because of the more indolent course of tuberculous osteomyelitis, bone destruction is greater at the time of diagnosis than in the case of pyogenic infection, and therefore the angular deformity is usually more pronounced (Fig. 7–11A.)

154 SURGERY OF THE LUMBAR SPINE

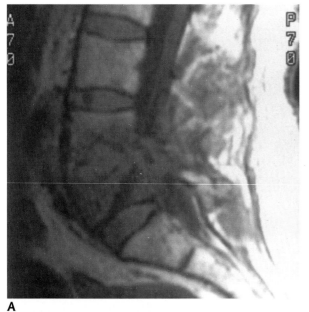
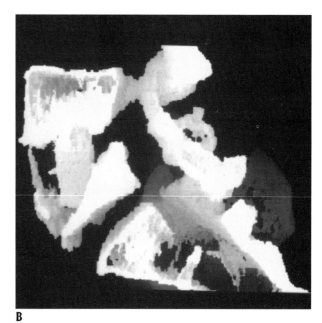
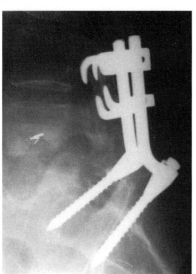
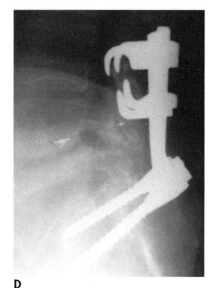

FIGURE 7–7
A MRI demonstrating L4–L5 osteomyelitis with encroachment on the spinal canal. **B** Three-dimensional CT scan done after lateral approach for resection at L4–L5 and placement of iliac crest graft. **C** Film taken shortly after posterior instrumentation. **D** Four months after surgery. Fusion has occurred at L4–L5.

FIGURE 7–8
A Osteomyelitis at L5–S1. **B** One year after the lateral approach for resection, interbody fusion at L5–S1 and subsequent posterior instrumentation from L4 to S2.

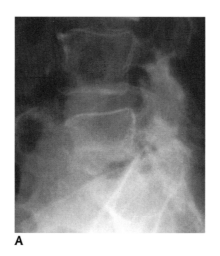
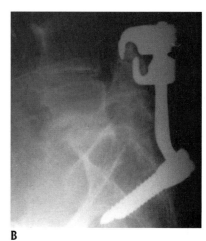

FIGURE 7-9

A Interspace infection at L3–L4. L4 is displaced posteriorly on L5 in extension with normal alignment in flexion. **B** Film 1 year after surgery demonstrates L3–L4 fusion.

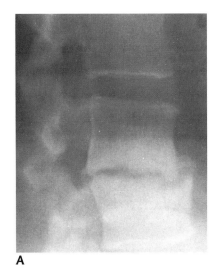

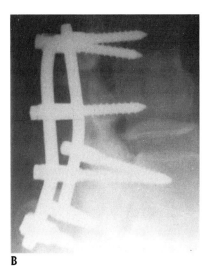

Management

If the patient is neurologically normal, chemotherapy is usually sufficient. However, if neurological deficit is present, surgical treatment is necessary.

Surgical treatment is much the same as for pyogenic infections. Appropriate chemotherapy should be administered for approximately 2 weeks prior to the operation. The surgical approach can be either lateral extracavitary, retroperitoneal, or transthoracic for resection of infected tissue and interbody fusion. Posterior instrumentation permits earlier mobilization, and a major advantage of the lateral approach is that it can be done at the same operation and through the same incision.

The patient in Figure 7–11A developed tuberculous spondylitis in early childhood, and a posterior fusion was done. She remained neurologically normal until age 54, when progressive paraparesis developed. Radiographic examination demonstrated deformity of the spinal cord at the level of the gibbus (Fig. 7–11B). A lateral approach was done to resect bone anterior to the dura, and neurological function returned to normal. The patient and her family had noticed increased thoracic kyphosis, which may have produced pathological tension in the spinal cord, resulting in myelopathy.

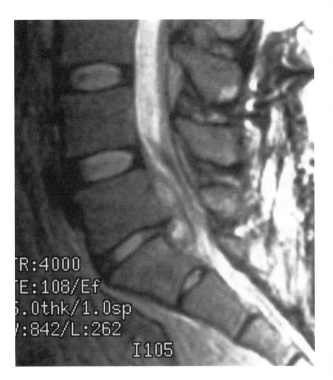

FIGURE 7-10 MRI demonstrating epidural abscess anterior to the dura in contrast to the usual posterior location. The abscess developed after a hemilaminotomy and removal of a herniated disc and was successfully treated by evacuation through the hemilaminotomy and primary closure with drainage.

Summary

To summarize, the basic principles in the treatment of vertebral infection, whether pyogenic or tuberculous, are immobilization, antibiotics, and, when necessary, resection of infected tissue and interbody fusion.

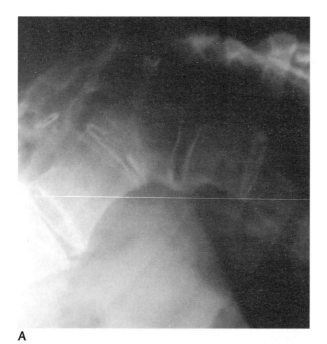

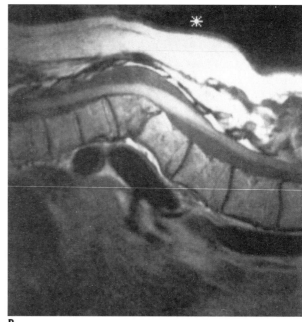

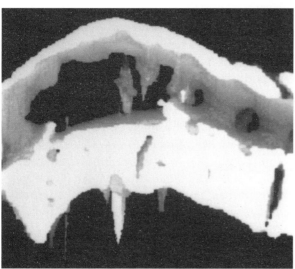

FIGURE 7-11
A Residual deformity from tuberculous spondylitis. **B** The spinal cord is stretched over the gibbus. **C** Postoperative 3-D CT scan. The "stalactites" are Hemoclip artifacts.

REFERENCES

1. Arnold PM, Baek PN, Bernardi RJ, et al: Surgical management of non-tuberculous thoracic and lumbar osteomyelitis: Report of 33 cases. Surg Neurol 47:551–561, 1997.

2. Eismont FJ, Bohlman HH, Soni PL, et al: Pyogenic and fungal vertebral osteomyelitis with paralysis. J Bone Joint Surg 65-A(1):19–29, 1983.

3. Fernand R, Lee CK: Post laminectomy disc space infection: A review of the literature and a report of three cases. Clin Orthop 209(Aug):215–218, 1986.

4. Fernandez-Ulloa M, Vasavada PJ, Hanslits ML: Diagnosis of vertebral osteomyelitis: Clinical, radiological and scintigraphic features. Orthopedics 8(9):1144–1150, 1985.

5. Fouquet B, Goupille P, Jattiot F, et al: Discitis after lumbar disc surgery: Features of "aseptic" and "septic" forms. Spine 17(3):356–358, 1992.

6. Graziano GP, Sidhu KS: Salvage reconstruction in acute and late sequelae from pyogenic thoracolumbar infection. J Spinal Disord 6(3):199–207, 1993.

7. Larson SJ: Infection of the spine. In Current Therapy in Neurological Surgery, ed. DM Long, B.C. Decker, Inc., Toronto, Ontario, pp. 200–201, 1989.

8. Lindholm TS, Pylkkanen P: Discitis following removal of intervertebral disc. Spine 7(6):618–622, 1982.

CHAPTER 8

Trauma

Pathology

Classification of Spine Fractures

Radiographic Evaluation

Management

Sacral Fractures

Gunshot Wounds of the Spine

Prognosis

Rehabilitation

Trauma

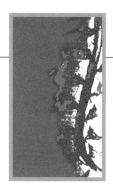

The thoracolumbar junction is the most common site for fractures in the lumbar spine, largely as a result of its biomechanics.

The most common level of injury is L1 (35%) in our series, followed by L2 (25%). There is approximately 10% incidence of injury at the other levels, and 10%—in the absence of osteoporosis—are multiple. Probably 2000 to 2500 lumbar fractures occur annually with permanent neurological deficit; there are probably 20,000 to 30,000 more non paralyzing injuries that produce either transient or only radicular neurological abnormalities.[93]

Pathology

The thoracolumbar junction is transitional, in that it is aligned in a neutral position between the thoracic kyphosis and the lumbar lordosis. The spine becomes more mobile caudal to the rib cage. The facet joints change their alignment, and disc shape is altered. In addition, the eccentric loading, which is anterior to the vertebra, tends to create a flexion moment.

Motor vehicle accidents are responsible for 50% of injuries and falls for another 25%. Over 75% of those injured are males. Considering the age distribution, patients tend to be slightly older than those with cervical spine fractures.

The most common pattern of neurological injury is the cauda equina syndrome, which involves some leg weakness and bowel and bladder paralysis; paralyzing lumbar fractures are uncommon, representing less than 10% of total instances of spinal cord injury, and are not most commonly incomplete.

Associated trauma is seen in over 70% of the patients in our series. A disproportionate number of these are fractures of the lower extremities and pelvis. Approximately one-fourth of patients with hyperflexion or shear injuries suffer intra-abdominal injury. Pelvic trauma is seen in about 20% of our series, and another 20% have suffered long bone fractures. In addition, 10 to 15% are found to have spine fractures elsewhere.

Furthermore, the most common consideration in lumbar fractures is spinal stability rather than neurological decompression. Thus, as will be noted later in this chapter, thought patterns regarding treatment are evolving.

Classification of Spine Fractures

There is no topic in the area of spinal surgery more difficult than the optimal classification of fractures. Indeed, there are probably as many classifications as there are surgeons treating these injuries. Schemes have been developed based on radiography,[26] biomechanics and pathophysiology,[52] and clinical outcome.

The most popular early proposal was that of Roaf, who proposed a two-column theory. As discussed in Chapter 2, this divides the spine into two separate environments; injuries of both are necessary for instability.[86] This classification, which is clearly biomechanically based, evolves much later into the three-column theory of Denis outlined in the biomechanics chapter.[26]

Possibly the most popular classification scheme currently in use is that of McAfee.[75] This attempts to unify anatomic and mechanistic considerations. Originally, it included five different classifications for five fractures; in recent years multiple subclassifications have been created. Several of McAfee's injury types, however, contradict the classification of Denis.[26] For example, what this author would call a flexion and compression fracture (that is, both compression and flexion forces causing vertebral compression and disruption of the posterior elements) is called a flexion-distraction injury by McAffe and compression fracture by Denis. However, if there is pedicle injury, the fracture becomes a burst fracture, although the forces producing injury are not associated with axial loading. It is no wonder that consistency in clinical decision making is difficult to obtain.

We prefer classifications that are mechanistic, that define injuries based on the major vectors that appear to produce the fracture. As discussed in Chapter 2, instability is considered a continuum proportional to the severity of injury to individual structures. Thus a 50% vertebral compression is often biomechanically stable; when compression increases to 60%, the fracture may be unstable, not because of increased vertebral injury, but because posterior element trauma becomes more likely.

Gertzbein developed a scheme that divides fractures into three basic types: compression (type A), distraction (type B), and injuries due to multiple force vectors, often with translation (type C). Fractures are subclassified from 1 to 3, based on increasing injury severity and deformity.[42]

This is an evolving area. There is increasing recognition that any classification should provide correlation between fracture type and results of management, especially neurological outcome. No available system does this. Certainly, our definition of unstable fractures is becoming more rigorous. In the absence of dislocation, most bone injuries-even unstable fractures, heal if immobilized. It remains to be seen if any currently available classification scheme will assist in determining appropriate treatment needs, rather than provide therapeutic license.

Radiographic Evaluation

Plain Radiographs

In the evaluation of lumbar spine fractures, plain radiographs are critical but often ignored. In addition to spinal alignment, accurate information regarding posterior element fractures and some vertebral body injury can be defined. Therefore, plain radiographs should be obtained early in the assessment of possible lumbar spine problems; this would seem obvious, but almost one-third of the fractures referred to our institution from outside hospitals in 1996 had lumbar fractures diagnosed on the basis of computed tomography (CT) of the abdomen or other incidental studies. Indeed, this author was recently informed that at a major trauma center (not ours), residents were likely to bypass plain radiographs altogether. Furthermore, the entire spine should be imaged in patients with any fractures, since multiple fractures occur in about 15%[51]; similarly, over 25% of sacral fractures and 7% of pelvic fractures are associated with thoracolumbar injury. The use of CT in managing fractures and trauma is discussed below.

Increased distance between spinous processes suggests disruption of the posterior ligamentous complex or facet joints, suggesting instability. Similarly, increased interpedicular distance or facet fractures are consistent with both ligamentous injury and fracture.[4]

Dynamic views contribute significantly to an accurate understanding of stability, predicting posterior element and ligament injury. However, they generally should not be performed before canal studies, which rule out significant neurological compression.

Plain radiography should not be used to define spinal canal status. Although frequently used postoperatively by spine surgeons to ensure that the canal has been decompressed, particularly following removal of canal masses by ligamentaxis, radiographs may not reflect central fragments compressing the spinal cord. Indeed, in trauma, large central fragments causing major thecal sac compression are missed on plain radiographs if the rest of the body is largely intact (Fig. 8–1). Thus canal studies are imperative.

Advanced radiographic studies of the lumbar spine should include accurate demonstration of the integrity of the spinal canal and its relationship to the neural elements, as well as bony elements of the spine. Even in the absence of neurological deficit, there may be critical injury to vertebrae or discs that puts neural elements at risk. Therefore, even trivial increases in deformity may cause later neurological deficit and contribute to deformity.

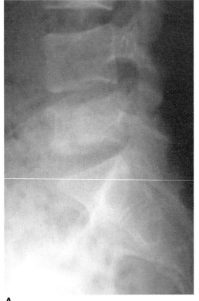
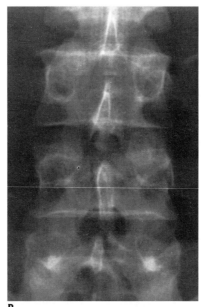

FIGURE 8–1

A–D Twenty-five-year-old male with severe cauda equina syndrome following a fall. **A, B** Lateral and anteroposterior radiographs suggest only a minor L5 fracture. **C, D** However, CT and myelogram images demonstrate a large central bone fragment compressing the thecal sac. The patient underwent an extracavitary approach with decompression and short-segment fixation.

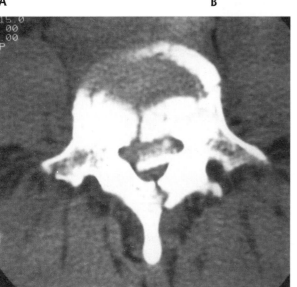
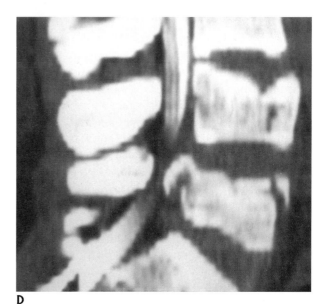

Magnetic Resonance Imaging

Our preference for canal imaging is magnetic resonance imaging (MRI). This technique allows accurate sagittal demonstration of bone and disc pathology and its relationship to neural elements. It is optimal for surgical planning. Furthermore, MRI provides valuable information regarding intrinsic spinal cord injury and the nature of masses within the spinal canal.

Both T1 and T2 sequences are essential, although some perform only the former in trauma. Certainly, T1 images are optimal for anatomic definition, particularly of the bone/disc interface with neural elements. However, we find T2 imaging useful for definition of disc and other soft tissue injury. Furthermore, gradient echo images can be helpful in defining intramedullary hemorrhage, if such a question exists (Fig. 8–2).

Recent iterations of the MRI scanner have improved imaging of disc and ligament injury, which can be helpful in assessing the potential for deformity, and may eventually be a tool for determining instability. Indeed, accuracy of over 90% for posterior ligament injury can be expected:[35] high signal intensity on T2 images usually represents ligament injury.

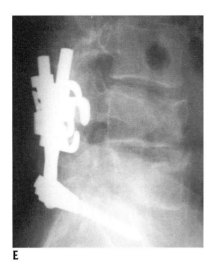 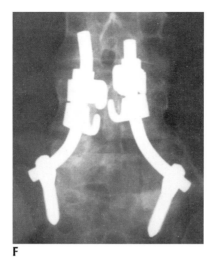 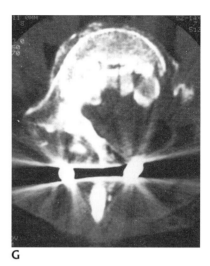

FIGURE 8–1 *(continued)* **E–G** Lateral and anteroposterior radiographs **E, F** and an axial computed tomogram **G** demonstrate good fixation and fusion, as well as complete decompression.

Contrary to the opinions of some, the quality of bone imaging in MRI remains inadequate for accurate surgical planning. Thus bone studies are necessary.

As discussed elsewhere in this book, myelography is used only if patients are unable to undergo MRI because of the presence of a pacemaker or obesity, for example. Because of the superior imaging provided by MRI, including ligament status, hematoma, and cord injury, we prefer to sedate the claustrophobic patient than accept a lesser study.

In patients with no or incomplete deficit undergoing surgery, spinal angiography is performed to locate the radiculomedullary artery of Adamkiewicz. It is found between T12 and L2 in about 20% of patients; disruption has been occasionally reported to cause paraplegia.[2,53,65]

Computed Tomography

Because plain radiographs cannot be relied upon to predict the severity of fractures, CT should be considered whenever even a minor fracture, whether of the vertebral body or other spine elements, is seen.[63] A series of patients with transverse process fractures, usually considered benign, underwent CT. Over 10 percent had other major fractures. CT is also necessary in the management of trauma. Although many consider the axial views produced by CT to be accurate in defining canal compromise,[38] we prefer MRI for this purpose. Rather, identification of the extent of bone injury is of critical importance in determining the nature of surgical treatment, if any, to be performed. In addition, the sagittal anatomy of the vertebral body is best determined with CT.

Evaluation of Neurological Status

Because lumbar fractures largely involve the cauda equina or nerve roots, two options are available: somatosensory evoked potentials (SEPs) and electromyography or nerve conduction studies (EMG). The latter may be useful when there is a fracture with nonradicular pain in an effort to answer the question of nerve root compromise.

In spite of decades of work and a significant number of publications in the area, the value of evoked potentials in the management of spinal fractures with neurological deficit is uncertain. Efforts to predict prognosis have been inconsistent. Several studies have shown that the more normal the amplitude of the SEP, the better the ultimate neurological status. However, our studies have suggested very little consistency; it may well be that evoked potential changes are consistent with the degree of ongoing distortion of neural elements but do not reflect the importance of impact.

For most clinicians treating spinal trauma, the primary role of evoked potentials, both motor and sensory, is in intraoperative monitoring. The SEP is

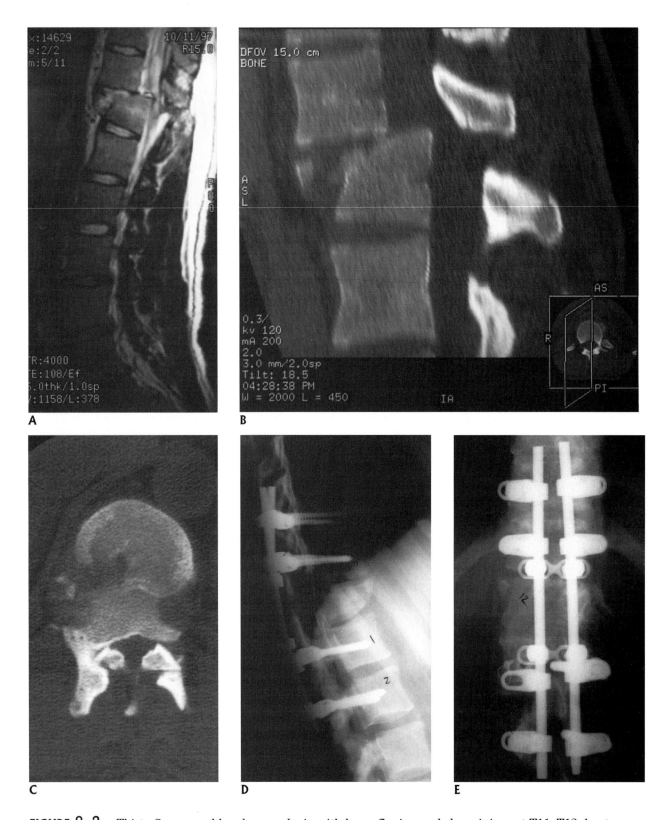

FIGURE 8-2 Thirty-five-year-old male paraplegic with hyperflexion and shear injury at T11–T12 due to a motor vehicle accident. **A** MRI demonstrates severe canal compromise, disruption of the posterior elements, and cord swelling, edema, and hemorrhage. **B, C** Sagittal and axial computed tomograms confirming the extent of bony injury. **D, E** Following reduction and instrumentation, a partial vertebrectomy was performed. Note that the right L1 pedicle would not hold a screw. Because the connector had already been placed, the surgeon elected to fixate that level to the transverse process via a hole in that structure. The patient demonstrated surprising motor improvement and is ambulatory with one brace; bowel and bladder function have not recovered.

independent of the level of consciousness, relatively resistant to ischemia, demonstrates predictable changes with anesthesia, and should provide a reasonably accurate assessment of what is going on within the spinal cord. Unfortunately, there are large percentages of false positives and negatives, which can negatively affect decision making in the operating room. We generally use intraoperative neurophysiology in operations performed for trauma when attempting reduction of dislocation without direct decompression (which is unusual in our practice).

Management

Appropriate evaluation and treatment of associated trauma generally takes priority over treatment of the fracture. Management of the fracture itself should include careful maintenance of spinal position when instability is suspected.[99] In unpublished data from our institution, the risk of deep vein thrombosis is equally high in both deficited and non deficited individuals: intermittent pneumatic stockings, elastic stockings, and judicious use of low-dose herapin decrease that incidence. Of great importance is regular ranging of the legs. In addition, in patients to be maintained at bedrest for any period of time, adequate attention to skin care and prevention of sores, nutrition, and psychosocial status are of paramount importance.

Currently, we rarely use rotating or air beds in spinal trauma patients. Instead, we prefer to log-roll and otherwise move patients at regular intervals. Indeed, again in unpublished data from our institution, the incidence of pressure sores in deficited patients is lower in those treated on conventional beds with regular log rolling than on kinetic beds.

The immediate involvement of a transdisciplinary rehabilitation team is imperative. The role of surgery in spinal cord injury remains unproved, but the value of rehabilitation is clear. Decreased morbidity and mortality, improved neurological and medical outcomes, and higher life satisfaction are associated with early and aggressive rehabilitation programs.

High-dose methylprednisolone (MPSS) should be given to patients with cord-related neurological deficit as soon as is reasonable following injury.[12] We generally do not use MPSS in patients with open injuries, such as gunshot wounds, nor in those with radicular abnormalities. Recent studies have recommended giving the bolus within 1 to 3 hrs from injury when feasible, followed by a steroid infusion for 23 hr more.

A common maxim is that patients should not be taken to the operating room for the management for associated trauma in the presence of an unstable fracture. However, with judicious handling, the risk of progressive deformity or neurological status is not increased in most circumstances. Therefore, unless a patient needs to be positioned prone for the management of associated trauma, it is generally permissible to allow other system injuries to be treated first.

Decision making in spinal trauma is extremely complex and is hampered by a lack of definitive data in certain critical areas. However, the following are true:

- Canal compromise does not correlate with neurologic status.[45,59,7,5,8,9]
- Static deformity does not lead to progressive neurological deficit.[6,23,39]
- Pain is not a consequence of deformity of less than 20 to 40 degrees.
- Complications of surgery may be higher than those of nonoperative treatment for many patients.

What are the goals of treatment of instability and deformity? Even those are not agreed upon. Classic orthopedic thinking is that fractures need to be perfectly aligned to consider an outcome acceptable. However, the spine is different than long bones: it is a heterogeneous structure that adapts to constantly varying loads, and it has internal mobility. Actually, the real goals are maximal neurological recovery and stability with alignment associated with the minimum long-term pain.

Non-Surgical Treatment

Nonoperative treatment of spinal fractures, even with neurological deficit, has been advocated for decades.[85] Guttmann reported on 142 patients treated nonoperatively, with a 20-year follow-up. Approximately half of the incomplete patients and 25% of the patients with complete injuries demonstrated substantial neurological improvement.[45a] Similarly, Stauffer noted that even patients with complete injuries tended to have at least nerve root recovery,[92] which contradicts our own findings in the cervical spine.[104] Patients with dislocations were reduced several weeks after the injury demonstrated the same ultimate recovery.

In Tator's large series of patients treated surgically or nonoperatively, the only difference was in mortality rates: patients in the surgical group had lower mortality rates.[95,96] More recently, Donovan suggested again that the role of surgical decompression is questionable, and that the timing of surgery for biomechanical instability is largely optional.[31]

These studies are not just of historical interest: recently, there has been an increased interest in nonoperative treatment of lumbar fractures.[49] In an unpublished work by Rechtine, matched groups were treated with surgery and with recumbence followed by orthoses. Contrary to older publications, the complication rate for nonoperative treatment was better than for surgical treatment. For example, there were two complications (1 deep vein thrombosis, 1 heel ulcer) in 32 nonoperative patients. In a series of 50 surgical patients, there were 8 complications related directly to the instrumentation, 3 infections, 1 progressive kyphosis, and 1 paraparesis. The length of stay was significantly higher in patients treated nonoperatively, with an average of 45 days, as opposed to a mean of 24 days in the surgical group. Costs were much lower in the nonoperative group. Neurological improvement was approximately the same, although patients treated nonoperatively had, on average, less canal compromise to start.[84]

Canal compromise, however, in and of itself, is not a surgical indicator. Bony remodeling following trauma is common.[24,57,88] In Krompinger's series, canal diameter returned to normal in half the patients with 25% canal compromise.[62] Mumford et al monitored resorption of retropulsed central fragments over a 2-year period in 41 patients with single-level fractures with retropulsed vertebral fragments. Patients were treated at bedrest from 7 to 68 days (fewer days in recent years), and then in a thoracolumbar orthosis (TLSO). Cobb angles were carefully monitored for development of deformity; the average increase was 7 degrees. Canal area improved an average of 22%. Neurological deterioration and other complications were uncommon.[78] However, other series have reported complication rates as high as one-third, including neurological deficit, and deformity requiring surgical treatment.[23]

In yet another anecdotal report of fractures treated nonoperatively, Singer reported on 73 British soldiers who suffered thoracolumbar fractures without deficit, and who were followed for an average of 5 years. Over three-fourths had an excellent outcome, defined as return to all preinjury activities with minimal pain, and another 15% had good outcomes. Outcome had nothing to do with fracture type, severity of injury, or treatment. Even fractures with presumed ligament injury healed acceptably well: minor deformities were tolerated quite well.[91]

Long-term results have been just as successful. A series of 42 patients with thoracolumbar fractures treated nonoperatively was followed for an average of 20 years. These patients had unstable "burst" fractures, based on the criteria of Roaf,[86] with vertebral body injuries and posterior element instability. Patients were questioned about pain, daily activities, employment, and self-perceived disability. The average patient complained of minimal or mild back pain. Almost 90% of the group were working in their preinjury capacity. Average kyphosis was 26 degrees in flexion; the amount of kyphosis did not correlate with pain or deficit. In addition, physical examination did not predict radiographic abnormalities.[105] This, of course, disagrees with previous efforts that suggested that pain is directly correlated with deformity.[56,81] In the latter series cited,[81] neurological results seemed better in patients treated surgically, although there was no compelling evidence for this. Weinstein et al found that costs are 60% lower with nonoperative treatment:[105] frankly, the results of surgery are not always 60% better.

Not all agree with a nonoperative approach.[34] Denis presented a series of patients with burst fractures: those treated operatively all returned to work and complained of little pain. Patients treated nonoperatively had more pain, and about 16% developed neurological deficit.[27] McEvoy and Bradford eventually operated on 6 of a group of 23 fracture patients who had been initially treated nonoperatively. This subset had developed deformity or complained of pain. Unfortunately, the authors' recommended criteria for nonoperative treatment were not discussed.[76]

More recently, Yazici et al compared a small series of thoracolumbar fractures treated nonoperatively with those treated with indirect reduction and short-segment transpedicular fixation. Patients were compared using CT initially and at follow-up visits: ultimate canal diameter and neurological status were similar between both groups. As would be expected, canal remodeling occurred more rapidly in the surgical group.[108]

Cantor et al limited nonoperative treatment to neurologically intact patients with intact posterior elements and less than 50% loss of vertebral body height; certainly, this is a group of patients that we would usually treat nonoperatively. Canal compromise was immaterial in exclusion from the study. Patients were ambulated early in TLSOs. Almost all patients resumed active lives, including full return to employment. Average initial kyphosis was 19 degrees; average final kyphosis was 20 degrees. CT demonstrated resorption of bone compromising the spinal canal in most patients.[17]

Is posterior column integrity the main criterion for successful nonoperative treatment? Our data suggest otherwise. Certainly, fractures of the laminae and/or facet joints without dislocation are not a contraindication for nonoperative treatment. Patients with posterior element fracture but without ligament injury can often be mobilized quickly in a TLSO.

Fractures identified as being stable should be considered for surgery only in the presence of neurological deficit; this is uncommon.[36] Our preference is to perform appropriate decompression and stabilization in patients with unstable injuries and paraparesis. However, many deficited patients with unstable injuries can be treated nonsurgically as well.[87] A combination of bedrest, effective bracing, and appropriate rehabilitation allows fractures to heal with an increased risk of deformity but no significant increase in the risk of neurological deficit.

Protocol

We consider this protocol to be "aggressive nonoperative" (note that we avoid the word *conservative*) treatment. Although bedrest is incorporated, the patient is physically active to the extent possible. During the early period of bedrest, techniques can be used to enhance alignment. For example, placing an extension roll under the spine can improve alignment (Fig. 8–3). Similarly, in some patients with complete dislocation, pelvic traction partially or even completely reduces deformity. Certainly, traction under these circumstances has its own risks, including skin breakdown. However, it may be useful in patients with associated trauma or problems obviating surgery.

For the average fracture with good alignment and intact ligaments, 1 to 2 days of bedrest are followed by immobilization in a TLSO that extends down over the pelvis; a hip spica is often used for fractures below L3. Even fractures with ligament injury can be treated nonoperatively if there is no dislocation, using our modification of Rechtine's protocol. Instead of maintaining patients in the hospital, we discharge them home at bedrest soon after it has been determined that surgery is unnecessary. Patients are taught a recumbent exercise program, to be performed several times daily, and are placed on low-molecular-weight heparin. A TLSO is provided in case of emergency (e.g., house fire). Obviously, patients and their families must be committed to the treatment plan. Home health services are usually necessary.

Radiographs can be performed at home by mobile radiology services, or patients can be brought in via ambulance monthly as indicated. When it is anticipated that ambulation is safe, typically at 6 to 8 weeks for patients with severe fractures, the patient is readmitted to the hospital and mobilized progressively in a TLSO with the aid of a transdisciplinary rehabilitation team. Alignment is monitored radiographically for a brief period while the patient is hospitalized. The TLSO is maintained for another 8 to 12 weeks, along with radiographic monitoring.

In the series of patients treated with this protocol, none have lost neurological function; the average increase in deformity has been 2 degrees (Fig. 8–4). Most patients are pain-free at 6 months, and all survivors have returned to full employment. One patient died 3 months post-trauma of undetermined causes thought to be due to pulmonary embolism. This 50-year-old man was already back at work and walking several miles daily. Following a 4-hour drive, he suffered what his wife thought was an acute asthma attack and succumbed.

The decision to use operative treatment purely for the purpose of obtaining stability needs to be very carefully considered. The significance of bone and, particularly, disc and ligament injury, associated trauma, and individual patient characteristics should all be considered carefully in the equation. It is likely that in years to come we will be using much more nonoperative treatment for thoracolumbar fractures.

The rest of this chapter considers surgical treatment.

Surgical Treatment

In spite of increasing conservatism, deformity is often an indicator for surgery. Although some have had success with postural reduction,[45b] we prefer stabilizing inpatients who develop kyphosis while immobilized in an orthosis, or those presenting with deformities over 14 to 15 degrees following the initial traumatic event in conjunction with se-

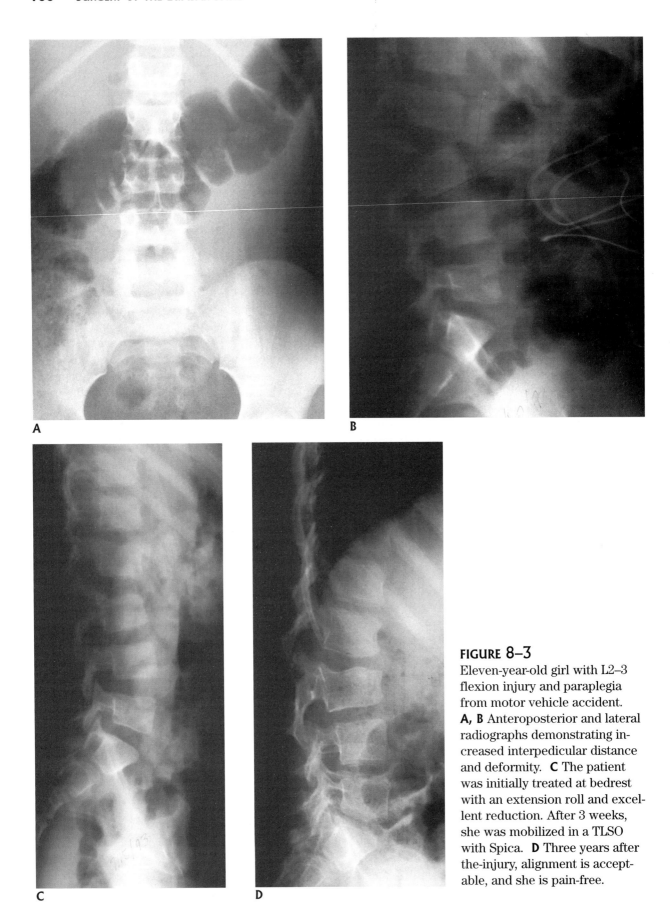

FIGURE 8–3

Eleven-year-old girl with L2–3 flexion injury and paraplegia from motor vehicle accident. **A, B** Anteroposterior and lateral radiographs demonstrating increased interpedicular distance and deformity. **C** The patient was initially treated at bedrest with an extension roll and excellent reduction. After 3 weeks, she was mobilized in a TLSO with Spica. **D** Three years after the injury, alignment is acceptable, and she is pain-free.

vere vertebral body fracture. Patients being treated nonoperatively with progressive deformity may require reconstruction as well. The difficult part, of course, is determining when: generally, loss of correction of a few degrees is common in this population during the first month after fracture. Further collapse or deformity beyond that point is viewed less sanguinely, especially as the kyphosis approaches 30 degrees.[42,43,72]

Rotational injuries, dislocations with major ligament trauma, and severe translational injuries typically require surgical stabilization.[64]

Surgery remains appropriate for decompression as well as stabilization in the patient with persistent neurological deficit. Decompression is based on the premise, often presented, that removal of masses distorting the spinal cord and nerve roots leads to improvement in ultimate neurological status. Certainly, there have been multiple anecdotal studies substantiating this hypothesis.[7–10,13,14,18,32,33,53,55,58,70,71,100,107] However, to our knowledge, no legitimate randomized prospective efforts comparing surgical and nonsurgical treatment have been made.

Others have considered morbidity and mortality between the two groups. Although there is no increase in neurological improvement associated with simple fixation or instrumentation plus laminectomy,[16,30,39,110] complications associated with recumbence and delay of entry into rehabilitation are decreased. Surgical stabilization decreases costs in the neurologically impaired population, but not in patients without deficit.

Epidural hematomas resulting from trauma are common, but rarely symptomatic (Fig. 8–8). They should be surgically decompressed if they are causing severe neurological deficit. In our experience, they are usually benign in the otherwise uncompromised patient.

Timing

Probably no greater controversy in spinal surgery exists than over the timing of surgery in the neurologically impaired patient. A significant body of contemporary but anecdotal literature recommends immediate surgery for spinal injury with or without neurological deficit.[46,54,66,67] The theory is that reduction is simpler before fibrosis takes place, which some argue occurs as early as several hours after injury. In addition, some believe that immediate decompression of distorted neural elements is imperative. There is inadequate scientific justification for both positions.

Fibrosis of injured ligaments and discs does not begin to occur for greater than 72 to 96 hours. Indeed, there is ultrastructural evidence that injured ligaments are weaker several days after injury; thus, if ligamentaxis is conceivable, delaying surgery a few days does not significantly affect outcome. However, Yazici et al[109] argue to the contrary. In a recent series, patients were operated on within 24 hours (early) or after 24 hours (late) from thoracolumbar "burst" injury. Short-segment pedicle fixation and indirect decompression were used. Early surgery was associated with improved canal decompression, but this was not related to improved long-term outcome. The authors suggested direct decompression after 24 hours.

The major argument for emergent surgery, however, is that neurological deficit becomes more reversible.[25] It is well beyond the scope of this chapter to discuss the relative roles of primary impact versus continuing mechanical compression versus "secondary injury"; suffice it to say that all three have a role that varies from case to case.

The immediate effects of impact are irreversible. The ill-thought-out and ineffective-indeed, often injurious-efforts at "decompression" via laminectomy have made it clear that attempting to improve neuronal survival by removing bone from the back of the spinal canal is pointless. Although our experimental work shows that preinjury canal size has an effect on the extent of neurologic injury produced by impact, opening the canal after the trauma is of no value.

Logic would dictate that reversing cord compression and/or deformity emergently would improve outcome.[32] Indeed, some animal studies suggest that there is a time window for decompression. However, some also suggest the converse. Virtually all animal studies fail to incorporate the impact component of injury: the wisdom of manipulating a recently injured spinal cord needs to be considered.

Similarly, the role of "secondary injury" should be critically examined. That biochemical phenomena occur as a result of impact is unquestionable; to be determined is the importance of this in human injury. In controlled animal models, secondary biochemical changes may be associated with neural injury. However, if indeed edema and other changes are maximal several hours after injury, irreversible neurological deterioration should be expected: this rarely occurs, and in the absence of severe contusion, can often be attributed to physical causes such as marginal immobilization.

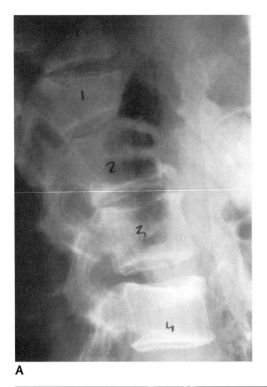
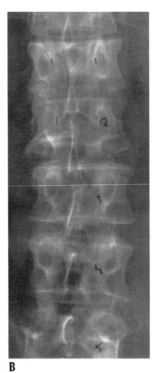
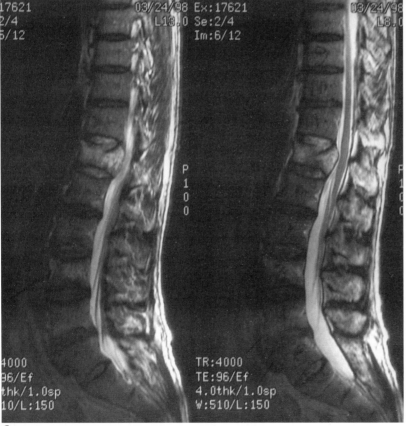

FIGURE 8–4

Forty-three-year-old man with unstable L1 fracture and no neurological deficit. **A, B** Lateral view shows 30% compression fracture; anteroposterior view with increased interpedicular distance. **C** MRI demonstrates 30% canal compromise, but attenuated and disrupted posterior ligaments. The patient was treated with 6 weeks of home bedrest and 3 months of TLSO. At 6 months, lateral

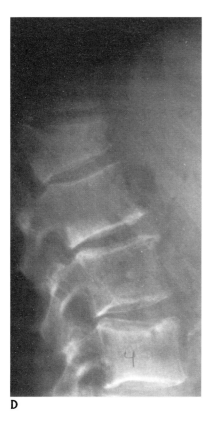
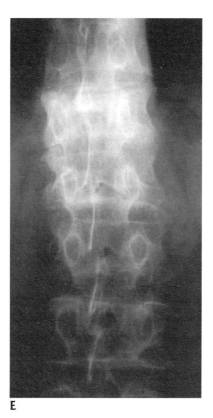

FIGURE 8–4 *(continued)* **D** and anteroposter **E** radiographs demonstrate good healing and acceptable alignment. Note the marked sclerosis in the latter view. The patient had no back pain.

We published a retrospective report in 1982, noting that decompression of masses distorting the spinal cord and cauda equina often led to significant neurological improvement even 5 years after the injury.[69] A similar series was published by Bohlman et al.[10] Both of these reports are unique in that the patients had plateaued neurologically prior to the decompression procedure, and could thus serve as their own controls. However, these series were nonrandomized, had relatively small numbers, and no nonoperated controls.

Numerous other retrospective clinical efforts appear in the literature to substantiate the positions of the senior authors of their manuscripts,[73] on both sides of the dispute. All of them, including those written by these authors, present a sizable number of cases, with a smaller number managed via the opposing position, and prove that the protagonist's approach is better. None are randomized, controlled, or even include an effective cohort. The reader is referred to a presentation by Baisden and Maiman for further discussion.[5] Suffice it to say that, all emotion and invective left aside, there is no compelling evidence to take one position or the other; those that choose to do so with vehemence do injustice to the topic. At the time of this writing, an effort is under way to perform a prospective, randomized study on surgical timing in spinal cord injury. Both of this book's authors strongly support this effort, confident that it will confirm their well-considered position.

Several others have reminded us that surgery as a treatment for spinal cord injury remains unproved altogether. A thoughtful retrospective study by Wagner and Chehrazi compared outcomes in a group of patients with traumatic spinal cord injury.[102] A significant percentage had suffered gunshot injuries to the cord; exclusion of this group would seem appropriate, since there is significant evidence that surgical treatment is rarely of benefit here.[65a] The most important factor predicting outcome was initial status. Of particular interest is that patients with cervical facet dislocations left unreduced did better neurologically than those who were reduced.

Techniques

Surgical procedures should be directed toward the pathology. This may seem trite: however, it bears mentioning because the most common procedure still performed for thoracolumbar trauma is laminectomy and its variants; ironically, anterior fixation to treat spinal instability with posterior dis-

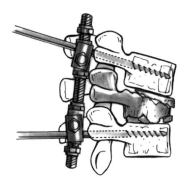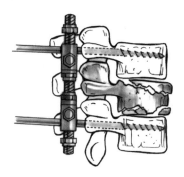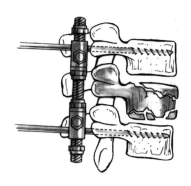
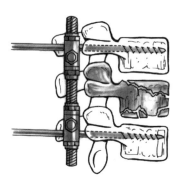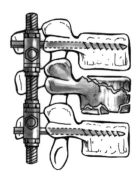

A

FIGURE 8–5 Fracture reduction using the Fixateur Internae. **A** Screw have been inserted through the pedicles, and the rods have been loosely placed. Rather than manually reducing the fracture by leveraging the Shantz screws, we prefer to twist down the turnbuckles until overcorrection is evident radiographically.

ruption is increasingly popular. Techniques for recommended procedures are presented in Chapter 13.

Ligamentotaxis Reduction (ligamentotaxis) has long been advocated as the technique of choice in many patients, the premise being that the tension applied to the posterior longitudinal ligament is enough to reduce fractures and decompress the thecal sac.[9,19,21,48,61,101,109] However, the strength of this ligament is marginal at best. Fredrickson et al recently demonstrated that the critical fiber is actually the oblique fiber of the disc annulus.[40] However, unless the fragment is somehow related to the annulus, reduction cannot be expected.

Relying on ligaments and the annulus to reduce retropulsed fragments may be unwise, since these are frequently disrupted. For example, Willen et al demonstrated 100% injury of the PLL, and 50% ALL disruption in patients having 50% canal compromise.[106]

We suspect that the critical factor in fragment reduction is creating the opposite of the forces that produced the trauma initially. Thus distraction in conjunction with restoration of the lumbar lordosis is typically necessary (Fig. 8–5).

In one prospective, randomized study, 67 patients with acute thoracolumbar burst fractures of T12 or L1 were operated on with Harrington distraction rods, AO fixateur internae, or another posterior pedicle fixation system. Reduction was accomplished indirectly by distraction applied using the fixation device. Harrington distraction rods produced the best reduction; however, all three devices restored much of the spinal canal.[101]

There may be neurological risks associated with this, however. When the spine is distracted, the spinal cord is as well.[68,72,97] Distracting the cord across an anterior compressing mass may be associated with neural injury.[14]

Even if the spine seems realigned on plain radi-

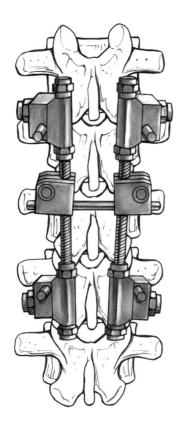

FIGURE 8–5 *(continued)* **B** The rod connectors are then tightened and a transverse connector is placed.

ography, central fragments may continue to occupy the spinal canal. Patients with suboptimal improvement should undergo a canal study and be considered for anterior decompression. Rather, we could recommend performance of vertebrectomy and appropriate fixation as the initial procedure.

Extracavitary Approach Our preferred approach for anterior decompression is the extracavitary approach to the lumbar spine,[64] as detailed in Chapter 13. It allows, in a logical sequence anterior decompression, posterior stabilization, and anterior fusion (Fig. 8–1 and 8–6).

Retroperitoneal Decompression In the occasional patient with vertebral body fracture, neurological deficit, and no need for fixation, retroperitoneal decompression and fusion with or without anterior fixation are appropriate (Fig. 8–7).[32,74] Many use anterolateral decompression and fusion with second stage posterior fixation. But must fracture patients be subjected to two separate operative procedures if definitive decompression and stabilization can be carried out under one anesthesia through one incision?

Instrumentation The purpose of instrumentation is to maintain alignment and promote fusion, regardless of the pathogenesis of instability. Several techniques, from the older Harrington rods and their variants, to sublaminar wiring,[94] and to more recent multilevel hook and pedicle screw constructs, are available. Optimal fixation incorporates the minimum number of vertebral levels and provides adequate stiffness to promote fusion.[1]

We rarely use Harrington rods alone for stabilization. First popularized in the 1960s for trauma, two points of fixation with intermediate distraction were used to stabilize the spine.[47] Unfortunately, failure due to hook dislodgement was common, and therefore the technique has since been modified to incorporate sublaminar or spinous process wiring,[15] increasing stiffness considerably.[72] This technique is still occasionally used, especially in osteoporotic patients. Other problems of Harrington rods include the difficulty in contouring them and appropriately restoring the lumbar lordosis. In addition, providing stability requires incorporating normal segments both above and below the fusion. In one small series, 6-year follow-up was provided on 33 patients who had undergone Harrington rodding and short fusion for thoracolumbar fractures. Thirty-one had no or minimal pain and 23 were employed. Initial kyphosis of 8 degrees had increased to an average of 13 degrees. There was no correlation between kyphosis and pain in this group.[29]

We prefer universal instrumentation with multilevel hooks and pedicle fixation. Hooks placed in the laminae or transverse processes provide excellent fixation in nonosteoporotic bone.[19,20] Transverse connection improves rotational stability in rods longer than 12 cm,[83a] and are attached inside of each claw. Rods are readily contoured to promote normal lordosis, and distraction and compression can be applied to improve alignment. Generally, two levels distal to the pathologic segment are necessary in the lumbar spine, with hooks configured in a claw. Rather than use three hooks on each side of the fracture, we often use just two, skipping a level between hooks. This is biomechanically equivalent to a claw plus a compressing or distracting hook. Generally, we prefer to perform "short fusions" to allow the option—exercised in about one-third of patients—to remove the instrumentation 24 months later.

We have at least 2-year follow-up in 136 patients who have undergone the extracavitary approach and hook/rod fixation for trauma. Neurological deficits improved in over 70% of deficited patients. Although correction initially was 12 degrees, at 2 years it was 8 degrees. Two hardware

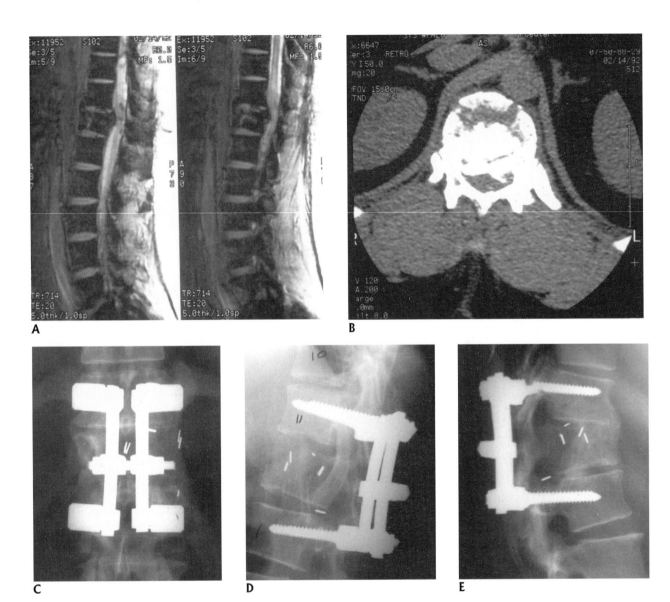

FIGURE 8-6 Forty-year-old firefighter with T12 fracture and conus injury following a fall. Sagittal MRI image **A** and axial computed tomogram **B** with canal compromise and conus injury. The patient underwent an extracavitary approach with single-level pedicle fixation. Anteroposterior **C** and lateral **D** radiographs were obtained one year after the injury, 6 months after he had returned to firefighting. **E** Routine follow-up radiographs were performed 2 years after the injury. There has been a loss of correction and the superior screws have fractured, but the fusion is well healed. The patient denied back pain or other problems.

failures occurred, and 47 patients had their hardware removed. There were 6 nonunions, including the 2 hardware failures. Additional complications included infection (4 patients), nonunions in 4, and unexpected pneumothoraces in 3. There were no neurological injuries.

Since 1986, we have incorporated transpedicular fixation in lumbar fractures when feasible. As identified elsewhere in this book, screw fixation provides excellent biomechanical stability. Because of that, many have advocated fixation only one level above and below the fracture.[80] In ca-

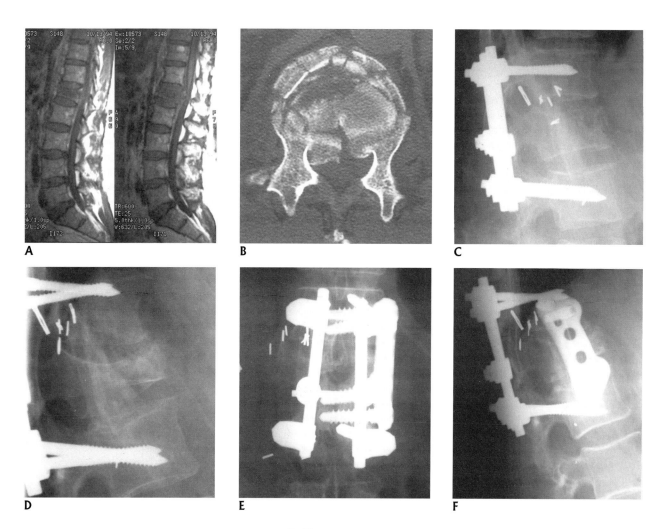

FIGURE 8–7 Fifty-one-year-old male with L1 fracture suffered in rollover accident, with cauda equina syndrome. MRI **A** and axial computed tomogram **B** show marked canal compromise. **C** Lateral radiograph following extracavitary approach and anterolateral grafting; the patient had some neurological improvement. **D** At 12 months, the patient complained of increasing back pain; radiographs show loss of correction, and nuclear scanning was consistent with nonunion. **E** The patient subsequently underwent a retroperitoneal anterior fusion with plating. Note the short plate, used to allow anterior fixation but to avoid the pedicle screws that the patient did not want removed.

daver studies, this provides excellent resistance to local forces.[3] However, our clinical experience has been less positive.

In 27 patients, single-level transpedicular fixation was incorporated. Neurological results were similar to results from other fixation techniques, and all but one patient fused. Average initial correction was 13; degrees at 1 year, however, it was 6 degrees (Fig. 8–6). This loss of correction with single-level fixation has been observed elsewhere as well.[77] If two levels were fixated above the fracture, most correction was maintained: since 1992, this has been our preferred technique for fracture fixation. Indeed, even in deformity, longer-segment pedicle fixation allows distraction and realignment (Figs. 8–2 and 8–8).

Anterior fixation is seldom used at our institution. It is reserved for fractures requiring surgery in which no posterior element injury has occurred, which is uncommon. In spite of some biomechanical evidence to the contrary, we do not believe it as stiff as posterior fixation. Indeed, a well-seated tricortical bone graft may impart just as much stiffness.

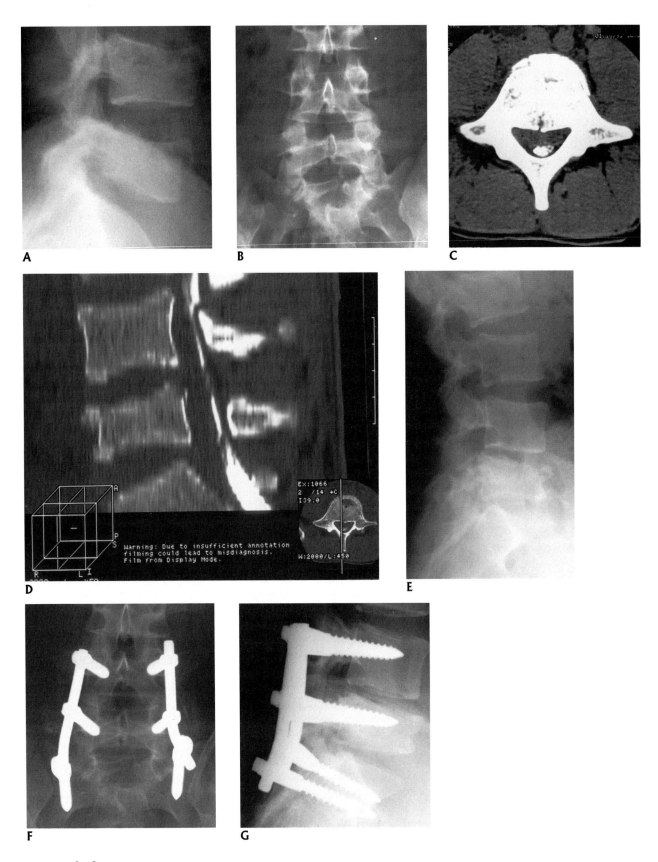

FIGURE 8–8 **A, B** Twenty-year-old male who suffered minor L5 fracture in a construction accident. **C, D** Because of an S1 radiculopathy, he underwent intrathecal computed tomography, which demonstrated a large epidural hematoma but little bone injury. The patient was treated nonoperatively in a TLSO for 4 months, without radiologic changes. **E** However, during rehabilitation after removal of the orthosis, the patient developed increasing back pain, and radiographs showed an unstable L5–S1 listhesis. **F, G** Following L4–S1 fusion, the patient did well. The surgeon elected to extend the fusion to L4 because of concerns about the integrity of L5, even though surgery was performed 6 months after the injury.

Sacral Fractures

Isolated sacral fractures represent less than 5% of spinal fractures and are commonly diagnosed quite late, as a consequence of late pain or bowel and bladder compromise. In our series, all were associated with direct impact, although others have reported them to be more common due to severely translated pelvic fractures. Indeed, some have suggested that as many as 50% of pelvic fractures extend into the sacrum.[28] This means, then, that most are the result of high-velocity impact, and the likelihood of life-threatening injury to the pelvic contents exists.

Sacral fractures have been classified by location, which may have prognostic value (Fig. 8–9).

- Type I fractures, the most common type, are through the ala, and may involve the L5 nerve root as it courses anterolaterally on the sacrum.
- Type II fractures (about 15% of the total) extend into the foramina, and cause, if anything, S1 abnormalities.
- Type III fractures are vertical and extend through the spinal canal.
- Type IV are vertical fractures through the spinal canal.

Type III and IV fractures may be associated with cauda equina injury.[11,28,44]

Evaluation should include careful physical examination of the rectum and neurological examination of the sacral roots. CT performed to rule out pelvic trauma may visualize the fracture but should not be assumed to be diagnostic. Diagnosis of sacral fracture, especially vertical fractures, is sometimes made on plain radiographs. More commonly, coned-down sacral views and high-resolution CT with reconstruction diagnose the fracture. We rarely even request the sacral views, preferring to proceed immediately to CT when sacral fracture is suspected clinically or on the basis of associated trauma.

CT is inadequate in patients with neurological deficit. Historically, we have used myelography and postmyelogram CT to define root compression due to bone fragments or hematoma. However, getting dye to flow into the sacral root sleeves may be difficult.[82] More recently we have found that MRI with specific attention to the sacrum to define nerve root compression is as effective.

In the absence of neurological deficit, most isolated sacral fractures are successfully treated with a few days of bedrest and immobilization in a hip Spica. Fractures with severe translation may require pelvic fixation; the limiting factor is the state of the pelvis.[41,79] Isolated sacral dislocations may be surgically stabilized with screw and plate reconstruction.[90] We use standard lateral mass plate systems with 30-mm screws entering lateral to the foramina, angled 30 degrees medially at L5 and S1, and 20- to 25-mm screws directed 20 degrees laterally at S2–S4.

Patients with cauda equina syndrome with vertical fractures are more likely to recover from surgi-

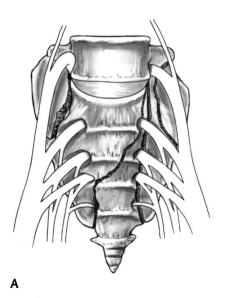
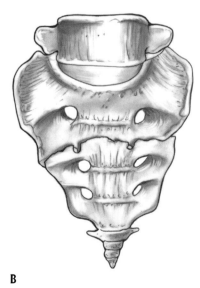

FIGURE 8–9

Sacral fractures: **A** vertical sacral fractures. Far left is a Type I fracture through the ala. The Type III fracture (also shown on the left) extends through multiple neural foramina. **B** A Type II midsacral fracture extends through sacral foramina.

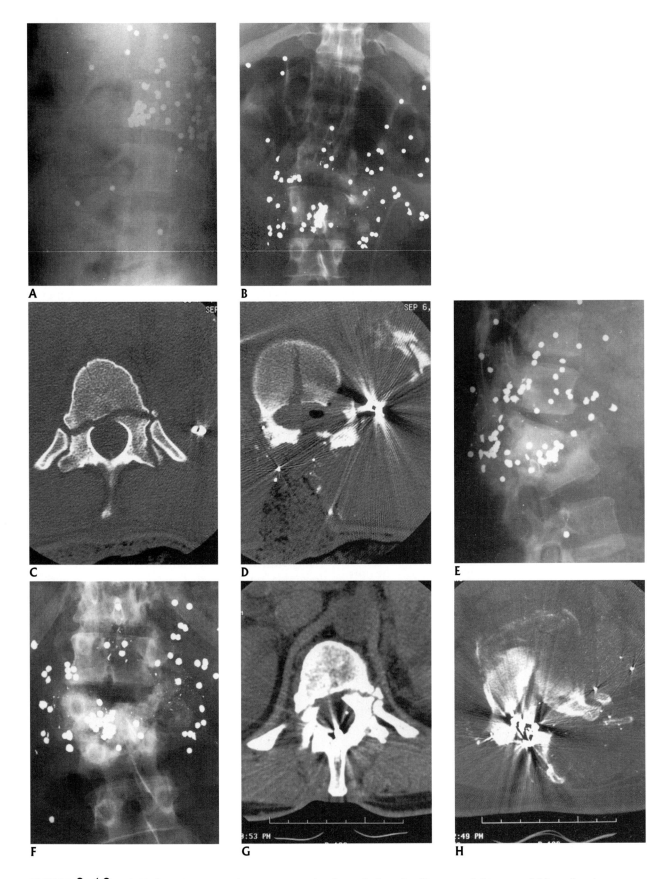

FIGURE 8–10 **A–H** Gunshot wound to spine causing later deformity. Twenty-eight-year-old female who sustained shotgun blast to the abdomen, with complete paraplegia. **A** A lateral radiograph and **B** Anteroposterior radiograph were taken shortly after admission. **C, D** Computed tomograms of L1 and L2: note that pedicles are intact at L1, and body fracture is in apposition. At L2, the right pedicle and lamina are intact. The patient was maintained in a TLSO for 6 months and was doing well at 1 year after the injury. **E, F** She returned 2 years after the injury with severe back pain and deformity. **G,** L1; **H,** L2 Computed tomography was unchanged.

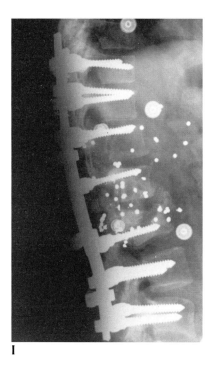 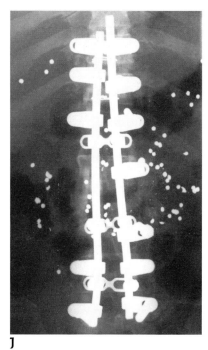

FIGURE 8–10 *(continued)*
I, J Following an extracavitary approach for anterior fusion and multilevel fixation with restoration of alignment, the patient was pain-free.

cal than expectant treatment. In the unusual patient with dislocations of the anterior sacrum, anterior sacral resection followed by posterior fixation is necessary (see Chapter 10). With posterior comminuted fracture or dislocation, laminectomy may result in significant improvement.[37] Again, fixation may be necessary in many of these patients.

Sacral laminotomy or foraminotomy is occasionally indicated for nerve root abnormalities, although we have seen very few persistent deficits from these lesions.

Gunshot Wounds of the Spine

Gunfire is now the third most common cause of neural injury of the thoracolumbar spinal contents. However, it is increasingly recognized that surgical indications are quite limited. Indeed, in our series, surgery failed to improve neurological outcome or decrease complications; it did, however, increase costs substantially.

Early evaluation and treatment are primarily directed toward associated trauma. Over 75% of patients with gunshot wounds of the chest and abdomen have injury to critical viscera. Thus appropriate surgical consultation and radiologic studies, including CT, sonography, and often angiography, should be obtained immediately.[60]

Initial treatment of the spinal injury is limited to antibiotics and debridement. We do not recommend high-dose methylprednisolone in most patients with cord or nerve root transection or open injury because there is no evidence for efficacy and risks are high. Rather, we limit steroids only to patients with no evidence of canal violation who have "blast" injuries or bone fractures causing neural compression. Such injuries are decidedly uncommon.

Radiologic studies typically include plain radiographs to determine the extent of bone fracture and canal violation. MRI is rarely useful because of metal fragments; rather, we recommend myelography and postmyelographic CT. We usually wait several days to allow dural tears to seal.

Surgical treatment is indicated only in patients with incomplete cord injury and a mass caused by bullet or bone, or radicular abnormalities due to root compression.[22,103] During the last five years, we have performed only four operations for decompression of patients in either category; one patient with root compression due to bullet fragment improved.[65a]

The second potential problem in gunshot patients is that of stability. Most injuries of the thoracolumbar spine are stable and do not require immobilization; indeed, without multiple insults, it is unlikely that sufficient structural components can be injured to put the stability at risk. Late deformity can occur, however (Fig. 8–10).

Prognosis

The prognosis for neurological recovery in spinal trauma is most related to admission status. Certainly, patients with residual function are more likely to improve than those without motor function. However, the natural tendency in neurological trauma is for improvement. Whether this is a consequence of the resolution of edema, neuronal recruitment, or resolution of spinal shock is irrelevant. Improvement is also unpredictable. Indeed, a small percentage of patients with apparent complete paraplegia demonstrate meaningful neurological improvement.[32]

Correlation with canal compromise is less consistent. Deformation of neural structures is as much a consequence of distortion by distraction, as discussed by Breig, as it of compression. This may explain why patients deteriorate during indirect decompression, whether by axial distraction during instrumentation or by laminectomy.[14,30]

For how long can recovery be expected to occur? Our unpublished observation is that maximum recovery tends to occur within 6 months in patients undergoing surgical treatment and 18 months in those treated nonsurgically.

The literature in the area of prognosis is difficult to interpret, because most of it regards the cervical spinal cord, which, of course, is different from the lumbar spine with its conus and cauda equina. Ranges reported extend from 6 months[98] to 3 years.[83] Occasional deterioration occurs: as is true for the cervical spine, it is most commonly due to mechanical reasons such as increasing deformity. However, on occasion in patients with severe canal compromise and contusion, progressive edema leads to inevitable deterioration and paraplegia. Emergent surgical decompression in an effort to reverse this process is rarely successful.

Rehabilitation

Certainly, this book is not the place to provide a meaningful discussion of rehabilitation. Rather, the authors again want to emphasize the importance of the early and definitive participation of a transdisciplinary team in the management of patients with neurological deficit. Such treatment is ideally provided in specialized spinal cord injury centers, rather than in general rehabilitation units.[50,93] Our present health care environment often makes appropriate rehabilitation difficult to access, but evidence remains clear that rehabilitation is probably more important than even surgery in promoting functional recovery.

REFERENCES

1. Akbarina BA, Crandall DG, Burkus JK, et al: Use of long rods and a short arthrodesis for burst fractures of the thoracolumbar spine: A long-term follow-up study. J Bone Joint Surg 76A:1629–1635, 1994.

2. Apel DM, Marrero G, King J, et al: Avoiding paraplegia during anterior spinal surgery: The role of somatosensory evoked potential monitoring with temporary occlusion of segmental spinal arteries. Spine 16S:365–370, 1991.

3. Ashman RB, Birch JG, Bone LB, et al: Mechanical testing of spinal instrumentation. Clin Orthop 112:27–43, 1988.

4. Atlas SW, Regenbogen V, Rogers LF, et al: The radiographic characterization of burst fractures of the spine. Am J Radiol 147:575–582, 1986.

5. Baisden JA, Maiman DJ: The argument for elective surgery in spinal cord injury. In Benzel EZ (ed): Controversies in spinal surgery. WB Saunders, in press 1998.

6. Bedbrook GM: A balanced viewpoint in the early management of patients with spinal injuries who have neurological damage. Paraplegia 23:8–15, 1985.

7. Benzel EC, Larson SJ: Functional recovery after decompressive operation for thoracic and lumbar spine fractures. Neurosurgery 19:772–778, 1986.

8. Bohlman HH, Andersen PA: Anterior decompression and arthrodesis of the cervical spine. Long-term motor improvement. J Bone Joint Surg 74:671–682, 1992.

9. Bohlmann HH: Treatment of fractures and dislocations of the thoracic and lumbar spine. J Bone Joint Surg 67A:165–169, 1985.

10. Bohlmann HH, Freehafer A: Late anterior decompression of spinal cord injuries. J Bone Joint Surg 57:1025–1028, 1975.

11. Bonnin JG: Sacral fractures and injuries to cauda equina. J Bone Joint Surg 27:113–127, 1945.

12. Bracken MB, Shepard MJ, Holford TR, et al: Administration of methylprednisolone for 24 or 48 hours or tirilizad mesylate for 48 hours in the treatment of acute spinal cord injury. Results of the Third National Acute Spinal Cord Injury Randomized Con-

trolled Trial. National Acute Spinal Cord Injury Study. JAMA 277:1597–1604, 1997.

13. Bradford DS, McBride GG: Surgical management of thoracolumbar spine fractures with incomplete neurologic deficits. Clin Orthop 218:201–216, 1987.

14. Breig A: Adverse mechanical tension in the central nervous system. Uppsala: Almquist and Wiksell, 1978.

15. Bryant CE, Sullivan JA: Management of thoracic and lumbar spine fractures with Harrington distraction rods supplemented with segmental wiring. Spine 8:532–537, 1983.

16. Burke DC, Murray DD: The management of thoracic and thoraco-lumbar injuries of the spine with neurologic involvement. J Bone Joint Surg 58B:72–78, 1976.

17. Cantor JB, Lebwohl NH, Garvey T, et al: Nonoperative management of stable thoracolumbar burst fractures with early ambulation and bracing. Spine 18:971–976, 1993.

18. Clohisy JC, Akbarnia BA, Bucholz RD, et al: Neurological recovery associated with anterior decompression of spine fractures at the thoracolumbar junction. Spine 17:S325–330, 1992.

19. Convery FR, Minteer MA, Smith RW, et al: Fracture/dislocation of the dorsal-lumbar spine: Acute operative stabilization by Harrington instrumentation. Spine 3:160–166, 1978.

20. Cotrel Y, Dubousset J, Guillaumat M: New universal instrumentation in spinal surgery. Clin Orthop 227:10–23, 1988.

21. Crutcher JP Jr, Anderson PA, King HA, et al: Indirect spinal canal decompression in patients with thoracolumbar burst fractures treated by posterior distraction rods. J Spinal Dis 4:39–48, 1991.

22. Cybulski GR, Stone JL, Kant R: Outcome of laminectomy for civilian gunshot injuries of the terminal spinal cord and cauda equina: Review of 88 cases. Neurosurgery 24:392–397, 1989.

23. Davies WE, Morris JH, Hill V: An analysis of conservative (nonsurgical) management of thoracolumbar fractures and fracture dislocations with neural damage. J Bone Joint Surg 62A:1324–1328, 1980.

24. de Klerk LWL, Fontijne PJ, Stijnen T, et al: Spontaneous remodeling of the spinal canal after conservative management of thoracolumbar burst injuries. Spine 23:1057–1060, 1998.

25. Delamarter RB, Sherman J, Carr JB: Pathophysiology of spinal cord injury. J Bone Joint Surg 77:1042–1049, 1995.

26. Denis F: The three column spine and its significance in the classification of acute thoracolumbar spinal injuries. Spine 8:817–831, 1983.

27. Denis F, Armstrong GW, Searls K, et al: Acute thoracolumbar burst fractures in the absence of neurologic deficit: A comparison between operative and nonoperative treatment. Clin Orthop 189:142–149, 1984.

28. Denis F, Davis S, Comfort T: Sacral fractures: An important problem. Restrospective analysis of 236 cases. Clin Orthop 227:67–81, 1988.

29. Devilee R, Sanders R, de Lange S: Treatment of fractures and dislocations of the thoracic and lumbar spine by fusion and Harrington instrumentation. Arch Orthop Trauma Surg 114:100–102, 1995.

30. Dickson JH, Harrington PR, Erwin WD: Results of reduction and stabilization of the severely fractured thoracic and lumbar spine. J Bone Joint Surg 60A:799–805, 1978.

31. Donovan WH: Operative and nonoperative treatment of spinal cord injury. Paraplegia 32:375–388, 1994.

32. Duh MS, Shepard MJ, Wilberger JE, et al: The effectiveness of surgery on the treatment of acute spinal cord injury and its relation to pharmacological treatment. Neurosurgery 35:240–249, 1994.

33. Dunn HK: Anterior spine stabilization and decompression for thoracolumbar injuries. Orthop Clin North Am 17:113–119, 1986.

34. Edwards CC, Rosenthal MS, Gellad F, et al: The fate of retropulsed bone following vertebral body fracture: Late stenosis or resorption? Orthop Trans 13:32–33, 1989.

35. Emery SE, Pathria MN, Wilber RG, et al: Magnetic resonance imaging of the post traumatic spinal ligament injury. J Spinal Dis 2:229–233, 1989.

36. Ferguson RL, Allen BL: An algorithm for the treatment of unstable thoracolumbar fractures. Orthop Clin North Am 17:105–112, 1986.

37. Fisher RG: Sacral fracture with compression of the cauda equina: Surgical treatment. J Trauma 28:1678–1680, 1988.

38. Fontijne WPJ, de Klerke, Braakman R, et al: CT scan prediction of neurological deficit in thoracolumbar burst fractures. J Bone Joint Surg 74:683–685, 1992.

39. Frankel HL, Hancock DO, Hyslop G, et al: The value of postural reduction in the initial management of closed injuries of the spine with paraplegia and quadriplegia. Paraplegia 7:179–192, 1969.

40. Fredrickson BA, Edwards WT, Rauschning W, et al: Vertebral burst fractures: An experimental, morphologic, and radiographic analysis. Spine 17:1012–1021, 1992.

41. Frederickson BC, Yuan HA, Miller HE: Treatment of painful long-standing displaced fracture-dislocations of the sacrum. Clin Orthop Rel Res 166:93–95, 1982.

42. Gertzbein SD: Spine update: Classification of thoracic and lumbar fractures. Spine 19:626–628, 1994.
43. Gertzbein SD, Court-Brown CM, Marks P, et al: Neurological outcome following surgery for spinal fractures. Spine 13:641–644, 1988.
44. Gibbons KJ, Soloniuk DS, Razack N: Neurological injury and patterns of sacral fractures. J Neurosurg 72:889–893, 1990.
45. Guerra J Jr, Garfin SR, Resnick D: Vertebral burst fractures: CT analysis of the retropulsed fragment. Radiology 153–772, 1984.
45a. Guttmann L: The conservative management of closed injuries of the vertebral column resulting in damage to the spinal cord and nerve roots. In Vinken PJ, Bruyn GW, Braakman R (eds): Handbook of clinical neurology, vol 25: Injuries of the spinal and spinal cord. Amsterdam, North Holland, 1975, pp 285–306.
46. Hanley EN, Simpkins A, Phillips ED: Fractures of the thoracic, theracolumbar and lumbar spine: Classification, basis for treatment, and timing of surgery. Serminar Spine Surg 2:2–7, 1990.
47. Harrington PR: The history and development of Harrington instrumentation. Clin Orthop 227:3–5, 1988.
48. Harrington RM, Budorick T, Hoyt T, et al: Biomechanisms of indirect reduction of bone retropulsed into the spinal canal in vertebral fracture. Spine 18:692–699, 1993.
49. Hartman MB, Chrin AM, Rechtine GR: Non-operative treatment of thoracolumbar fractures. Paraplegia 33:73–76, 1995.
50. Heinemann AW, Yarkony GM, Roth EJ, et al: Functional outcome following spinal cord injury: A comparison of specialized spinal cord injury center versus general hospital short-term care. Arch Neurol 46:1098–1102, 1989.
51. Henderson RL, Reid DC, Saboe LA: Multiple noncontiguous spine fractures. Spine 16:128–131, 1991.
52. Holdsworth FW: Fractures, dislocations, and fracture-dislocations of the spine. J Bone Joint Surg 52A:1534–1551, 1970.
53. Hollowell J, Maiman DJ: Management of thoracolumbar trauma. In Rea GL, Miller CA (eds): Spinal trauma. Am Assn Neurol Surg Joint Sec Disorders Spine Peripheral Nerves, 1994, pp. 180–197.
54. Horsey WJ, Tucker WS, Hudson AR, et al: Experience with early anterior operation in acute injuries of the cervical spine. Paraplegia 15:110–122, 1977.
55. Hu SS, Capen DA, Rimoldi RL, et al: The effect of surgical decompression on neurologic outcome after lumbar fractures. Clin Orthop Rel Res 288:166–173, 1993.
56. Jacobs RR, Asher MA, Snider RK: Thoracolumbar spinal injuries: A comparative study of recumbent and operative treatment in 100 patients. Spine 5:463–477, 1980.
57. Johnsson R, Herrlin K, Hagglind G, et al: Spinal canal remodeling after thoracolumbar fractures with intraspinal bone fragments. Acta Orthop Scand 62:125–127, 1991.
58. Kaneda K, Abumi K, Fujiya M: Burst fractures with neurologic deficits of the thoracolumbar-lumbar spine: Results of anterior decompression and stabilization with anterior instrumentation. Spine 9:788–795, 1984.
59. Keene JS, Fischer SP, Vanderby R Jr, et al: Significance of acute posttraumatic bony encroachment of the neural canal. Spine 14:799–802, 1989.
60. Kihtir T, Ivatury RR, Simon R, et al: Management of transperitoneal gunshot wounds of the spine. J Trauma 31:1579–1583, 1991.
61. Knight RQ, Stornelli DP, Chan DP, et al: Comparison of operative versus nonoperative treatment of lumbar burst fractures. Clin Orthop Rel Res 293:112–121, 1993.
62. Krompinger WJ, Fredrickson BE, Mino DE, et al: Conservative treatment of fractures of the thoracic and lumbar spine. Orthop Clin North Am 17:161–170, 1986.
63. Krueger MA, Green DA, Hoyt D, et al: Overlooked spine injuries associated with lumbar transverse process fractures. Clin Orthop 327:191–195, 1996.
64. Larson SJ: Unstable thoracic fractures: Treatment alternatives and the role of the neurosurgeon. Clin Neurosurg 27:624–640, 1980.
65. Lazorthes G, Gouaze A, Zadeh JO, et al: Arterial vascularization of the spinal cord. J Neurosurg 35:253–262, 1971.
65a. Lemke DM, Hollowell JP, Maiman DJ: Civilian firearm spinal cord injury. In Frontiers in head and neck trauma: Clinical and biomechanical. Yoganandan N, Pintar FA, Larson SJ, Sances A Jr (eds). IOS Press, The Netherlands, pp 88–91, 1998.
66. Lemons VR, Wagner FC, Montesano PX: Management of thoracolumbar fractures with accompanying neurologic injury. Neurosurgery 30:667–671, 1992.
67. Levi I, Wolf A, Rigamonti D, et al: Anterior decompression in cervical spine trauma: Does timing of surgery affect outcome? Neurosurgery 29:216–222, 1991.
68. Maiman DJ, Barolat G, Larson SJ: Management of bilateral locked facets of the cervical spine. Neurosurgery 18:542–547, 1986.
69. Maiman DJ, Larson SJ, Benzel EC: Neurological improvement associated with late decompression of the thoracolumbar spinal cord. Neurosurgery 14(3):302–307, March 1984.

70. Maiman DJ, Sypert GW: Management of trauma of the thoracolumbar junction: Part I. Contemp Neurosurg 11 (4):1–6, 1989.

71. Maiman DJ, Sypert GW: Management of trauma of the thoracolumbar junction: Part II. Contemp Neurosurg 11 (5):1–6, 1989.

72. Malcolm BW, Bradford DS, Winter RB, et al: Posttraumatic kyphosis: A review of forty-eight surgically treated patients. J Bone Joint Surg 63A:891–899, 1981.

73. Marshall LF, Knowlton S, Garfin SR, et al: Deterioration following spinal cord injury. J Neurosurg 66:400–404, 1987.

74. McAfee PC, Bohlman HH, Yuan HA: Anterior decompression of traumatic thoracolumbar fractures with incomplete neurological deficit using a retroperitoneal approach. J Bone Joint Surg 67:89–104, 1985.

75. McAfee PC, Yuan HA, Fredrickson BE, et al: The value of computed tomography in thoracolumbar fractures: An analysis of one hundred consecutive cases and a new classification. J Bone Joint Surg 65A:461–473, 1983.

76. McEvoy RD, Bradford DS: The management of burst fractures of the thoracic and lumbar spine: Experience in 53 patients. Spine 10:631–637, 1983.

77. McLain RF, Sparling E, Benson DR: Early failure of short-segment pedicle instrumentation for thoracolumbar fractures: A preliminary report. J Bone Joint Surg 75A:162–167, 1993.

78. Mumford J, Weinstein JN, Spratt KF, et al: Thoracolumbar burst fractures: The clinical efficacy and outcome of nonoperative management. Spine 18:955–970, 1993.

79. Nagi ON, Dhillon MS, Gill SS: Bilateral fracture dislocation of the sacrum without injury to the anterior pelvis. Orthopedics 16:215–217, 1993.

80. Olerud S, Karlstrom G, Sjostrom L: Transpedicular fixation of thoracolumbar vertebral fractures. Clin Orthop 227:44–51, 1988.

81. Osebold WR, Weinstein SL, Sprague BL: Thoracolumbar spine fractures: Results of treatment. Spine 6:13–34, 1981.xs

82. Phelan ST, Jones DA, Bishay M: Conservative management of transverse fractures of the sacrum with neurological features. J Bone Joint Surg 73B:969–71, 1991.

83. Piepmeier JM, Jenkins NR: Late neurological changes following traumatic spinal cord injury. J Neurosurg 69:399–402, 1988.

83a. Pintar FA, Maiman DJ, Yoganandan N, KD, Hollowell JP, Woodard E: Rotational stiffness of a lumbar spinal pedicle screw/rod system. J Spinal Disord 8:49–55, 1995.

84. Rechtine G: Non-surgical treatment of thoracolumbar trauma. Presented at Am Spinal Injury Assn Ann Mtg, Houston, TX, April 1997.

85. Reid D, Hu R, Davis L, et al: The nonoperative treatment of burst fractures of the thoracolumbar junction. J Trauma 28:1188–1194, 1988.

86. Roaf R: A study of the mechanics of spinal injuries. J Bone Joint Surg 42B:810–823, 1960.

87. Roberts JB, Curtis PH Jr: Stability of the thoracic and lumbar spine in traumatic paraplegia following fracture-dislocation. J Bone Joint Surg 52A:1115–1130, 1970.

88. Scapinelli R, Candiotto S: Spontaneous remodeling of the spinal canal after burst fractures of the low thoracic and lumbar region. J Spinal Dis 8:486–493, 1995.

89. Shuman WP, Rogers JV, Sickler ME, et al: Thoracolumbar burst fractures: CT dimensions of spinal canal relative to post-surgical improvement. Am J Neuroradiol 6:337–341, 1985.

90. Simonian PT, Routt C, Harrington RM, et al: Internal fixation for the transforaminal sacral fracture. Clin Orthop Rel Res 323:202–209, 1996.

91. Singer BR: The functional prognosis of thoracolumbar vertebrae fractures without neurological deficit: A long-term follow-up study of British army personnel. Injury 26:519–521, 1995.

92. Stauffer ES: Neurologic recovery following injury to the cervical spinal cord and nerve roots. Spine 9:532–534, 1984.

93. Stover SL, DeLisa JA, Whiteneck G (eds): Spinal cord injury: Clinical outcomes from the model system. Gaithersburg, MD: Aspen Publishers, 1995.

94. Sullivan JA: Sublaminar wiring of Harrington distraction rods for unstable thoracolumbar fractures. Clin Orthop 189:178–185, 1984.

95. Tator CH, Duncan EG, Edmonds EV, et al: Comparison of surgical and conservative management in 208 patients with acute spinal cord injury. Can J Neurol Sci 14:60–69, 1987.

96. Tator CH, Duncan EG, Edmonds VE, et al: Neurological recovery, mortality and length of stay after acute spinal cord injury associated with changes in management. Paraplegia 33:254–262, 1995.

97. Tencer AF, Ferguson RL, Allen BL Jr: A biomechanical study of thoracolumbar spine fractures with bone in the canal: The effect of flexion angulation, distraction, and shortening of the motion segment. Spine 10:586–589, 1985.

98. Tominaga S: Periodic, neurologic-functional assessment for cervical cord injury. Paraplegia 27:227–236, 1989.

99. Toscano J: Prevention of neurological deterioration before admission to a spinal cord injury unit. Paraplegia 26:143–150, 1988.

100. Transfeldt EE, White D, Bradford DS, et al: Delayed anterior decompression in patients with spinal cord and cauda equina injuries of the thoracolumbar spine. Spine 15:953–957, 1990.

101. Vornanen MJ, Bostman OM, Myllynen PJ: Reduction of bone retropulsed into the spinal canal in thoracolumbar vertebral body compression burst fractures: A prospective randomized study between Harrington rods and two transpedicular devices. Spine 20:1699–1703, 1995.

102. Wagner FC, Chehrazi B: Early decompression and neurological outcome in acute cervical spinal cord injuries. J Neurosurg 56:699–705, 1982.

103. Waters RL, Adkins RH: The effects of removal of bullet fragments retained in the spinal canal. Spine 16:934–939, 1991.

104. Weinshel S, Maiman DJ, Baek P, et al: Neurologic recovery in quadriplegia following operative treatment. J Spinal Disord 3:244–249, 1990.

105. Weinstein JN, Collalto P, Lehmann TR: Thoracolumbar burst fractures treated conservatively: A long-term follow-up. Spine 13:33–38, 1988.

106. Willen J, Uttam HG, Kakulas BA: Burst fractures in the thoracic and lumbar spine: A clinico-neuropathological analysis. Spine 14:1316–1323, 1989.

107. Wilmont CB, Hall KM: Evaluation of the acute management of tetraplegia: Conservative versus surgical treatment. Paraplegia 24:148–153, 1986.

108. Yazici M, Atilla B. Tepe S, et al: Spinal canal remodeling in burst fractures of the thoracolumbar spine: A computerized tomographic comparison between operative and nonoperative treatment. J Spinal Disord 9:409–913, 1996.

109. Yazici M, Gulman B, Sen S, et al: Sagittal contour restoration and canal clearance in burst fractures of the thoracolumbar junction (T12–L1): The efficacy of timing of surgery. J Orthop Trauma 9:491–498, 1995.

110. Zou D, Yoo JU, Edwards WT, et al: Mechanics of anatomic reduction of thoracolumbar burst fractures. Comparison of distraction versus distraction plus lordosis, in the anatomic reduction of the thoracolumbar burst fracture. Spine 18:195–203, 1993.

CHAPTER 9

Benign Tumors of the Spine

Osteoid Osteomas

Osteochondromas

Osteoblastomas

Giant Cell Tumors

Vascular Tumors/Hemangiomas

Aneurysmal Bone Cysts

Benign Tumors of the Spine

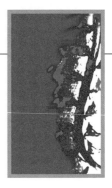

The lumbar spine is the preferred location for a variety of benign tumors of the spine that can produce a full range of clinical syndromes and may mimic malignancy.

Several of the processes considered in this chapter may not even be true neoplasms, but represent the development of masses in response to inflammation. Diagnosis for all of them tends to be rather late in their course. Furthermore, symptoms are often intermittent.

We have elected to focus only on tumors of bone: intramedullary and extramedullary lesions, epidural, and other pathologic processes not affecting the skeletal elements are not presented in this volume, since the spine itself is the emphasis of this book.

Osteoid Osteomas

Pathology

The pathogenesis of osteoid osteoma is uncertain.[57] It may represent a nidus of residual inflammation from previous trauma, with subsequent atypical growth of osteoid tissue. However, inflammatory cells are not commonly seen in or around the mass. Therefore, some investigators have proposed that osteomas arise from an infectious focus that resolves but leaves a pathologic zone of osteogenesis that grows slowly, shows immature bone cells in the nidus, and demonstrates marginal sclerosis. Lesions tend to be well vascularized and to have a self-contained blood supply, substantiating independence from the surrounding tissue. These, of course, represent the criteria for a true neoplasm.[58]

Histologically, the lesions initially present with an osteoblastic zone, which is later followed by the development of calcified osteoid. These two pictures may be mixed throughout the tumor; the histologic picture does not correlate with the clinical picture or duration of symptoms prior to surgical removal.

Clinical Presentation

Although osteoid osteomas are among the most common benign osteoblastic tumors of the spine, the overwhelming majority are located elsewhere in the skeleton: according to Delamarter et al[15], only 1.5% of them are found in the spine. Typically, they are diagnosed during the late teenage or young adult years and are rarely reported in patients over 35 years old. They are more common in men, although there appears to be no hormonal relationship.[57,58] Over half of osteoid osteomas of the spine are located in the lumbar region, and approximately 3% are in the sacrum.

In Maiuri's series of 110 spinal osteoid osteomas, 60% were in the lumbar spine. Most patients had had pain for over a year, more severe at night and during motion. The most common neurological abnormality was sciatica caused by nerve root compression produced by pedicle enlargement. Scoliosis was seen in 70% of reported cases.[44] Most patients responded very well to surgery; therefore, surgical treatment of symptomatic lesions was recommended.[46]

The lesions typically arise in a single pedicle (Fig. 9–1);[56,77] occasionally, they present in the other elements of the spine, particularly the lamina and vertebra.[56,77] Patients have had several months of mechanical back pain, with increases noted during ambulation or other physical activities.[31] Neuro-

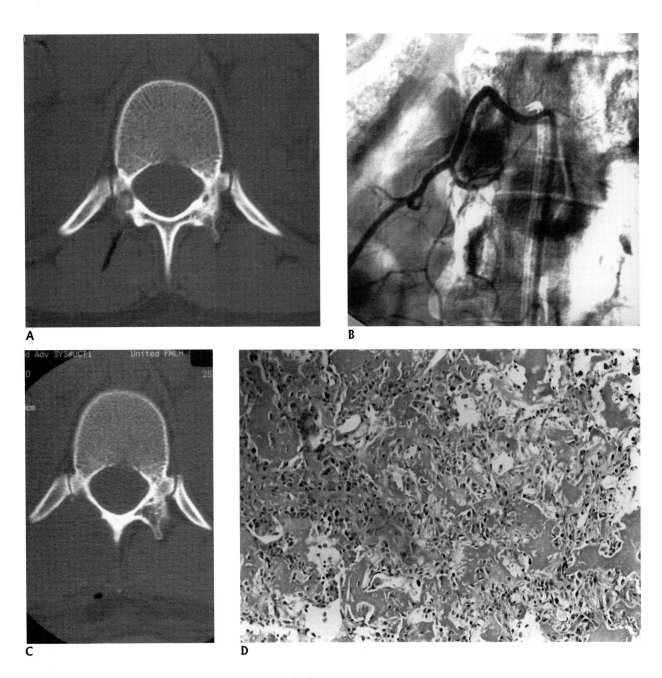

FIGURE 9-1 Osteoid osteoma in a 23-year-old female with back pain and scoliosis not responsive to antiinflammatory agents. **A** Axial CT with lesion of right T12 pedicle. **B** Spinal angiogram demonstrating vascular nidus. **C** Axial CT following surgery. The osteoid osteoma has been excised, and the residual pedicle drilled to the cortical surface. **D** Typical histology with mixed inflammatory elements and some osteoid.

logical deficit, particularly radiculopathy, occurs in approximately one-third of reported cases. Osteoid osteomas often produce local scoliosis, with the convex side of the curve away from the affected pedicle. This scoliosis is produced by local muscle spasm.[58,62]

Radiographic Evaluation and Diagnosis

Conventional radiographs in more advanced cases demonstrate a radiolucency in the affected area that is surrounded by sclerosis. Rarely, the lesion may appear dense. Radionuclide scanning demonstrates a focal area of increased activity with a halo of less obvious uptake.[79] Before magnetic resonance imaging (MRI), this was the most important study used to screen for osteoid osteomas. Unfortunately, it is not very specific and will not help define the growth rate, staging, or specific location in the vertebra. Computed tomography (CT) is critical for defining the extent of bony lesions for surgical planning (Fig. 9–1). The CT scan demonstrates no unique characteristics but is more specific in defining the extent and type of osseous abnormality, and thus aids in surgical planning.[7,25,83]

Isolated pedicle hypertrophy with a narrowed neural foramen may simulate osteoid osteoma. Thus the differentiation between tumor and local congenital changes or degenerative disease will require a careful review of the arch. One must look for abnormalities of the pars articularis, scoliosis (which is characteristic), and sclerosis to make the diagnosis of osteoid osteoma.[57]

In recent years, MRI has become quite popular for evaluating osteoid osteomas. Although it is not effective in characterizing the nature of the bony abnormalities, it readily demonstrates the calcified nidus and the less dense area around it.[83] It is, of course, critical for precisely defining spinal cord or nerve root compression in the presence of a neurological deficit.

Management

Most patients with osteoid osteomas obtain excellent or very good pain relief with aspirin or antiinflammatory drugs.

Surgical indications remain uncertain: in the presence of neurological deficit, intractable pain, or (rarely) spinal instability, surgical excision is indicated; osteomas need not be removed out of a fear that clinical phenomena will suddenly progress. The presence of progressive scoliosis is an indication for excision because the deformity may become permanent if surgical treatment is delayed beyond 1 year.[62] In our experience, this is a more important, although uncommon, indication for excision than local pain.

Total excision of an osteoid osteoma is quite feasible using direct exposure of the pedicle and radical removal (Fig. 9–1).[31] Malignant degeneration has not been reported, but regrowth will occur with incomplete excision. Thus subtotal removal, which has occasionally been recommended, is undesirable. Because of the well-localized nature of osteomas, surgical removal can often be accomplished through minimally invasive surgical approaches.[36] Recently, techniques have been described to incorporate radionuclide labeling of the tumors to assist in total extirpation. These techniques use sterilized probes that detect radioactivity.[80]

Some recommend spinal angiography prior to surgical excision.[13] This will help identify key feeding radiculospinal vessels, presumably making surgery easier. Embolization may be attempted for hypervascular lesions. We use angiography only occasionally for osteoid osteomas, since they are typically well localized, although we do use angiography for most other vascular tumors.

Osteochondromas

Osteochondromas—often incorrectly considered variants of osteoid osteomas—usually arise from the posterior elements and appear as mutifocal calcified masses with defined borders (Fig. 9–2). Although they are probably the most common bone tumor, they are uncommon in the lumbar spine and represent less than 5% of the total of these tumors.[52,70] They produce local pain and nerve root compression, the latter due to foraminal narrowing.[71] Treatment is surgical, and recurrence is uncommon. Degeneration to chondrosarcoma occurs rarely.[21]

Osteoblastomas

Osteoblastomas are much less common than osteoid osteomas, but are important benign tumors. Many consider them to be transitional lesions, between benign and malignant.[8,34,65] Osteoblastomas are more aggressive than osteoid osteomas and tend to grow by direct extension. They will recur if incompletely excised.[30]

The lumbar region is the site of approximately one-third of all spinal osteoblastomas. They typically arise in the pedicle and are likely to extend into the posterior elements. Epidural extension of the tumor is common.[8]

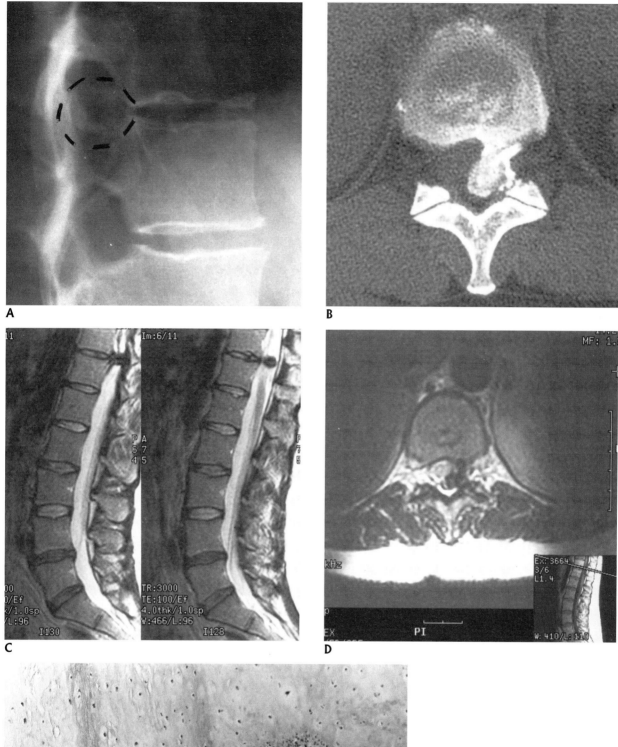
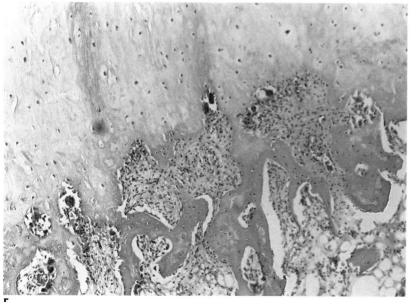

FIGURE 9–2

Osteochondroma: 41-year-old female with back pain and large T12 mass. **A** Lateral radiograph showing mass. **B** Axial CT showing large left pedicle and/or posterior element mass. **C** Lateral sagittal MRI. **D** Axial MRI with mass deviating the thecal sac. **E** Histologic sections showing obvious chondral tissue at margins (160×).

Clinical Presentation and Diagnosis

At the time of diagnosis, most patients have had symptoms for at least 1 year. Like osteoid osteomas, osteoblastomas produce painful scoliosis and present in the first decades of life, most commonly in males.[2] Pain is mechanical and associated with weight bearing. It is accompanied by localized tenderness and scoliosis with the convex side away from the vertebra.[17] Radiculopathy and even myelopathy are more common than in other types of benign bone tumors.[2]

Radiographic Evaluation

On plain radiography, an expansile lesion is typically seen (Fig. 9–3).[35] Sclerosis is not nearly as common as in the osteoid osteoma,[1] but a calcified shell is occasionally seen. Occasionally, an "ivory vertebra" is reported on plain radiography because of diffuse sclerosis; scoliosis suggests the diagnosis of osteoblastoma as opposed to, for example, a metabolic bone disease such as Paget's disease.[1,66] Radionuclide scanning is highly accurate and universally demonstrates significantly increased uptake.

Again, CT represents the optimal technique for imaging the extent of bone involvement (Fig. 9–3).[37] MRI is critical for defining soft tissue involvement and, more importantly, epidural extension. It may also suggest areas of creeping bone and periosteal involvement not seen on CT.[34]

Surgical Management

Little is known of the natural history of the osteoblastoma. Considering its typical clinical course, it is better considered a low-grade malignancy than a benign tumor.[8,22,47] It is locally aggressive and destructive of normal bone while maintaining a histologically benign picture.[30] This tumor recurs if incompletely removed, but is typically cured when aggressively resected along with judicious margins of normal bone.[34] Although there have been occasional cures following repeat incomplete resections, more commonly recurrence occurs quickly.[47,48]

For these reasons, it is critical that complete surgical excision is achieved at the first operation.[30] Excision should be extensive enough to provide an unaffected bone margin of at least 20% of the tumor diameter. Because of the extensive removal required, instrumentation to produce stability is often required. We typically place autograft across the defect when appropriate. Contrary to occasional opinion, there is no evidence that the tumor will penetrate fusion masses.

Successful surgical excision is associated with pain relief and neurological recovery. Although some older reports have suggested that radiotherapy be incorporated in treating patients following incomplete resection, more current data suggest that it be used only for patients with unresectable disease, which should rarely be the case in the lumbar spine. In nonresectable tumors, chemotherapy may also be beneficial.[6]

Giant Cell Tumors

Pathology

The giant cell tumor, much like the osteoblastoma, represents a clinical spectrum. Although usually considered benign, it has malignant variants and may behave as a malignancy even if histologically benign.[11,60,69] The giant cell sarcoma, which is extremely malignant and typically includes scattered giant cells, often occurs at the site of a previous partially removed giant cell tumor, but occasionally arises spontaneously from a typical benign giant cell tumor.[11,69] Indeed, the histology of locally aggressive giant cell tumors may demonstrate malignant characteristics (mitotic figures, loss of adhesiveness) at the margins, even as the main body of the tumor appears characteristically benign.[11,63]

The classic giant cell tumor has a 30 to 50% local recurrence rate even with radical excision, and may metastasize even when it appears benign on histology or radiography.[12,51] Alternatively, it may be multifocal.[33] There is a high (15–30%) malignant degeneration rate after radiation therapy.

Clinical Presentation

Giant cell tumors are most commonly found in the sacrum, followed by the lumbar spine. They typically originate from the vertebral body and are destructive to the point that the site of origin is often indeterminable (Fig. 9–4).[5] They are more com-

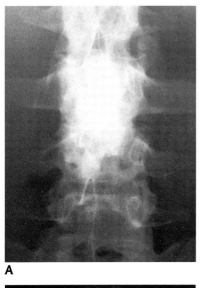
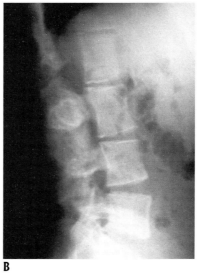
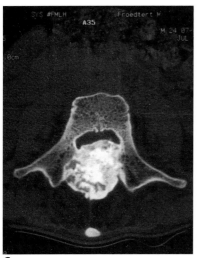
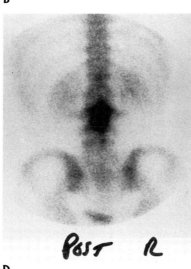
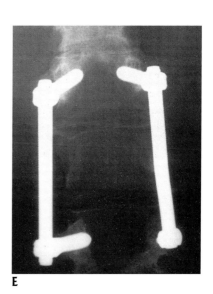

FIGURE 9-3
Osteoblastoma in young man with back pain. **A** Anteroposterior lumbar spine radiograph showing nonspecific sclerosis. **B** Lateral radiograph showing laminar thickening. **C** Axial CT image of mass expanding and filling the posterior elements. **D** Radionuclide scan showing marked uptake. **E** Postoperative radiograph. Because of the wide laminectomy and bilateral pedicle removal, spinal instrumentation has been performed.

monly seen in females under the age of 30. The most common clinical presentation is local pain, mechanical in nature, following a minor traumatic event. Rarely, neurological deficit—especially bowel and bladder deficit—will occur early.[19]

Radiographic Evaluation and Diagnosis

Lesions are easily defined radiographically. Routine radiographs will demonstrate a circumscribed lytic mass that often extends into adjacent soft tissue. There may be cystic enlargement of the vertebral body. Typically there is a minimally sclerotic pseudocapsule around the tumor. CT will accurately define the degree of vertebral body erosion. MRI is critical for evaluating the spinal canal, neural elements, and the soft tissue extent of the lesion.[78] Prior to any surgical consideration, angiography is important. These tumors are frequently quite vascular, and embolization is a valuable surgical adjunct.

In the sacrum, giant cell tumors present as lytic lesions with indistinct margins on CT. Because of the anatomy of the sacrum, plain radiographs are often inaccurate.

Management

Surgical Treatment

Accurate radiologic staging is critical to exactly define the lesion's extent. Since radical surgical excision is imperative, destabilization—which can be

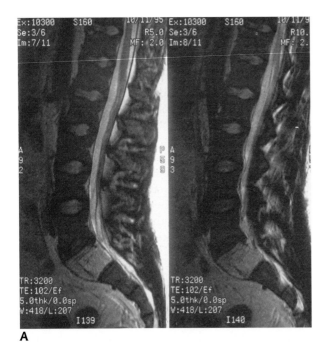
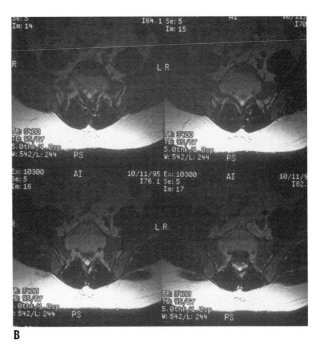
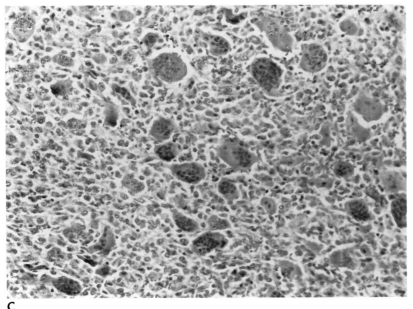

FIGURE 9–4
Atypical giant cell tumor.
A Sagittal MRI image demonstrates an expansile mass in the sacrum. In contrast to the typical lesion, which is destructive and has poorly defined margins, this tumor is well defined. **B** Axial MRI shows an expansile mass causing compromise of the spinal canal. **C** Diagnosis was not confirmed until the typical histologic picture of giant cell was seen (200×).

corrected—is of little concern. Following diagnosis either by radiography or, rarely, directed needle biopsy, aggressive, and often staged, surgical treatment should be performed.

Our preference is to employ embolization 24 hours prior to the surgical procedure to decrease blood loss. Two-stage excision of the sacrum can be accomplished, in conjunction with stabilization, as discussed below and in Chapter 10, "Primary Malignant Tumors."[26] In the distal lumbar spine, which is the most common location of giant cell tumors of the mobile spine, a bilateral extracavitary approach allows for complete resection of the vertebral body and pedicles, anterior fusion, and spinal instrumentation, which is critical.

Others have recommended two-stage procedures, performing anterior decompression and fusion at one sitting and posterior excision and instrumentation at another.[42] Stener also has reported significant success with total spondylectomy, which is more typically used for malignant tumors.[72,73] However, soft tissue extension, which may be purely lateral, may be harder to define and eliminate. Morbidity is also increased with two separate procedures.

Historically, we have used the Galveston procedure for stabilization in both lumbar and sacral tumors; recently, we have begun using Jackson screw fixation to the pelvis if bone density allows. Bone grafting is preferred over the use of methylmethacrylate: first of all, fusion will likely occur. In addition, it may be difficult to image recurrence if methylmethacrylate is used.[59]

Some have attempted radical removal of sacral giant cell tumors via transabdominal approaches alone: as noted earlier, however, local extension into adjacent vertebral bodies is common, and instability is a result of decompression. Therefore, posterior decompression, instrumentation, and fusion are usually imperative.[67,68] We recommend the modifications of the two-stage procedure presented by Gokaslan et al:[26] first, a transabdominal or bilateral anterior retroperitoneal approach is used to dissect the great vessels and viscera off the presacral space. The iliac veins should be ligated, and the L5–S1 disc excised to define the sacrum. Aggressive debulking can occur. Following closure with two drains, the patient is positioned prone, and L5 laminectomy and ligation of the thecal sac performed. The ilium is incised bilaterally lateral to the tumor, and the sacrum excised en mass. Instrumentation from L1 or L2 into the pelvis is imperative.

Loss of voluntary bowel and bladder function is often the consequence of this approach.[19] Hesitation on the part of the surgeon to perform such radical removal is ill advised because of the high rate of local recurrence; loss of bowel and bladder function in sacral tumors is largely inevitable in these patients anyway. Indeed, planned subtotal resection is of little value, since morbidity is high, prognosis similar to that of nonoperative treatment, and neurological results the same.

Our preference for radical excision is disputed by Dahlin,[14] who argues that because of the more benign characteristics of giant cells in the spine (as opposed to those in long bones), limited resections with curettage of lesions may be advisable. He recommends the use of adjunctive radiation therapy with 4000 to 5000 cGy for tumor control, and has observed few recurrences. However, the high risk of malignant sarcomatous degeneration following radiation must be considered, and hence we suggest that radical surgical excision represents optimal treatment. Furthermore, others have demonstrated a much higher rate of local recurrence and metastasis with local curettage of long bone lesions, even when the tumors had similar histological pictures.[40] Aggressive removal may also decrease the incidence of pulmonary metastasis, which occurs even in tumors that have not undergone malignant degeneration.[69]

This emphasis on careful radiographic staging and aggressive resection was validated in a major multicenter study,[28] which resulted in a spine tumor classification scheme referred to as the Weinstein-Boriani-Biagini staging system for spine tumors.[9] The authors observed that giant cell tumors isolated to the vertebrae are typically more aggressive biologically and have a much higher recurrence rate than those in the posterior elements. Similarly, recurrence rates were dramatically higher in patients treated surgically prior to referral to tertiary care centers. In many cases, this reflected inadequate staging and limited surgical approaches. Furthermore, patients with giant cell lesions that extended into the posterior musculature or the spinal canal also did more poorly.

Adjunctive Therapy

Little exists on the appropriate treatment of metastases. Chemotherapy is beneficial in selected patients, in conjunction with resection.[53,74] Metastases appear to share histologic and biologic characteristics with the primary tumor. Cheng et al recommend resection of pulmonary metastases and found that patients enjoy long-term survival even if these are incompletely resected.[12] This would appear a logical choice for management of other metastatic disease, as well.[69] The authors note, but do not emphasize, that three of four patients suffering pulmonary metastases had been treated with curettage primarily; all the metastases recurred. The question becomes, then, whether the metastatic lesions derived from the original tumor or the more malignant local recurrence.

Vascular Tumors/Hemangiomas

Pathology

The primary vascular tumor of the spine is the hemangioma. There is significant controversy as to whether or not this is even a neoplasm, since many consider hemangiomas to be hamartomas. However, some studies have indicated that they are truly neoplasms and develop de novo in the vertebra. Again, as is true for benign spinal tumors, secondary scoliosis and deformity are common. These lesions may occur anywhere in the vertebra, including the body, posterior elements, and pedicles. Approximately 25% of spinal hemangiomas are in the lumbar spine. Neural compression may occur through vertebral body collapse and associated epidural extension. Rarely do hemangiomas compress the cord primarily. Although it is strongly suspected that the involved bone is significantly weakened, there are few biomechanical data that consider the strength of the bone. The surviving bone trabeculations are probably strong enough to provide support within the lesion area.

Clinical Presentation

Hemangiomas are most commonly asymptomatic (indeed, one author has suggested that they may be found in as many as 11% of the population at autopsy[45]); when symptoms do occur, they are typically related to local pain and spasm (Fig. 9–5). Lesions tend to occur in adults, and they affect multiple vertebral levels in approximately one-third of affected individuals.

Fox and Onofrio presented a series of 59 patients with vertebral hemangiomas, of which 35 were asymptomatic. The development of neurological deficit usually followed the initial presentation of pain by an average of 4.4 months. No patients had neurological deficit without preexisting pain. On the basis of this experience, annual radiographic evaluation was recommended to follow thoracic—but not lumbar—lesions.[23] This is not our practice, since pain is almost always present prior to loss of function: we recommend that patients be cognizant of the development of back pain and report it promptly. Furthermore, painful lesions with no posterior element involvement or cortical disruption do not tend to progress rapidly.[23,38,39] Thus, rather than performing annual or periodic radiograph we wait until symptoms develop. Fox and Onofrio recommend decompressive laminectomy or minimal anterior decompression without stabilization for neurologic deficit.[23] Our more aggressive approach is discussed below.

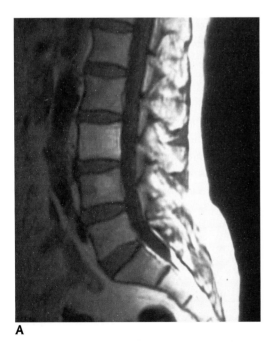
A

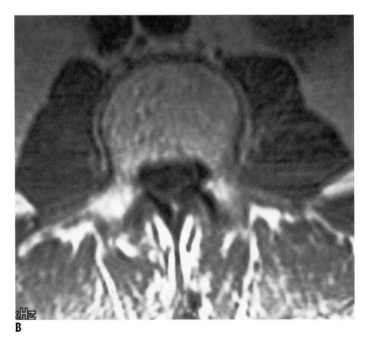
B

FIGURE 9–5 Hemangioma presenting as low back pain in a 50-year-old male. Sagittal **A** and axial **B** MRI slices show typical picture. The patient responded to antiinflammatory agents.

Radiographic Evaluation and Diagnosis

Plain radiographs typically demonstrate coarse trabeculated bone with a classic honeycomb appearance and an expanded vertebral body and, often, the arch as well (Figs. 9–5 and 9–6). Disc spaces and end plates are not usually involved. CT will demonstrate the typical striations, and may create a spoke-wheel trabecular pattern (Fig. 9–6).[81]

MRI is used to define the spinal canal, but it also presents a characteristic pattern: because there is adipose or soft tissue within the pathologic trabeculae, increased signal intensity within the bone will be seen on T1-weighted images.[61] Increased signal intensity within cellular components is observed on T2-weighted images.[24,45] The fat-density material within the lesion is of pathologic significance: these lesions tend to be clinically inactive and are associated with less hypervascularity than those containing soft tissue.[39]

Angiography is not needed to make the diagnosis. If surgery is contemplated, selective angiography is critical to define the source of the tumor's blood supply and for preoperative embolization (Fig. 9–6).[49]

Management

Drug Therapy and Immobilization

The overwhelming majority of symptomatic hemangiomas do not require surgical treatment. Pain often resolves with antiinflammatory agents and rigid immobilization for 3 to 6 months.[20] Although Fox and Onofrio recommend annual radiography,[23] their results and our series suggest that expectant follow-up is the most appropriate way of managing asymptomatic lumbar hemangiomas.

Radiotherapy

In an early series, pain and myelopathy were successfully treated with radiotherapy ranging from 3000 to 4000 Gy.[18] In spite of effective pain relief, resolution of radiologic abnormalities did not occur. Yang et al reported a series of patients with severely symptomatic hemangiomas treated with radiation only.[82] Two-thirds of these were in the thoracic spine, and 8 out of 21 were lumbar. Most patients were treated for severe pain and mild myelopathy. Of patients with severe spinal cord compression, most improved with radiation and did not require surgical treatment. The patients were followed for at least 5 years. There was no significant recurrence except in 1 patient. In a more recent series, 17 patients were treated. Pain was relieved almost completely, and most had dramatic relief of neurological deficit. Many authors, then, recommend radiotherapy as the treatment in patients considered to be poor surgical risks, or with large tumors.[4] Radiotherapy has also been recommended following incomplete excision.[10]

There is no current evidence that malignant degeneration follows radiation therapy; similarly, it is uncertain whether hemangiomas may not become malignant decades after radiation. Therefore, we reserve radiotherapy for patients with intractable pain who are poor surgical candidates, or older individuals who accept the long-term risks.

Embolization

Another nonsurgical option is embolization, since malignant degeneration will not occur and infarction has not been reported. Decreased venous engorgement may actually lead to healing in conjunction with immobilization.[27] Some have used radiation therapy in preoperative patients in lieu of embolization.[20] Increased infection and decreased fusion rates would preclude this in our practice.

Surgical Treatment

Surgical treatment is indicated in the presence of neurological deficit and deformity due to vertebral collapse or remodelling, and occasionally in patients with intractable pain.[27] Rarely does neural compression due to soft tissue extension occur in the lumbar spine, although it may occur in the thoracic region. Occasionally, during the third trimester of pregnancy, venous engorgement will cause functional neural compression and myelopathy. This process does not respond to radiation or embolization and typically requires surgical treatment.[23] Alternatively, an ischemic syndrome has

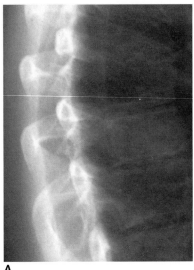

A

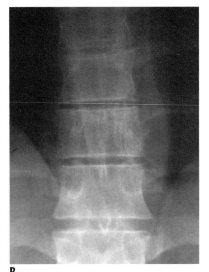

B

FIGURE 9–6
A–F Hemangioma producing progressive paraparesis in 42-year-old male. Plain lateral **A** And AP **B** Radiographs showing subtle vertebral lesion. **C** Sagittal CT scan demonstrating characteristic striations. **D** These are better seen on the axial view **E** Preembolization angiogram showing significant tumor vascularization. **F** Following embolization, the tumor's blood supply is largely obliterated.

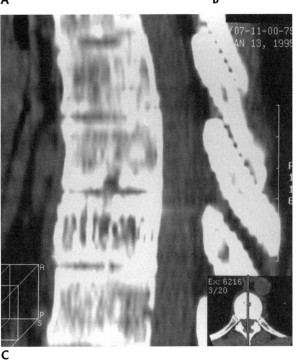

C

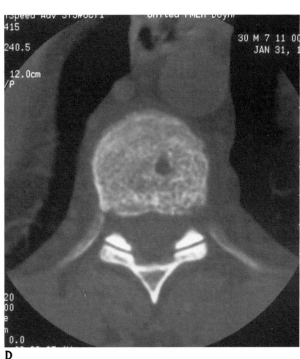

D

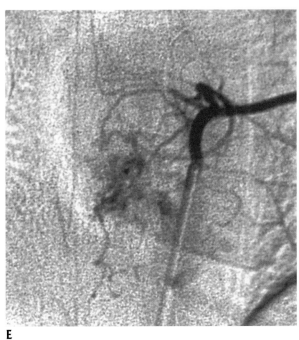

E

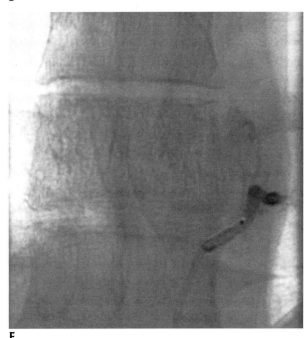

F

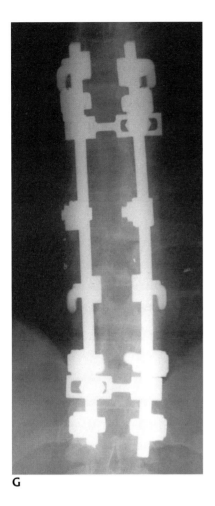
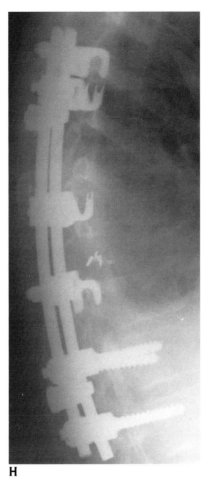

FIGURE 9-6 *(continued)*
G and H Postoperative AP
G And lateral **H** Radiographs.
The patient has undergone an extracavitary approach to the spine with vertebrectomy, removal of involved posterior elements, and anterior and posterior fusion with multilevel posterior fixation.

been observed during pregnancy; presumably vascular steal occurs due to rapid tumor enlargement.[41]

Since neurological deficit is most commonly a consequence of vertebral collapse, some have attempted vertebroplasty to solidify the body, usually using methylmethacrylate injected under pressure. This allows "decompression" to be accomplished via laminectomy and removal of epidural tissue, rather than via vertebrectomy, decreasing surgical blood loss and morbidity.[29] Two-year follow-up is available on a small number of patients, with no evidence of progression or neurological change.

We use selective angiography and embolization prior to surgical treatment.[16] As is true for other tumors, direct approaches allowing total excision should be used when possible. In cases of pedicle or posterior element involvement, transpedicular decompression and laminectomy may be useful.[50] However, in the more typical situation with vertebral body involvement, either a retroperitoneal approach or an extracavitary approach should be considered. In single-level lesions, vertebrectomy, anterior grafting, and anterior plating may be effective. However, if deformity is present, posterior instrumentation is desirable, and then the extracavitary approach is recommended. The latter will allow for effective excision even if the pedicle and posterior elements are involved in addition to the vertebral body. With complete excision, follow-up radiation is unnecessary and long-term results are excellent.

At times, and particularly in the presence of vertebral body collapse without neural compression in poor-risk patients, surgical treatment will consist of simple stabilization and fusion. This avoids the significant blood loss and morbidity of the largely anterior procedure.

Aneurysmal Bone Cysts

Aneurysmal bone cysts are actually benign neoplasms, similar in biological characteristics to

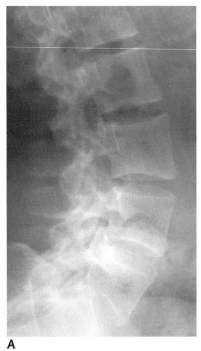
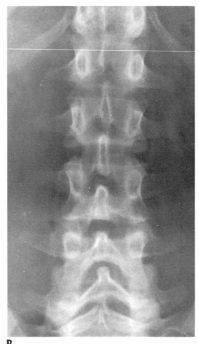
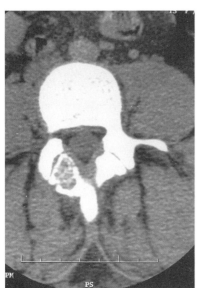
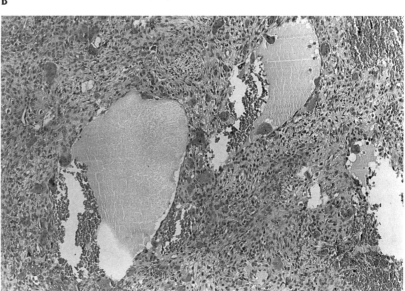

FIGURE 9–7
Aneurysmal bone cyst in 19-year-old female with persistent back pain following a fall. **A** The lateral radiograph suggests laminar thickening. **B** However, AP view appears normal. **C** Axial CT scan showing a lytic lesion. **D** Typical pathology with large venous areas.

osteoblastomas.[43] They consist of intracystic cavernous cavernomas.[3,26,76]

tients present with neurological deficit; on questioning, most have histories of local pain.[33,35]

Clinical Presentation

Aneurysmal bone cysts are typically seen in teens and more commonly in females. In our series, they have been diagnosed most frequently in young adults following minor trauma (Fig. 9–7). However, others have found local pain to be the most common presenting complaint.[54] About one-fifth of pa-

Radiographic Evaluation and Diagnosis

Although aneurysmal bone cysts are cavernous in nature, they are often not vascular at angiography.[76] In spite of that, they are the source of significant hemorrhage.[43] Typically, a lytic lesion is seen on plain radiographs and CT; a common radiographic picture following minor trauma is that of a collapsed or expanded vertebra with defective cortical bone (Fig. 9–7). Posterior element involvement is ubiquitous but may not be seen on plain radiographs. Almost one-half involve more than one vertebra.[54] MRI may demonstrate the cavernous tissue within the lesion.[78,84]

Biopsy for diagnosis is undesirable because of the hemorrhage that may occur; thus the diagnosis is often by exclusion. In addition, the diagnosis often can be made radiographically, and therefore the risks of biopsy may not be worth it.[75] The pathologic picture is of vascular tissue with small areas of bone. Large amounts of fibrous tissue in and about the trabecular bone are seen as well. Hemorrhage and hemosiderin production within the lesion are often present.

Surgical Management

Surgical treatment is indicated for pain or deformity.[55] Rarely does compression of neural structures occur, but in those circumstances, radical resection is necessary. Preoperative embolization will decrease bleeding dramatically in many instances, and in rare cases will suffice as treatment.[32] Surgical treatment should consist of complete resection of the affected portion of the spine usually by intralesional curettage of small lesions and fusion and stabilization when indicated for correction of deformity or maintenance of alignment. Incomplete surgical resection is likely to lead to recurrence. Radiation therapy is undesirable, since it is rarely effective and has been reported to result in sarcomatous degeneration.[33,55]

REFERENCES

1. Akbarnia BA, Rooholamini SA: Scoliosis caused by benign osteoblastoma of the thoracic or lumbar spine. J Bone Joint Surg 63A:1146–1155, 1981.
2. Amacher AL, Eltomey A: Spinal osteoblastoma in children and adolescents. Childs Nerv Syst 1:29–32, 1985.
3. Ameli NO, Abbassioun K, Saleh H, et al: Aneurysmal bone cyst of the spine: Report of 17 cases. J Neurosurg 63:685–690, 1985.
4. Asthana AK, Tandon SC, Pant GC, et al: Radiation therapy for symptomatic vertebral hemangioma. Clin Oncol 2:159–162, 1990.
5. Bidwell JK, Young JWR, Khalluff E: Giant cell tumor of the spine: Computed tomography appearance and review of the literature. J Comput Assist Tomogr 11:307–311, 1987.
6. Berberoglu S, Oguz A, Aribal E, et al: Osteoblastoma response to radiotherapy and chemotherapy. Med Pediatr Oncol 28:305–309, 1997.
7. Bilchik T, Heyman S, Siegel A, et al: Osteoid osteoma: The role of radionuclide bone imaging, conventional radiography, and computed tomography in management. J Nucl Med 33:269–271, 1992.
8. Boriani S, Capanna R, Donati D, et al: Osteoblastoma of the spine. Clin Orthop 278:37–45, 1992.
9. Boriani S, Weinstein JN, Biagini R: Primary bone tumors of the spine. Spine 22:1036–1044, 1997.
10. Bremnes RM, Hauge HN, Sagsveen R: Radiotherapy in the treatment of symptomatic vertebral hemangiomas: Technical case report. Neurosurgery 39:1054–1058, 1996.
11. Brien EW, Mirra JM, Kessler S, et al: Benign giant cell tumor of bone with osteosarcomatous transformation: Report of two cases. Skeletal Radiol 26:246–255, 1997.
12. Cheng JC, Johnston JO: Giant cell tumor of bone: Prognosis and treatment of pulmonary metastases. Clin Orthop 338:205–214, 1997.
13. Crouzet G, Mnif J, Vasdev A, et al: Osteoid osteoma of the spine: Radiological aspects and value of arteriography. Four cases. J Neuroradiol 16:145–159, 1989.
14. Dahlin DC: Giant cell tumor of the vertebrae above the sacrum: A review of 31 cases. Cancer 39:1350–1356, 1977.
15. Delamarter RB, Sachs BL, Thompson GH, et al: Primary neoplasms of the thoracic and lumbar spine. Clin Orthop 256:87–100, 1990.
16. Djindjian M, Nguyen JP, Gaston A, et al: Multiple vertebral hemangiomas with neurological signs. J Neurosurg 76:1025–1028, 1992.
17. Fakharani-Hein M, Griss P, Ludke A, et al: Rapidly developing scoliosis in an adolescent due to spinal osteoblastoma. Arch Orthop Trauma Surg 107:259–262, 1988.
18. Faria SL, Schlupp WR, Chiminazzo H Jr: Radiotherapy in the treatment of vertebral hemangiomas. Int J Radiat Oncol Biol Phys 11:387–390, 1985.
19. Feldenzer JA, McGauley JL, McGillicuddy JE: Sacral and presacral tumors: Problems in diagnosis and management. Neurosurgery 25:884–891, 1989.
20. Feuerman T, Divan PS, Young RF: Vertebrectomy for treatment of vertebral hemangioma without pre-

operative embolization. J Neurosurg 65:404–406, 1986.
21. Fischgrund JS, Cantor JB, Samberg LC: Malignant degeneration of a vertebral osteochondroma with epidural tumor extension: A report of the case and review of the literature. J Spinal Dis 7:86–90, 1994.
22. Floman Y, Milgrom C, Kenan S, et al: Spongious and cortical osteoblastoma of the axial skeleton. Orthopedics 8:1478–1484, 1985.
23. Fox MW, Onofrio BM: The natural history and management of symptomatic and asymptomatic vertebral hemangiomas. J Neurosurg 78:36–45, 1993.
24. Friedman DP: Symptomatic vertebral hemangiomas: MR findings. AJR 167:359–364, 1996.
25. Gamba JL, Martinez S, Apple J, et al: Computed tomography of axial skeletal osteoid osteomas. AJR 142:769–772, 1984.
26. Gokaslan ZL, Romsdahl MM, Kroll SS, et al: Total sacrectomy and Galveston L-rod reconstruction for malignant neoplasms. J Neurosurg 87:781–787, 1997.
27. Graham JJ, Yang WC: Vertebral hemangioma with compression fracture and paraparesis treated with preoperative embolization and vertebral resection. Spine 9:97–101, 1984.
28. Hart RA, Boriani S, Biagini R, et al: A system for surgical staging and management of spine tumors: A clinical outcome study of giant cell tumors of the spine. Spine 22:1773–1782, 1997.
29. Ide C, Gangi A, Rimmelin A, et al: Vertebral haemangiomas with spinal cord compression: The place of preoperative percutaneous vertebroplasty with methyl methacrylate. Neuroradiology 38:585–589, 1996.
30. Jackson RP, Reckling FW, Mantz FA: Osteoid osteoma and osteoblastoma: Similar histologic lesions with different natural histories. Clin Orthop 128:303–313, 1977.
31. Kirwan EO, Hutton PA, Pozo JL, et al: Osteoid osteoma and benign osteoblastoma of the spine. J Bone Joint Surg 66B:21–26, 1984.
32. Konya A, Szendroi M: Aneurysmal bone cysts treated by superselective embolization. Skeletal Radiol 21:167–172, 1992.
33. Kos CB, Taconis WK, Fidler MW, et al: Multifocal giant cell tumors in the spine: A case report. Spine 22:821–822, 1997.
34. Kroon HM, Schurmans J: Osteoblastoma: Clinical and radiological findings in 98 new cases. Radiology 175:783–790, 1990.
35. Kumar R, Guinto FC, Madewell JE: Expansile bone lesions of the vertebra. Radiographics 8:749–769, 1988.
36. Labbe JL, Clement JL, Duparc B, et al: Percutaneous extraction of vertebral osteoid osteoma under computed tomography guidance. Eur Spine J 4:368–371, 1995.
37. Lanzieri CF, Solodnik P, Sacher M, et al: Computed tomography of solitary spinal osteochondromas. J Comput Assist Tomogr 9:1042–1044, 1985.
38. Laredo JD, Reizine D, Bard M, et al: Vertebral hemangiomas: Radiologic evaluation. Radiology 161:183–189, 1986.
39. Laredo JD, Assouline E, Gelbert F, et al: Vertebral hemangiomas: Fat content as a sign of aggressiveness. Radiology 177:467–472, 1990.
40. Lausten GS, Jensen PK, Schiodt T, et al: Local recurrences in giant cell tumour of bone: Long-term follow up of 31 cases. Int Orthop 20:172–176, 1996.
41. Lavi E, Jamieson DG, Granat M: Epidural hemangiomas during pregnancy. J Neurol Neurosurg Psychiatry 49:709–712, 1986.
42. Lubicky J, Patel NS, Dewald RL: Two-stage spondylectomy for giant cell tumor of L4. Spine 8:112–116, 1983.
43. MacCarty CS, Dahlin DC, Doyle JB Jr, et al: Aneurysmal bone cysts of the neural axis. J Neurosurg 18:671–677, 1961.
44. Maiuri F, Signorelli C, Lavano A, et al: Osteoid osteomas of the spine. Surg Neurol 25:375–380, 1986.
45. Masaryk TJ: Neoplastic disease of the spine. Radiol Clin North Am 29:829–845, 1990.
46. Maclellan DI, Wilson FA: Osteoid osteoma of the spine. J Bone Joint Surg 49A:111–121, 1987.
47. Merryweather R, Middlemiss JH, Sanerkin NG: Malignant transformation of osteoblastoma. J Bone Joint Surg 58B:381–384, 1980.
48. Myles ST, MacRae ME: Benign osteoblastoma of childhood. J Neurosurg 68:884–888, 1988.
49. Ng VW, Clifton A, Moore AJ: Preoperative endovascular embolisation of a vertebral haemangioma. J Bone Joint Surg 79B:808–811, 1997.
50. Nguyen JP, Djindjian M, Gaston A, et al: Vertebral hemangiomas presenting with neurologic symptoms. Surg Neurol 27:391–397, 1987.
51. Nojima T, Takeda N, Matsuno T, et al: Benign metastasizing giant cell tumor of the spine. Skeletal Radiol 23: 583–585, 1994.
52. O'Connor GA, Roberts TS: Spinal cord compression in a patient with multiple osteochondromatosis. J Neurosurg 60: 420–423, 1984.
53. Osaka S, Toriyama M, Taira K, et al: Analysis of giant cell tumor of bone with pulmonary metastases. Clin Orthop 335:253–261, 1997.
54. Papagelopoulos PJ, Currier BL, Shaughnessy WJ, et al: Aneurysmal bone cyst of the spine: Management and outcome. Spine 23:621–628, 1998.

55. Parrish FS, Pevey JK: Surgical management of aneurysmal bone cyst of the vertebral column: A report of three cases. J Bone Joint Surg 49A:1597–1604, 1987.
56. Patel NP, Kumar R, Kinkhabwala M, et al: Lumbar vertebral pedicles: Radiologic anatomy and pathology. CRC Crit Rev Diagn Imaging 28:75–132, 1988.
57. Pettine KA, Klassen RA: Osteoid-osteoma and osteoblastoma of the spine. J Bone Joint Surg 68A:354–361, 1986.
58. Raskas DS, Graziano GP, Herzenberg JE, et al: Osteoid osteoma and osteoblastoma of the spine. J Spinal Disord 5:204–211, 1992.
59. Remedios D, Saifuddin A, Pringle J: Radiological and clinical recurrence of giant-cell tumour of bone after the use of cement. J Bone Joint Surg 79B:26–30, 1997.
60. Rios-Martin J, Otal-Salaverri C, Vazquez-Ramirez FJ, et al: Fine needle aspiration diagnosis of aggressive giant cell tumor of bone: A case report. Acta Cytologica 39:550–554, 1995.
61. Ross JS, Masaryk TJ, Modic MT: Vertebral hemangiomas: MR imaging. Radiology 165:165–169, 1987.
62. Saifuddin A, White J, Sherazi Z, et al: Osteoid osteoma and osteoblastoma of the spine: Factors associated with the presence of scoliosis. Spine 23:47–53, 1998.
63. Sakkers RJ, van der Heul RO, Kroon HM, et al: Late malignant transformation of a benign giant-cell tumor of bone: A case report. J Bone Joint Surg 79A:259–262, 1997.
64. Savini R, Martucci E, Prosperi P, et al: Osteoid osteoma of the spine. Ital J Orthop Trauma 14:233–238, 1988.
65. Schajowicz F, Lemos C: Malignant osteoblastoma. J Bone Joint Surg 58B:202–211, 1976.
66. Sherazi Z, Saifuddin A, Shaikh M, et al: Unusual imaging findings in association with spinal osteoblastoma. Clin Radiol 51:644–648, 1996.
67. Shikata J, Yamamuro T, Kotoura T, et al: Total sacrectomy and reconstruction for primary tumors. J Bone Joint Surg 70A:122–141, 1988.
68. Shikata J, Yamamuro T, Shimizu K, et al: Surgical treatment of giant-cell tumors of the spine. Clin Orthop 278:29–36, 1990.
69. Siebenrock KA, Unni KK, Rock MG: Giant-cell tumour of bone metastasizing to the lungs: A long-term follow-up. J Bone Joint Surg 80B:43–47, 1998.
70. Sluis R, Gurr K, Josheph M: Osteochondroma of the lumbar spine. Spine 17:1519–1521, 1992.
71. Spaziante R, Irace C, Gambardella A, et al: Solitary osteochondroma of the pedicle of L4 causing root compression: Case report. J Neurosurg Sci 32:141–145, 1988.
72. Stener B: Complete removal of vertebrae for extirpation of tumors. Clin Orthop 245:72–82, 1989.
73. Stener B, Gunterberg B: High amputation of the sacrum for extirpation of tumors: Principles and technique. Spine 3:351–366, 1978.
74. Stewart DJ, Belanger R, Benjamin RS: Prolonged disease-free survival following surgical debulking and high-dose cisplatin/doxorubicin in a patient with bulky metastases from giant cell tumor of bone refractory to "standard" chemotherapy. Am J Clin Oncol 18:144–148, 1995.
75. Tillman BP, Dahlin DC, Lipscomb DR, et al: Aneurysmal bone cyst, an analysis of 95 cases. Mayo Clin Proc 43:478–495, 1968.
76. Vergel De Rios AM, Bond JR, Shives TC, et al: Aneurysmal bone cyst: A clinicopathologic study of 238 cases. Cancer 69:2921–2931, 1992.
77. Villas C, Lopez R, Zubieta JL: Osteoid osteoma of the lumbar and sacral regions: Two cases of difficult diagnosis. J Spinal Dis 3:418–422, 1990.
78. Wetzel LH, Levine E: MR imaging of sacral and presacral lesions. AJR 154:771–775, 1990.
79. Winter PF, Johnson PM, Hilal SH, et al: Scintigraphic detection of osteoid osteoma. Radiology 122:177–178, 1977.
80. Wioland M, Sergent-Alaoui A: Didactic review of 175 radionuclide-guided excisions of osteoid osteomas. Eur J Nucl Med 23:1003–1011, 1996.
81. Yamada K, Whitbeck MG Jr, Numaguchi Y, et al: Symptomatic vertebral hemangioma: Atypical spoke-wheel trabeculation pattern. Radiat Med 15:239–241, 1997.
82. Yang ZY, Zhang LJ, Chen ZX, et al: Hemangioma of the vertebral column. Acta Radiol Oncol 24:129–132, 1985.
83. Zimmer WD, Berquist TH, McLeod RA: Bone tumors: MRI versus CT. Radiology 155:709–718, 1985.
84. Zimmer WD, Berquist TH, Sim FH: MRI of aneurysmal bone cysts. Mayo Clin Proc 59:633–636, 1984.

CHAPTER 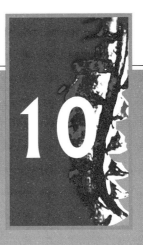 10

Primary Malignant Tumors

Diagnostic Biopsy

Plasma Cell Lesions

Chordomas

Sarcomas

Sacral-Coccygeal Tumors

Conclusions

Primary Malignant Tumors

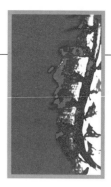

Primary tumors of the vertebral column are uncommon and present significant diagnostic and therapeutic challenges. Indeed, in a large series of almost 2,000 musculoskeletal tumors, only 1.5% originated in the thoracolumbar spine.[19,45]

Typically, back pain is the most common presenting complaint in lumbar spine and sacral tumors;[28] approximately one-half of patients have neurological abnormalities, including mild motor weakness or sensory changes, spasticity, and occasional bowel and bladder abnormalities. On physical examination, the only typical findings are paravertebral muscle spasm and local tenderness. Because of the nonspecific nature of the symptoms, late diagnosis is common.

In Delamarter's series, lesions were always visible on plain radiographs.[42] Of the 29 tumors, most underwent open biopsy; the rest, needle biopsy. Chondrosarcomas, lymphomas, chordomas, and one vascular tumor were seen. The authors recommended open biopsy for safe diagnosis prior to attempted surgical excision, considering that many tumors respond best to adjunctive therapy.

Dreghorn and colleagues similarly found a very low incidence of primary spine tumors, as compared to the entire population of patients with spine masses. Chordoma, which they often considered benign, was the most common tumor in the axial skeleton.[45] However, 70% of the chordomas in the lumbar spine were malignant; the next most common was osteosarcoma found in preexisting Paget's disease of bone.[67] Most others have reported plasmacytoma or myeloma to be the most common tumor.[42]

Prognosis, in many cases, is directly related to the extent of the surgery performed. Although these lesions are rarely cured by surgery alone, long-term survival for many of the lesions presented in this chapter is improved dramatically by securing tumor-free margins.[131] This, however, requires accurate imaging and appropriate preoperative preparation such as angiography and embolization.[20,93]

Diagnostic Biopsy

Selected patients benefit from CT-directed biopsy of spinal masses.[1,3,39,53,106] In patients for whom the histological diagnosis has not been made, and there is not a need for immediate decompression or stabilization, CT-directed biopsy has a high accuracy rate.[6,44,56,107] The success rates are approximately equal for massess located in the vertebral body, posterior elements, or paraspinal masses.[107,133] Generally, trocar needles are used for sclerotic lesions, and thin spinal needles for lytic or soft tissue masses.[39,106,141]

This technique is not ordinarily used in tumors for which the radiographic picture is diagnostic, such as hemangioma, or in lesions that are highly vascular.[102] Furthermore, as is discussed in the section on sacral tumors, we do not recommend transrectal biopsy, since this may spread tumor and create the need for a colostomy.[70]

The advantage of closed biopsy, of course, is that in patients who are relatively asymptomatic, major surgical procedures may be avoided for some time.[53] In addition, radiosensitive tumors can be pretreated or alternatively treated, avoiding the risks of an open procedure.

Kornblum et al recently reported a series of 103 successful CT biopsies of the spine; of these, 53 were lumbar and 14 sacral. Ninety of these provided enough material for pathologic evaluation, and 67 of 94 were diagnostic. These results are substantially better than those reported by others; furthermore, open diagnostic biopsies were avoided in several patients.[73]

Of particular significance is that, in many patients undergoing successful biopsy, metastatic tumor with an unknown primary is diagnosed.[92] Complication rates are low in most series, and most are performed on an outpatient basis. Even the minimal complications reported may not be justified if surgery is to be undertaken for neurological deficit or deformity. Several have reported better results for osteolytic than for osteosclerotic or blastic lesions.[27,73]

Plasma Cell Lesions

Among the most common tumors of the lumbar spine are solitary plasmacytomas. These are most commonly seen in men over the age of 50. They are composed of proliferation around a cluster of malignant plasma cells and often demonstrate a recent and specific immunoglobulin fragment.[144] Unpredictable in growth and behavior, they may progress to disseminated multiple myeloma of the spine, also to be considered here. However, evidence is sketchy that this relationship is a true continuum.

Solitary Plasmacytomas

Histologic and Clinical Characteristics

These are often seen in the thoracic and lumbar spine, as well as in extramedullary sites such as the airway, GI tract, and spleen. They are occasionally associated with Bence-Jones proteinuria, but are more commonly nonsecretory.[97] Indeed, many authors have indicated that the criteria for solitary plasmacytoma is that there be normal serum protein electrophoresis and absence of Bence-Jones proteins in the urine.[11,33,87] Cervoni et al observed that the M component (on immunoglobulin electrophoresis) is almost always associated with disseminated disease.[32]

In the presence of lytic lesions with negative radionuclide scanning, serum and urine electrophoresis as well as immunoelectrophoresis are recommended. These are often diagnostic, with evidence of serum M component assisting in the laboratory diagnosis. Similarly, monoclonal immunoglobulins are sometimes identified, particularly IgG. In addition to being helpful initially, some have suggested that local recurrence or dissemination are associated with a reappearance of the monoclonal immunoglobulin.[87]

Histology is characteristic. Plasma cells throughout the wide range of differentiation may be seen in a single mass. The cells generally demonstrate basophilic cystoplasm and pyknotic chromatin in the eccentric nucleus.[11]

Early clinical presentation typically includes back pain and radiculopathy.[144] Because of the nonspecific nature of the pain, and thus late presentation, myelopathy is common and is seen in approximately two-thirds of patients.[97] Early diagnosis is of value because long-term survivals are often observed with aggressive therapy: 85% plus 10-year survival can be expected with aggressive treatment.[11,33]

Radiographic Evaluation

Radiographically, the lesions are lytic with sharply margined, occasionally sclerotic borders (Fig. 10–1). Radionuclide scanning is typically negative, and can be used to help distinguish solitary plasmacytomas from metastatic lesions.[33] Computed tomography (CT) demonstrates low-density replacement of the vertebral body, and MRI shows compression fracture, abnormal signal in the vertebral body, and paraspinal soft tissue masses.[60] MRI is also essential to rule out additional foci of plasmacytoma not otherwise visible, since it may show disease in as many as one-third of patients so studied.[90,91] Because these tumors are so vascular, angiography is often incorporated into radiographic evaluation even before biopsy.[93] Indeed, deaths due to injury of tumor vessels have been reported during biopsy of this very vascular tumor. If angiography is performed before open surgery, embolization should be considered.

Treatment

Optimal treatment is controversial. Delauche-Cavallier et al have recommended surgery as the

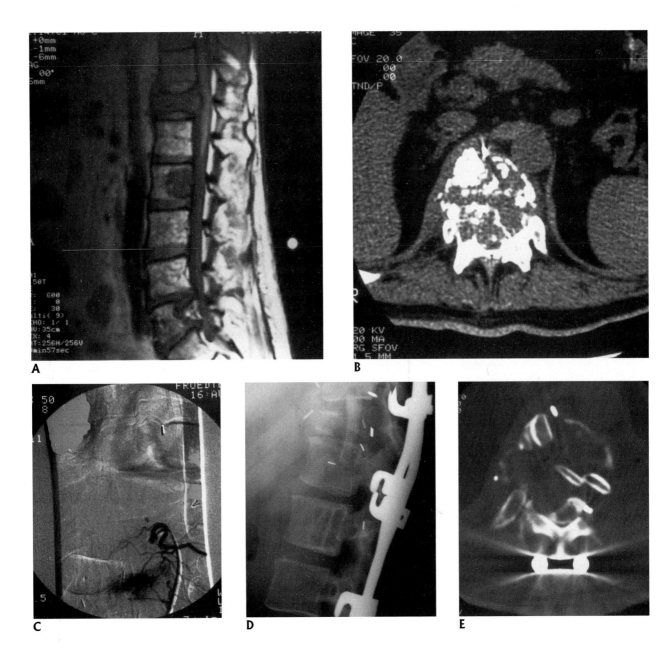

FIGURE 10–1 Plasmacytomas in a 50-year-old man with back pain and rapidly progressive paraparesis. **A** T12 compression fracture with cord compromise. There is an early lytic lesion at L2, not evident on plain radiography. **B** Computed tomogram demonstrating vertebral replacement and peripheral sclerosis. **C** Spinal angiogram immediately prior to embolization. The lesion is intensely vascular. **D** Lateral radiograph following surgery using the extracavitary approach and radiotherapy. **E** Computed tomogram 1 year later. The position of the rib grafts is evident. There is evidence of soft tissue in the spinal canal opposite the original decompression.

first line of treatment, followed by radiation therapy and often chemotherapy.[43] Wollersheim et al, on the other hand, noted that there is no evidence that any treatment is more effective than any other.[144] There may be no relationship between the aggressiveness of surgical treatment and long-term survival.

Surgery Sundaresan et al suggest that surgical treatment be carried out following radiation therapy for treatment of bone destruction with destabilization and/or neurological deficit.[122] In our experience, surgery is primarily for patients presenting with rapid onset of paraparesis.

Surgical treatment, when appropriate, should consist of aggressive radical excision of the tumor.[33] This should be predicated, as is always the case, on the level and location of involvement. In the absence of proof that surgery improves survival, one wonders whether such aggressive treatment should be recommended. However, since progression to destabilization often occurs with minimalist procedures, if surgery is to be incorporated, it is best to perform aggressive anterior decompression, fusion, and stabilization to decrease the morbidity of repeated surgeries.

In patients who are neurologically intact, and without evidence of vertebral collapse, we recommend surgery only if radiotherapy fails to cure the tumor.

Radiation Therapy and Chemotherapy In patients presenting with spinal pain or slowly progressive neurological changes, the results of radiation therapy plus immobilization to prevent further vertebral collapse can be gratifying. Regardless of when it is provided, radiation therapy should be incorporated into the treatment paradigm. This typically means the use of fractionated doses totaling 35 to 50 Gy, depending on the author.[89]

Little information exists in the literature regarding increased morbidity following radiation therapy. Some have recommended the simultaneous use of chemotherapy to prevent the expected and dreaded progression to myeloma. However, the agents used can lead to the development of leukemia.[16] It appears appropriate to reserve the use of chemotherapy for patients who have more malignant lesions initially and for those who have developed multiple myeloma.

Prognosis

The prognosis for solitary plasmacytoma depends on the characteristics of the patient as well as the tumor itself.[38,82] Bataille noted that older patients with spinal involvement and persistence of monoclonal proteins have poor prognoses and are likely to go on to dissemination.[11] Patients with multiple plasmacytomas typically go on to the development of multiple myeloma; this is not necessarily the case for patients with local recurrence or a second isolated plasmacytoma after aggressive therapy.[38] Soft tissue extension seems to indicate more aggressive disease with the likelihood of early development of myeloma.

Multiple Myeloma

Histologic and Clinical Characteristics

Multiple myeloma is a generalized bone marrow disease caused by plasma cell infiltration. Spinal spread is not always symptomatic but is virtually always present.[2,22] Patients often complain of back pain; subsequently, involvement of multiple vertebrae is noted, often with soft tissue involvement. Most patients demonstrate monoclonal immunoglobulins in either serum or urine; levels can often be titrated to the tumor mass present. In addition, Bence-Jones proteinuria is quite common. Bone marrow biopsy is usually pathologic and is diagnostic if more than 30% plasma cells are present. Although most myeloma patients will not have been previously diagnosed as having a solitary plasmacytoma, approximately 50% of patients with multiple plasmacytomas will have had a prior solitary lesion.[2]

Radiographic Evaluation

MRI is more successful in detecting myeloma-associated focal bone lesions than other techniques (Fig. 10–2).[98,99] One particular advantage of MRI is the ability to determine medullary abnormalities, which is not typically possible with other studies (Fig. 10–3).[51,60,83] Atypical neoplastic lesions appear on T1-weighted images, which show reduced signal

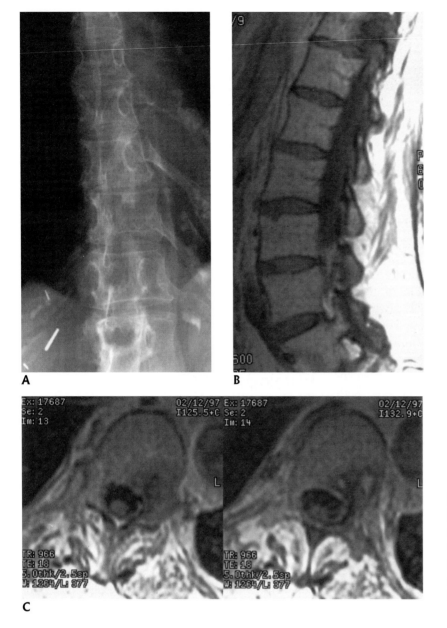

FIGURE 10-2
Multiple myeloma in a 60-year-old woman. **A** Plain radiograph with "pedicle sign." **B, C** Sagittal and axial magnetic resonance images with pedicle involvement extending into posterior elements.

intensity and occasionally soft tissue abnormalities.[40,83] This allows early radiotherapy prior to spinal pain or neurological deficit.[22,112] Indeed, the accuracy of MRI diagnosis may be equal to biopsy, and it can be used to monitor the success of treatment.[51,99] The only value of plain radiography in the early diagnosis is for determining minor vertebral compression fracture.

Treatment

The primary treatment of the disease is radiotherapy and chemotherapy.[80] The latter primarily involves the use of alkylating agents.[9,80] Recent protocols include autologous bone marrow transplant.[8,54] Unfortunately, the likelihood of long-term survival is low, regardless of treatment.[16]

Indications for surgery in myeloma are few. Occasionally, biopsy is necessary if immunoglobulin studies and bone marrow biopsy are negative. Instead, surgical treatment should be reserved for the patient with neurological deficit due to bony compression of the spinal cord, or spinal deformity due to vertebral collapse that does not respond to steroids, radiation, and immobilization.[14] Occasionally, severe and uncontrollable pain due to vertebral involvement requires stabilization.[115] However, this should rarely

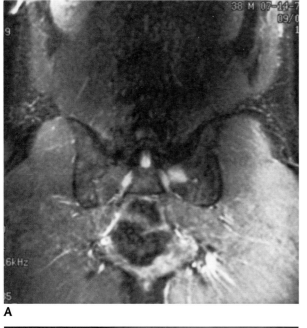
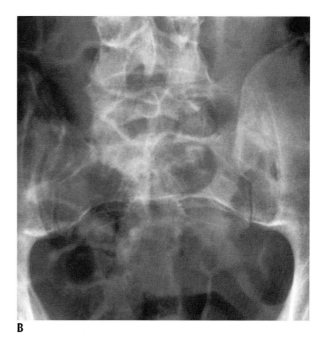
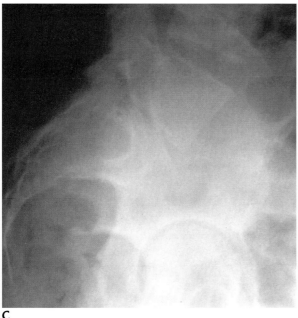

FIGURE 10-3
Plasmacytoma in a 38-year-old man with back pain. **A** Axial magnetic image demonstrate sacral medullary lesion. **B, C** Plain radiographs are normal.

be the case. Vertebroplasty has been employed in recent years, with improvement in pain in selected patients.[37] Needless to say, the systemic condition of the patient should be carefully considered in therapeutic decisionmaking. Thus the primary role of the surgeon may be to monitor the success of nonoperative treatment by following the sequential MRI scans as well as the immunoglobulin studies, and to ensure appropriate spinal stability.

Chordomas

Histologic and Clinical Characteristics

Although chordomas are uncommon malignant tumors of bone (only 4% of the total), they are extremely relevant to the lumbosacral spine. Over 50% of those affecting the spine occur in the sacrum, and roughly 10 to 20% affect the lumbar spine.[4] They arise from residual notochord cells along the spinal axis. These residual notochord rests have been commonly reported in autopsy series in 1 to 2% of autopsies, both in the clivus and around the sacrum. In the adult human, only the centrum of the pulposus derives from notochord. The vertebrae, on the other hand, are formed from surrounding mesochyme. Based on recent histochemical analyses, chordomas are divided into three groups:[46,96]

1. Classic chordomas are epithelial neoplasms with cords and nests of recessive cells in a mucinous matrix. These are typically of intermediate malignancy.
2. Those with spindle cell components or dedifferentiated chordomas are fully malignant.[34,66]
3. The third type, which is poorly defined, has been identified as the chondroid chordoma. This demonstrates focal cartilaginous differentiation with a matrix that stains for Type II collagen, and seems to be less aggressive clinically.[61,143]

In recent years, the classical thinking of Ribbert and Congdon that chordomas result from disc tissue has come into question.[35,100] For example, Sundaresan has suggested that chordomas rise from within the vertebra itself. Indeed, nonneoplastic microscopic notochord remnants are often seen in vertebral bodies of patients with chordomas.[128]

Le Pointe et al have noted that lumbar spine chordomas are typically confined to a single level, as opposed to those of the cervical spine. They hypothesize that this is primarily because of the slow growth of the tumor and the relatively large size of the vertebra; in the thoracic and lumbar spine, chordomas are typically located centrally in the body. Furthermore, in the lumbar spine, lesions are uncommonly osteolytic. They are more typically mixed osteosclerotic and osteoblastic, along with the osteolytic areas.[79]

Lesions of the lumbar spine and sacrum tend to appear in males during the fifth to seventh decades.[18] Spine cell tumors often occur in a younger age group and, as indicated earlier, are more aggressive.

The most common clinical presentation is of back and coccygeal pain. The diagnosis may be made as a consequence of unexpected and persistent back pain following a history of mild trauma. Feldenzer et al found a significant incidence of atypical sciatica. A change in bowel habits, bleeding, or rectal pain are also common. In sacral tumors, presacral masses are often identified.[49]

Less common are tumors of the lumbar spine presenting with radicular pain or, occasionally, cauda equina syndrome.[4] The relative rarity of this presentation often leads to error: the tumor is misdiagnosed as a metastatic lesion and is only partially removed, and subsequent histological diagnosis proves the lesion to be a chordoma. In recent years, however, improvements in radiologic diagnoses have made this phenomenon less likely.

Radiographic Evaluation

Plain radiography is characteristic, although rarely diagnostic. In sacral tumors, an expansile mass is typically seen, frequently involving multiple regions of the sacrum; presacral masses are usually seen late.[102,104,114] In the mobile lumbar spine, destructive lesions that may occasionally extend over multiple segments are often seen (Fig. 10–4). Sundaresan suggests that peripheral sclerosis at the tumor margins is diagnostic;[128] this has not been our experience. More helpful, but again not specific, is a prevertebral mass at the level of maximum involvement.

Accurate bone imaging requires *computed tomography* (CT).[77,88] In tumors of the mobile spine, vertebral body destruction is the most common finding.[41,114] Occasionally, chordomas spread from the posterior elements, in addition to the typical prevertebral soft tissue extension.[36] These soft tissue masses are more likely to be seen on CT than on plain radiography.[114] Occasionally, blastic lesions are seen in conjunction with the obvious lytic ones.[50] CT may also demonstrate epidural masses, but this should not be considered diagnostic.[62,77] Tumor calcification is typically peripheral and may demarcate the boundaries of the tumor.

Magnetic resonance imaging (MRI) is ideal for the evaluation of tumor spread and epidural involvement. There is a characteristic but nonspecific low-intensity signal on T1 and high intensity on T2-weighted images.[102] The sensitivity in determining tumor spread is exceptional. In addition to defining bone and disc involvement, as well as cord compression, MRI is superior to CT in examining the paraspinal tissues.[60] Intravenous gadolinium during MRI further aids in the definition of epidural tumor. Be-

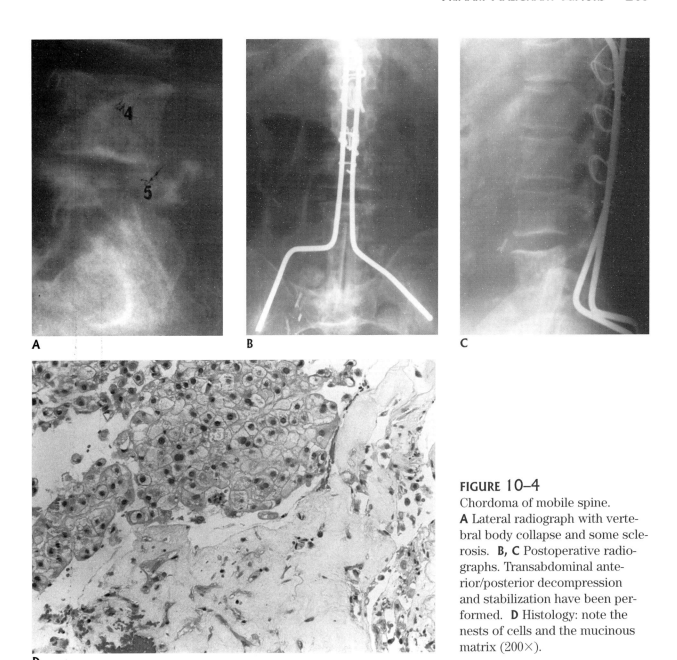

FIGURE 10–4
Chordoma of mobile spine.
A Lateral radiograph with vertebral body collapse and some sclerosis. B, C Postoperative radiographs. Transabdominal anterior/posterior decompression and stabilization have been performed. D Histology: note the nests of cells and the mucinous matrix (200×).

cause total excision with tumor margins is highly desirable, multiplanar imaging can be very helpful in precise tumor definition.[119] The value of imaging-guided surgery here remains to be determined.

Furthermore, MRI can accurately demonstrate cystic changes within the tumor, existence of the pseudocapsule, as well as fibrous bands within the tumor itself.[36] These cystic areas are also hypodense on contrast-enhanced CT.[50] Chondroid chordomas have shorter T1 and T2 relaxation times than classic chordomas; the former were also less intense on T2-weighted spin echo images than classic chordomas.[130] Such diagnostic accuracy on MRI should reduce the need for tumor biopsy in many instances.

There is little role for *nuclear imaging*, except for searching for distant—and rare—metastasis. Indeed, bone scanning has a 50% false-negative rate.[78,120]

Treatment

Patient Preparation

Prior to surgical treatment, careful planning is required, particularly in lesions of the sacrum. With improved imaging, diagnosis can often be made radiologically. Biopsy, which often must be performed transrectally and thus carries the risk of hemorrhage, rectal injury, and tumor invasion, can be avoided.[84] A thorough evaluation of the abdomen, colon, and rectum should be carried out via CT of the abdomen and pelvis, intravenous pyelogram, as well as a barium enema. We strongly recommend terminal colonoscopy to ensure that there has been no erosion through the mucosa. This is uncommon but has the potential to be surgically devastating. We also recommend urodynamic studies in patients with evidence of bladder dysfunction. Involvement of the S2 and S3 nerve roots is not uncommon, and sectioning is often necessary for curative surgery. Because a significant percentage of these tumors are vascular, preoperative embolization is quite valuable.[23]

Sacral tumors

Several approaches to large sacral tumors have been recommended, many of which are presented later in this chapter. Older procedures include radical sacrectomy via a posterior approach.[85,105] Unfortunately, the anatomy from a dorsal approach is often ill-defined, and it is difficult to remove anterior masses through this approach. Thus we do not recommend posterior sacrectomy for curative treatment of large tumors; instead, it is used primarily for palliation in conjunction with posterior instrumentation, or for smaller tumors with no anterior sacral mass.[139] It is imperative before using these procedures that there is no extension of the tumor anterior to the sacral periosteum.

Gennari et al, however, continue to use high sacral resection through S2 for curative surgery, and have reported excellent results.[55] The S2 roots can often be preserved, and surgical morbidity is lower than for combined procedures. Median survival has been 3 years.

For potentially curable lesions, the preponderance of evidence is that combined or staged anterior/posterior decompression and fusion are optimal.[17,94] Aggressive treatment is valuable: although long-term survival in the face of recurrence is quite low, long-term survival can be seen in as many as 60% of patients with successful complete resection.

Some have performed anterior/posterior procedures during a single anesthesia in the lateral decubitus position. An oblique incision is made across the perineum between the iliac and costal margins. A retroperitoneal approach is performed and the retroperitoneal contents mobilized, including the ureters and iliac vessels. The middle sacral arteries and veins and lateral sacral veins are taken and the tumor resected in both directions via both a laminectomy and an anterior approach. Unfortunately, we find instrumentation difficult in this position; in addition, the significant operative time and blood loss may add risk.

An alternative technique for sacrectomy has also been proposed by Stener that requires amputation of the sacrum through the first sacral vertebra and requires unilateral sectioning of all sacral nerve roots. This procedure, although quite radical, allows end block resection of sacral chordomas and has yielded actual cures without radiation.[117]

Our preferred technique for large sacral lesions is a staged anterior/posterior approach.[49,58,113,136] In this procedure, an anterior retroperitoneal exploration is performed by a general surgeon, with bilateral mobilization of the iliac vessels, ureters, and the rectum. The soft tissue mass protruding into the abdominal cavity as well as the anterior sacral tumor is grossly resected. As soon as is medically acceptable, the patient undergoes a posterior approach with radical resection of the sacrum, typically from the L5–S1 disc space to the coccyx. The sacrum is unroofed, nerve roots are carefully protected whenever possible, and the residual sacrum is removed. Typically, the dural sac is ligated.

Spinal fixation is accomplished as part of this posterior procedure. For sacral lesions, this includes pelvic fixation using the Galveston technique as described elsewhere in this book, or lumbar and pelvic fixation using transpedicular fixation, including Jackson screws into the ilium.

Chordomas of the Mobile Spine

An aggressive approach is also recommended for chordomas of the mobile spine,[21,48,118,135] although some have argued that the historically poor prognosis makes this approach optional.[4] Above L5, we have satisfactorily used a bilateral extracavitary approach for total excision of affected vertebral bodies, as well as removal of the posterior elements. A full 360-degrees decompression can be performed, with both anterior and posterior fusion and instrumentation. Although technically challenging, the extracavitary approach can also be used at L5. In this circumstance, the exposure to the side of the spine is provided by resection of the iliac crest, as discussed in Chapter 13. Certainly anterior vertebrectomy can be performed; this must be performed via a true anterior approach to allow complete vertebral resection, and requires mobilization and retraction of the aorta and/or iliac arteries and veins.[48] In addition, a second procedure for posterior resection and instrumentation is necessary. Regardless of the approach, primary fusion can be performed from the adjacent vertebra into the sacrum or coccyx as indicated. Our preference is to use bank bone, as opposed to methylmethacrylate, since fusion may occur.

Spinal instrumentation is critical regardless of tumor size.[110] Radiation is often indicated, as discussed below, and radical surgical excision produces significant instability. Preferred techniques include transpedicular fixation over at least two segments above and below the affected segment. In upper lumbar tumors, therefore, instrumentation may consist solely of transpedicular fixation. In tumors extending to but not including the sacrum, we recommend pelvic fixation using the Galveston technique or Jackson screws.

For both sacral and vertebral tumors, incomplete excision is to be assiduously avoided.[109] In an effort to avoid radical extirpation and protect bowel and bladder function, several have suggested tumor debulking followed by radiation. Unfortunately, the results are marginal: long-term control is not improved by partial removal and then radiation therapy. Instead, progression-free curves for incomplete surgery versus biopsy and radiation are quite similar.[102] Indeed, many radiation oncologists recommend preoperative radiotherapy, an interval to allow tumor shrinkage, and then gross resection.

In the presence of neurological deficit, particularly bowel and bladder abnormalities, nerve root section is often necessary and desirable following careful informed consent. Several patients in our series have required multiple operative procedures because of local recurrence, with undesirable results. Performing subtotal resections because of fears of instability is rarely indicated, since stabilization, although challenging, is typically effective. Attempting to preserve bowel and bladder function in patients with curable lesions is often self-defeating. Local regrowth will eventually cause loss of function anyway. Rather, subtotal resection should be performed only in patients with unresectable tumors and normal bowel and bladder function. The surgeon is again advised that repeat procedures are that much more challenging than the first, and are rarely gratifying.

Adjunctive Therapy

Radiation therapy is often recommended following subtotal resection or recurrence. Most patients obtain satisfactory local control at doses of 55 cGy or above.[52,78,121] In one series, patients treated with doses higher than 55 cGy were significantly more likely to be free of tumor at 5 years.[52] Others recommend doses of greater than 65 cGy for effective local control, still with low morbidity;[101] results for the palliation obtained for high-dose radiotherapy are the same for patients undergoing incomplete resection and preradiotherapy needle biopsy.[52,78,101] Ion beam therapy allows higher doses than conventional radiotherapy, with minimal morbidity.[106] However, in Catton et al's large series, the technique of radiotherapy employed did not affect outcome.[31]

It is unusual to see reversal of the bone and soft tissue changes, although pain and neurological deficits typically stabilize.[46] Occasionally, brachytherapy with direct interstitial implantation of low-activity seeds reduces tumor bulk even in previously irradiated patients.[78] On rare occasions, chordomas degenerate into grossly malignant tumors such as histiocytomas or undifferentiated malignant chordomas following radiation therapy.[13,68]

Repeat radiotherapy is often recommended for local recurrence. Unfortunately, this may be associated with spinal cord infarction. Instead, surgical salvage procedures are typically employed after postradiotherapy progression, but are associated with a high incidence of fistulae and serious skin coverage problems.

Prognosis

Distant metastases are seen in 10 to 15% of patients with sacral lesions.[34,52,137] These are typically pulmonary and respond poorly to nonsurgical treatment.

With aggressive multidisciplinary treatment, 5-year survival rates of over 50% overall can be expected; 10-year survival of 40% in sacral lesions can be expected.[46,52] Patients with chondroid elements within their tumors can expect survival of over 15 years with curative treatment.[18,123,125,128]

Sarcomas

Most sarcomas in our series have been secondary: arising in vertebrae affected by metabolic conditions such as Paget's disease, or arising in previously irradiated bone.[147] The latter tend to occur in patients previously treated for curable lesions, such as Hodgkin's disease. In one large series, onset of the second malignancy averaged 10 years after treatment of the first cancer. These sarcomas tend to be quite aggressive, with survivals of less than 1 year even with aggressive treatment.[124,126] Some specific tumor types are considered below.

Osteosarcomas (Osteogenic Sarcomas)

These are said to be among the more common bone tumors, although they are quite uncommon in our series.[15] Most of the osteosarcomas treated at the Medical College of Wisconsin were secondary to Paget's disease (over 50%) or postradiation exposure for other tumors.[7,24,67,86,145]

Osteosarcomas typically arise from medullary bone, although occasionally they originate in paravertebral soft tissue.[7,10,95] Rarely, they may arise in the posterior elements.[74] Isolated spinal involvement in primary osteosarcoma is unusual. When it occurs, it often causes clinical, if vague, symptomatology. Prognosis is poor, with median survivals averaging 1 year.[15]

Patients typically present with local pain and low-grade radiculopathy or myelopathy.[10] When primary, osteosarcomas occur principally during the growth spurt; oncogenesis is probably related to rapid bone growth.[10] Shives et al reported prolonged duration of symptoms prior to diagnosis;[111] we usually have seen severe myelopathy due to epidural tumor.

Radiographic Evaluation

Plain radiographs demonstrate a sclerotic or osteolytic vertebral body; there may be an exuberant calcified soft tissue mass extending from the vertebra.[95] Unfortunately, this picture is nonspecific, and may be confused with giant cell tumors. In older patients, the lesions may mimic active Paget's disease, or even certain metastatic tumors.

MRI defines the extent of spinal cord compression and exophytic soft tissue tumor growth. CT also accurately demonstrates soft tissue extension, and is probably more accurate than MRI for that purpose.[12] Radionuclide scanning is important to define metastasis and to monitor results of subsequent radiation and chemotherapy. It is thus imperative in pre surgical evaluation: certainly the surgical planning and the goals of therapy will be altered if there is evidence of disease elsewhere.

Treatment

In the patient with contained disease, radical surgical excision is recommended. Because of the relative accuracy of radiographic diagnosis, vertebral biopsy is rarely useful, although it is recommended by Tigani et al to distinguish osteosarcoma from osteoblastoma, which may have a similar radiologic appearance.[134] The vascularity of osteosarcoma may make biopsy undesirable. Rather, careful imaging and the neurological picture should determine treatment.

Before surgery, spinal angiography should be performed. Since osteosarcomas are typically quite vascular, embolization is important; we also use angiography to define the artery of Adamkiewicz, as is discussed in Chapter 13.[23,116]

It is imperative that the correct surgery be performed initially. There is very little role for laminectomy even in the presence of acute myelopathy, since laminectomy accomplishes little in what is primarily an anterior mass, although posterior elements are also often invaded. Rather, the initial procedure—in the patient who does not have disseminated disease—should be designed to allow aggressive and comprehensive resection as well as stabilization.[48] It seems undesirable to subject patients to two procedures if they are avoidable.

We use a modified extracavitary approach to the spine. A circumferential osteotomy, bilateral pedicle removal, and full removal of the posterior elements can be accomplished simultaneously. Following radical resection, spinal stabilization and anterior grafting with methylmethacrylate and/or bone or coral can be accomplished. Although technically demanding, if hemostasis is acceptable, this procedure will accomplish the goals with less morbidity and certainly allow more rapid mobilization and entry into subsequent therapy. Another option is en bloc spondylectomy, as advocated by Kawahara et al.[71] However, this alternative may require multiple operations for posterior instrumentation as well as circumferential decompression.

Adjunctive Therapy Radiotherapy is started within days of surgery because of the rapid growth of the tumor. Our skin complications have been minimal with meticulous hemostasis and closure. Aggressive combination chemotherapy may improve the outlook in many patients; certainly, without it rapid recurrence is inevitable.[64,134]

In one of the largest clinical series reported to date, Sundaresan et al compared the results for limited tumor removal and external radiation (used from 1949 to 1977) with a protocol incorporating radical excision, brachytherapy, and combination chemotherapy (1978 to 1984). Almost half of the second group were long-term survivors, and only one patient developed metastatic disease while being treated.[127]

Chondrosarcomas

Chondrosarcomas are the third most common primary tumor of bone.[30] They arise primarily from the pelvis and long bone, and solitary or initial spinal involvement is rare, although metastatic deposits in the spine are not. The malignant chondrocytes produce cartilage without bone, although lower-grade lesions may occasionally calcify and can be confused with endochondromas.[76] Characteristically, chondrosarcomas are invasive, however.[29,30] Tumors with atypical cells, more mitotic figures, and increased nuclear DNA content as well as polyploidy have a worse prognosis.[76]

Chondrosarcomas are most commonly seen in middle-aged males. Patients typically present with local pain that is worse at night and is gradually progressive. Neurological deficit is unusual and is associated with advanced disease. Many patients diagnosed with this lesion have a distant history of radiotherapy for childhood cancer.[81]

Radiographic Evaluation

Imaging should include plain radiographs, CT, and MRI, (Fig. 10–5). Plain films and tomography demonstrate a radiolucent lesion with intralesion bone destruction and soft tissue expansion.[62,63] Islands of discrete calcification are observed: the less calcium, the more malignant the lesion. MRI accurately defines soft tissue expansion, as well as spinal cord and nerve root compression. It can also be helpful in defining the biology of the tumor, including the use of contrast to imply vascularity.[12] Radionuclide imaging should be performed to rule out the existence of lesions elsewhere.[30] Again, it is particularly uncommon for these to arise primarily in the spine: all the chondrosarcomas in our series arose from the pelvis or femur.

Treatment

We rarely perform tumor biopsies, since most tumors are widely excised anyway. However, less malignant chondrosarcomas respond well to intracapsular removal or cryosurgical curettage as described below for sacral tumors, which may be less morbid and more technically feasible than radical excision. Therefore, needle biopsy is occasionally helpful, especially in tumors with minimal enhancement, which is typically the case.[30]

More malignant tumors should be subjected to wide and radical excision, whenever possible, through aggressive spondylectomy either via a lateral extracavitary or anterior approach, as described in the techniques chapters.[29] If needed, surgery can be staged. Tumor-free margins should be obtained whenever possible, since recurrence or residual tumor significantly affects survival. Radiotherapy and chemotherapy are not typically helpful, although they are usually provided postoperatively, sometimes successfully.[59,72] Stabilization is characteristically necessary for spinal tumors.

Although the prognosis for patients with spinal or sacral involvement is worse than for long bone tumors, complete resection of lower-grade lesions can result in 50% 5- to 10-year survival. Prognosis worsens dramatically with residual tumor. Thus the importance of radical excision cannot be overemphasized. However, excision of local recurrence may be useful.[65]

Sacral-Coccygeal Tumors

This section focuses primarily on the treatment of primary tumors of the sacrum other than chordo-

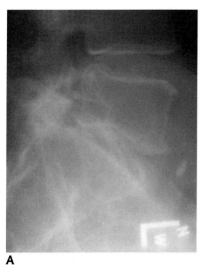
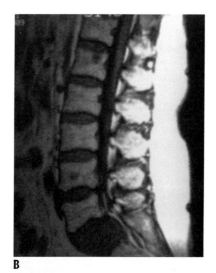
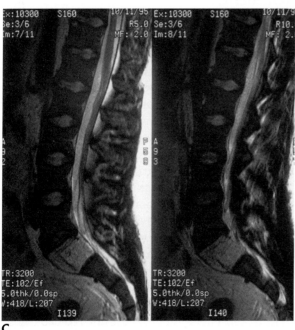
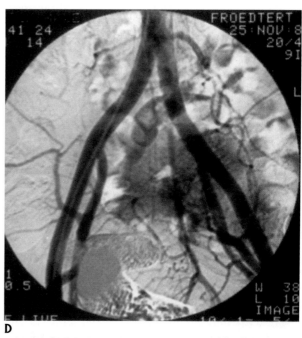
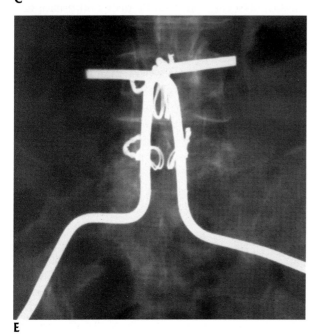
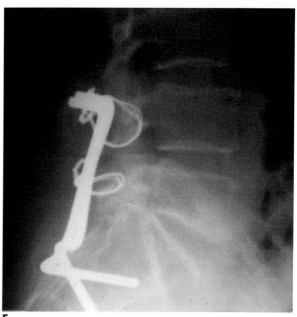

FIGURE 10–5 Chondrosarcoma in a 50-year-old man. **A** Lateral radiograph with trivial vertebral expansion but some increased soft tissue evident, even on plain radiography. **B, C** Sagittal magnetic resonance image with homogeneous expansile lesion of L5. **D** Spinal angiogram documenting a highly vascular lesion. **E, F** Anteroposterior and lateral radiographs performed 2 year postoperatively. Note that, with intact posterior elements and a tumor contained to the vertebra with complete excision, the surgeon has elected to place wires at L5.

mas. Sacral tumors, although uncommon, have been extensively examined because of their unique therapeutic requirements. They represent significant clinical challenges because of their location in the pelvis and their close relationship to the uterus, major pelvic blood vessels, rectum, and nerve roots. Stabilization has classically been felt to be difficult. Additionally, they typically require multidisciplinary treatment: although surgical resection is rarely complete, the tumors are rarely radiosensitive. Furthermore, diagnosis can be difficult and is often late because initial clinical findings are nonspecific and radiographic pictures are similar across multiple types of lesions. Indeed, many tumors are not diagnosed until they extend into the presacral space and cause symptoms due to compression of retroperitoneal and abdominal contents.

Benign tumors have been discussed elsewhere. Giant cell tumors (which are transitionally malignant), osteoblastomas, aneurysmal bone cysts, and osteoid osteomas together represent a significant percentage of the tumors seen in the sacrum. Neurilemomas are usually seen proximal in the sacrum but originate medially and grow laterally. They typically have well-defined bony margins.

The rest of this section considers malignant tumors.

Malignant Tumors of the Sacrum

Pain in the buttock and/or atypical radiculopathy are among the first presenting symptoms and are often associated with sacral tenderness. Particularly with low-grade malignancies such as chordomas, symptoms are present for years before they are diagnosed. The latter tend to be located centrally in the sacrum, and thus are quite large by the time they create neurological deficit. More aggressive tumors such as sarcomas, on the other hand, present more dramatically with pelvic structure abnormalities and occasionally bowel and bladder incontinence. Pain when positioning the hip in external rotation is often seen with involvement of the sacroiliac joint. Atypical sciatica may indicate an upper sacral tumor.

In most series, the most common malignancy of the sacrum is metastasis, especially adenocarcinoma directly invading the sacrum. These tumors are typically eccentric and proximal. Treatment considerations are, of course, related to the extent of the primary tumor. Radical excision of a sacral metastasis is rarely indicated, since typically sacral metastasis represents a focus of disseminated disease.

Sarcomas of the Sacrum

These often arise from the pedicle. Presentation with myelopathy typically occurs shortly after onset of symptoms.

Ewing's sarcoma is typically seen in adolescents and young adults. Symptoms are the rapid onset of a toxic picture with fevers, weight loss, and debilitation.[142] On occasion, this tumor is seen in older adults and therefore must be part of the differential diagnosis in sacral lesions, especially when systemic symptoms are present.[6,26,140] There may be lower abdominal and pelvic pain and bowel and bladder abnormalities, but rarely is neurological deficit an early finding.[140,142] Plain radiographs may show only a minor osteolytic lesion, but CT and MRI demonstrate a soft tissue mass extending into the pelvis but often contained by the presacral fascia, which is typical for sarcomas.[75,148] This fascia should be preserved for surgical planning: yet another reason to avoid diagnostic transrectal biopsy.

A similar picture is seen in *osteosarcoma*, which is rarely seen in the sacrum. Again, radiographic studies may show only a nonspecific soft tissue mass with minimal bony changes. Alternatively, there may be new bone formation around the eroded sacral margins, with occasional calcification in the tumor itself.

Chondrosarcomas are slow-growing but locally aggressive. They may arise from within endochondromas or from exocytic bone. They typically arise in the upper portion of the sacrum, and often involve the sacroiliac joint. Diagnostic radiographic studies include plain radiographs and radionuclide scanning. The latter demonstrates increased uptake. MRI and CT define the soft tissue component as well as bone destruction.

Treatment Aggressive treatment of all of these lesions can be gratifying. Following treatment with radical surgery, adjuvant radiotherapy (mean 5000 cGy), and chemotherapy, almost one-third can be expected to have survival without recurrence at 5 years.[132,138] Evans et al performed high-dose intermittent multiagent chemotherapy on patients with incomplete resections; at 5 years, disease-free survival was 55%, and survival with or without metastasis was 63%, compared to 23% and 35%, respectively, without combination chemotherapy.[47] Similar results are expected for other sacral sarcomas.

Surgical Treatment of Sacral Tumors

In addition to the imaging studies discussed earlier, we generally perform selective angiography because of the vascular nature of many sacral tumors. Embolization can be extremely helpful in decreasing hemorrhage.[23,25,93]

Biopsy is selectively useful. Again, we feel that transrectal biopsy should usually be avoided. With many tumor types, transrectal biopsy results in tumor seeding, necessitating major abdominal procedures with excision of the rectum and subsequent colostomy. Often a CT-directed biopsy can be performed anteriorly, or through a posterior approach if the posterior sacrum is involved. It is usually necessary to excise the biopsy tract at surgery; this is a consideration in the choice of biopsy procedure.

For patients who are to undergo resection of sacral tumors, advance preparation should be as for laparotomy. Meticulous bowel cleansing should be performed, since unexpected bowel involvement may be found at the time of surgery. Some authors also recommend preoperative radiation, which may shrink the tumor mass and decrease vascularity.

Following are several approaches to sacral tumors; there is some redundancy in the presentation, in that two or more of the operations presented can be used for multiple tumor locations. However, there are enough differences between them to justify the effort. The principles are the same: for lesions entering the body of the sacrum, some type of anterior/posterior approach is optimal.

Posterior Approaches

Laminectomy and curettage represent an effective approach to removing posterior sacral tumors that do not extend to or through the anterior cortex of the sacrum, and can even be curative. However, they are only recommended for more proximal and dorsal lesions.[69] A vertical incision is made from the upper margins of the iliac crest to the sacralcoccygeal junction. The lumbodorsal fascia is elevated and the muscle retracted laterally. If the lesion is only on one side, we recommend a unilateral subperiosteal dissection. The bony cortex over the tumor is then carefully removed to normal margins (Fig. 10–6). We recommend that the nerve roots be carefully mobilized and retracted away from the tumor to allow exposure of the anterior sacral margins. With a combination of high-speed drill, curettage, and meticulous dissection, large tumors of the sacrum proper can be carefully excised. We have been able to successfully remove tumors that even extend through the anterior cortex of the sacrum, although do not generally use this approach if there is a soft tissue mass anterior to the sacrum.

If the surgeon violates the anterior cortex, or if there is a wide lower lumbar laminectomy, spinal instrumentation is recommended using the Galveston technique or transpedicular fixation with pelvic fixation. Meticulous wound closure is critical. Cerebrospinal fluid fistula remains one of the most common complications of posterior sacral approaches.

There is an high rate of wound infection and hemorrhage in posterior sacral resections. Infection rates approach 20 to 40%, especially in irradiated patients. This emphasizes the importance of myocutaneous flaps and careful surgical repair. If the surgeon is unsuccessful in preserving at least one of the S2 nerve roots, bowel and bladder paralysis can be expected to occur. This may well be

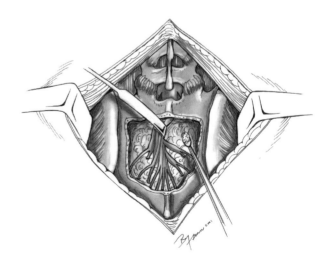

FIGURE 10–6 Laminectomy for dorsal sacral tumor 2 (see text).

The tumor is then carefully removed, with attention to homeostasis. This may be particularly difficult because of the vascular nature of the tumors and the large size that they achieve in this often clinically silent area. Strategies for decreasing blood loss include using cutting electrocoagulating loops, and sequentially freezing and removing the tumor with liquid nitrogen. Neither can be used near nerve roots.

Low Sacral Resection Techniques for low sacral resection via a posterior approach are available. We recommend this procedure only for tumors below S3, as suggested by Sung et al.[129] A horizontal or vertical incision (Fig. 10–8A) is made. If a horizontal incision is used, it should be one level higher than the anticipated site of the tumor. A skin flap is developed and retracted to expose the gluteus. This is then transected from the iliac crest. The piriformis muscle, ligaments, pudendal nerve, and gluteal vessels are exposed and the muscle and ligaments transected near their insertion (Fig. 10–8B). The gluteal vessels are ligated, but an effort should be made to protect the pudendal nerve. The sacroiliac joints are identified and exposed and the border at the lateral margins of the sacrum identified with blunt dissection (Fig. 10–8C).

The carefully identified presacral fascia is used as a plane to protect the rectum and the retroperitoneal contents. Blunt dissection is used to dissect this fascia away from the sacrum and the tumor. The sacrum is transected with osteotomes one segment above the proximal limits of the tumor (Fig. 10–8D), the peroneal levator muscles are cut, and the sacrum elevated (Fig. 10–8E). Distal transection is then carried out below the tumor. A large tumor bed will be left, which is typically closed with rotational flaps (Fig. 10–8F).

The sacrifice of sacral nerve roots is quite controversial. Most authors recommend that the first three sacral nerve roots be preserved whenever possible, at least unilaterally. Sundaresan has suggested that the salvage of the S2 root is enough to preserve most bowel and bladder function.[125] For benign tumors, therefore, the S3 nerve root should be preserved. For malignant tumors where excision is necessary for a cure, sacrifice of these nerve roots should be considered.

The morbidity of this procedure is considerable, with extensive blood loss. Mortality rates approaching 5% have been reported for radical sacral resection. For lower sacral resection, instrumentation is typically unnecessary.

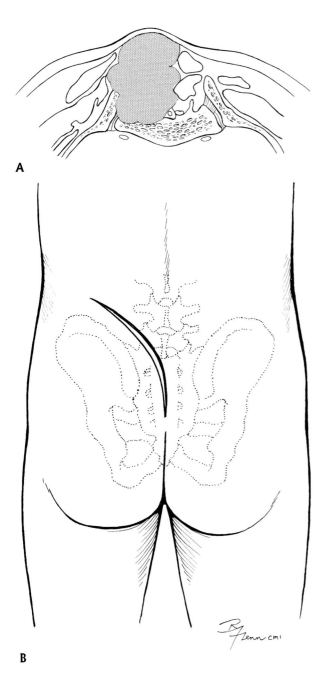

FIGURE 10–7 Approach to paramedian or sacroiliac tumors (see text).

inadvertent, but it should be prevented whenever possible.

Paramedian Tumors Paramedian tumors and those involving the sacroiliac joint require an alternative approach (Fig. 10–7A). A curvilinear incision is marked from the sacral-coccygeal junction over the iliac crest on the involved side (Fig. 10–7B). The gluteus is detached from the iliac crest and reflected distally, which should expose the tumor.

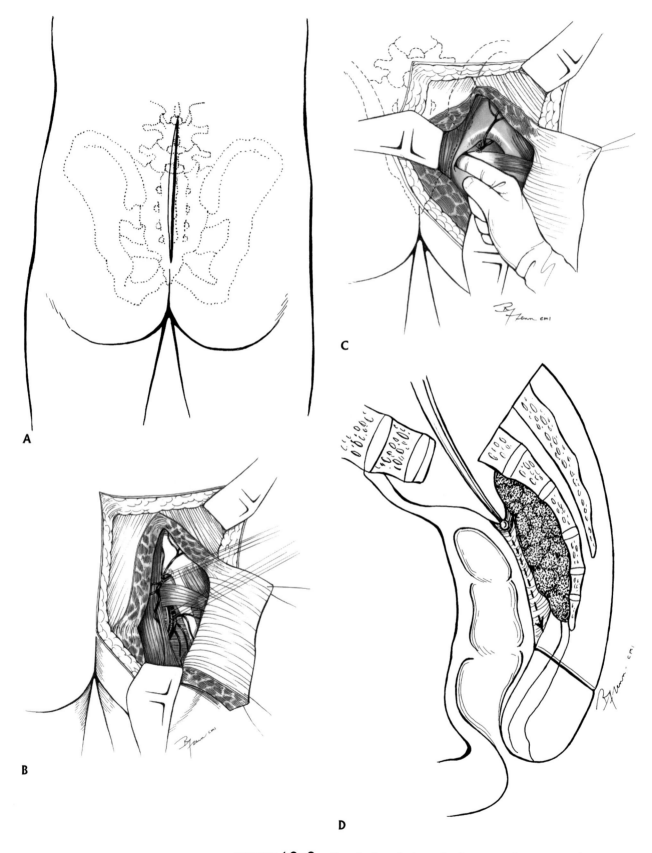

FIGURE 10–8 Surgical technique for low sacral resection (see text).

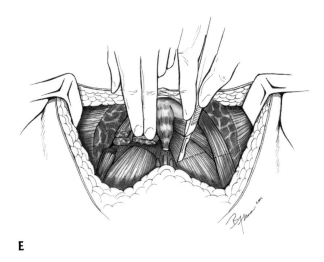

E

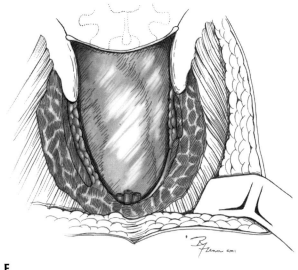

F

FIGURE 10-8 *(continued)*

Anterior/Posterior Resection

One of the controversies in the surgical treatment of larger malignant sacral tumors is whether to stage anterior/posterior approaches or to carry them out simultaneously.[146] The simultaneous anteroposterior approach to malignant tumors of the sacrum is preferred not only because of the efficiency and obvious benefits of earlier mobilization, but also because it decreases blood loss by allowing ligation of appropriate anterior vessels before one attempts sacral resection, protects major pelvic blood vessels, and allows better direction of the osteotomy to be made in the sacrum.[57,94,109] Similarly, Sundaresan et al prefer combined approaches even for chordomas and most benign lesions.[123,128] Technical difficulties can be daunting, however.

The patient is placed in the right lateral position, and an oblique incision is made parallel to the inguinal ligament, as for the retroperitoneal approach discussed in Chapter 13; a flap is rotated and the ureter mobilized. This allows dissection to the pelvis and exposure of the tumor with its capsule. The waldaris fascia and rectal plane can be dissected and the iliac vessels mobilized. We mobilize but avoid, if possible, ligation of the hypogastric arteries, although some feel that that is imperative. The major arterial supply of the anterior body of the tumor is ligated, and the tumor is freed from the rectum.

Alternatively, the patient is positioned supine on a turning, or Jackson, frame. A vertical incision is made (Fig. 10-9A). The peritoneum and contents are reflected laterally to expose the tumor behind the presacral fascia. Following excision of the fascia in the region of the tumor, the lesion is debulked (Fig. 10-9B), and the capsule carefully resected (Fig. 10-9C). Although a posterior approach will soon be performed, we recommend placement of a fascial graft (Fig. 10-9D). Laporotomy pads (which are removed later) are placed to protect the contents, and the anterior wound is closed primarily.

The posterior incision is then made. We recommend a curved, horizontal incision with the concave side toward the tumor, based at the spinous process of L5 (Fig. 10-9E). A skin flap is developed that includes the percutaneous fat. The gluteus maximus is then stripped off the iliac crest bilaterally and cut. The sacrotuberous and sacrospinous ligaments are cut, thus freeing the sacrum (Fig. 10-9F). It is imperative that the sciatic nerve be identified and protected. A sacral laminectomy is then performed to identify the dural sac; the decompression is carried laterally to mobilize the S1 and S2 nerve roots, as in Figure 10-6.

Osteotomy can then be safely performed and should extend well cephalad of the tumor. The iliac vessels are temporarily occluded during the resection of the sacrum: while the abdominal surgeons, from within the abdominal cavity, monitor the placement of the osteotomes and protect the abdominal contents as well as the iliac vessels, the spinal surgeon, from behind, uses osteotomes or a high-speed saw for en bloc resection of the tumor and normal surrounding bone. Once the cuts are made, the entire mass is elevated. Additional Marlex mesh is placed into the defect to prevent rectal herniation (Fig. 10-9G). Because of poor healing of

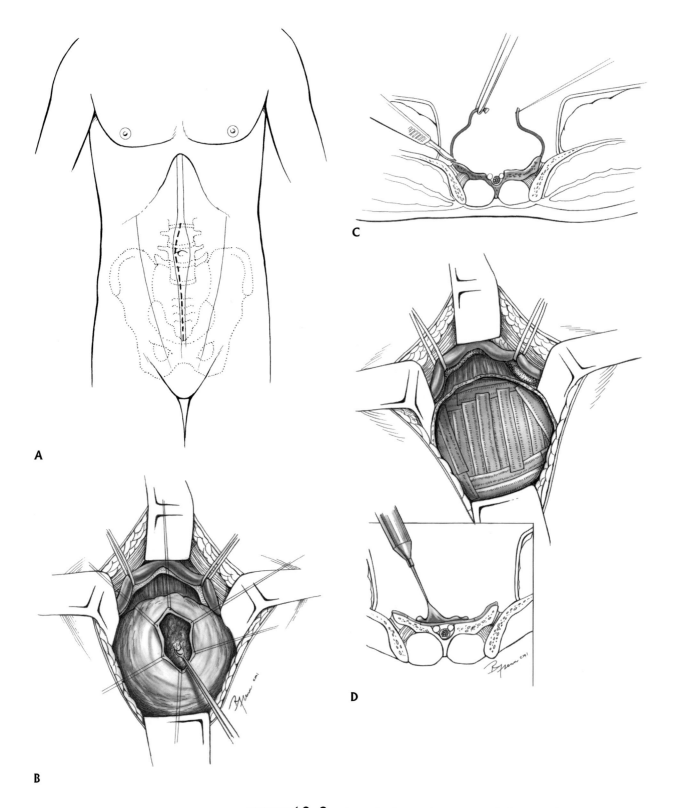

FIGURE 10–9 Anterior/posterior approach for sacral resection (see text).

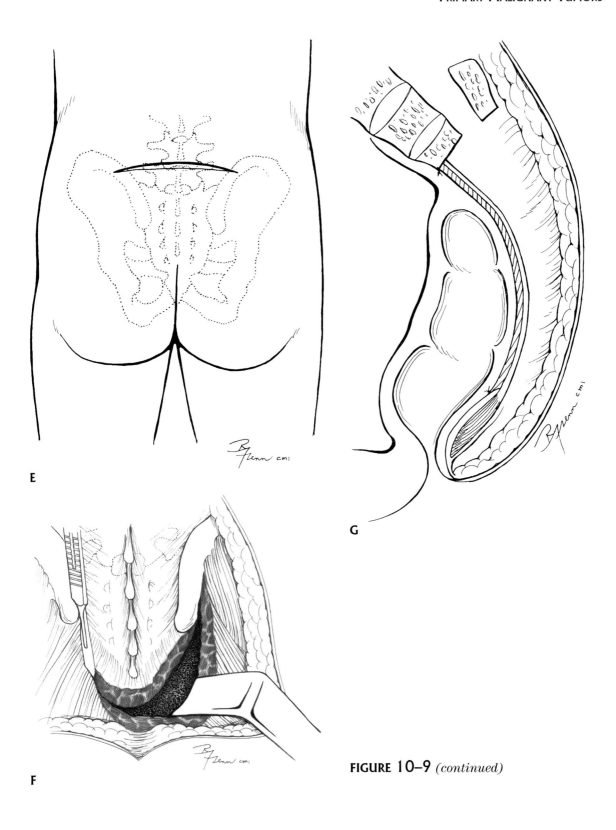

FIGURE 10–9 (continued)

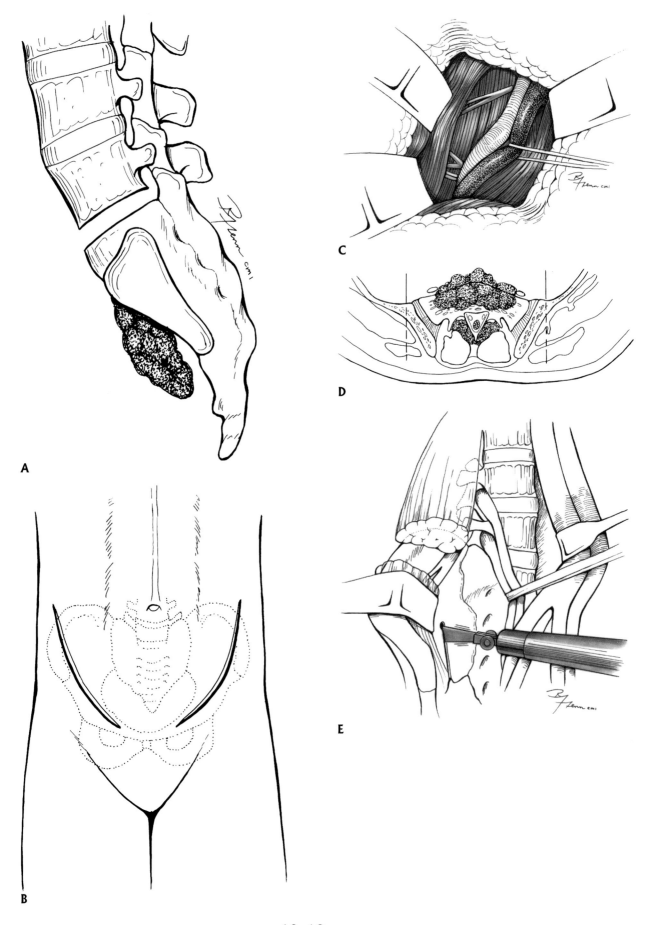

FIGURE 10–10 High sacral resection via anterior/posterior approach (see text).

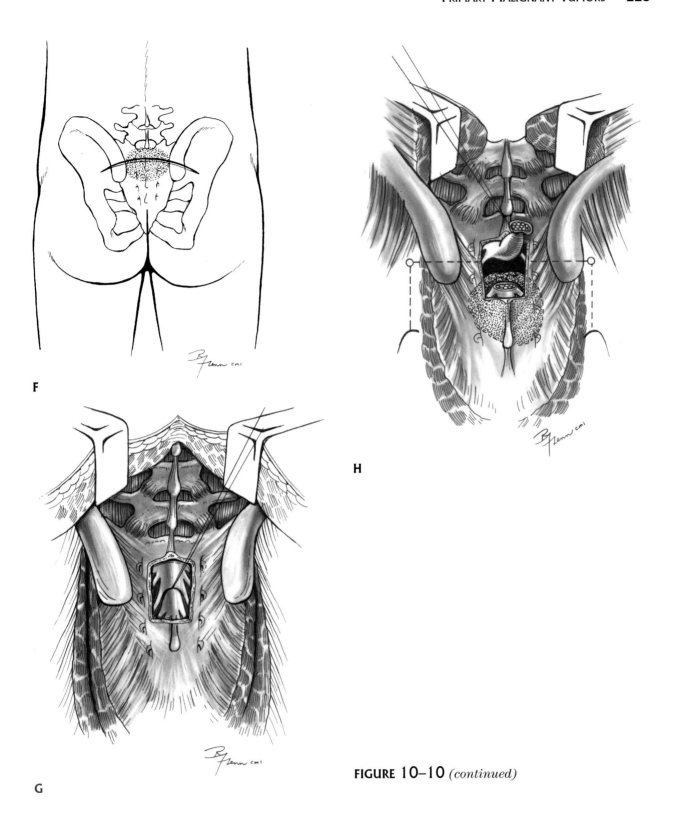

FIGURE 10–10 (continued)

High Sacral Resection via Anterior/Posterior Approach

There are few procedures more technically demanding than high sacral resection. However, this procedure is often indicated for tumors that extend up into the upper sacrum such as chordomas, which frequently go to the L5–S1 disc space (Fig. 10–10A). Both anterior and posterior approaches are required, although the order is optional. Some prefer to first perform the posterior procedure, we recommend carrying out the anterior approach first to protect the abdominal contents.

Stage One The patient is positioned supine and a bilateral retroperitoneal incision or approach is performed (Fig. 10–10B). Remaining in the retroperitoneal space provides exposure with minimal risk of tumor contamination of the peritoneal cavity, and also allows optimal visualization of the great vessels and the iliolumbar nerves. Following incision and exposure of the retroperitoneal space, the iliac arteries and veins are identified. The hypogastric arteries and veins are ligated and cut (Fig. 10–10C). To facilitate ligation of the multiple venous channels and other vessels that are typically in the field, femoral-venous bypass is often helpful.

The iliopsoas muscle is transected to visualize the sacroiliac joint as well as the lumbar nerve roots. The superior level of the tumor is identified both radiographically and visually: markers are inserted into the spine from anterior to posterior (Fig. 10–10D), using osteotomy cuts with edges kept separate by metal wedges, or more commonly, short Steinmann pins. If the tumor is below S1, the L5–S1 disc space can be used as the defining superior marker. The iliac crests are then cut vertically using osteotomes to the transverse junction of the Steinmann pins (Fig. 10–10E). The presacral space is then bluntly dissected and laparotomy pads are placed between the tumor/sacrum and the presacral fascia; this is done to protect the retroperitoneal contents from the posterior osteotomes that are performed later. The wounds are then closed in layers over two large surgical drains. The sponges that were left are removed during the sacral excision. Caution is advised: it is easy to lose even several laporotomy pads in this big cavity.

Stage Two The second stage of the procedure is performed under the same anesthesia when possible, because Steinmann pins or metal wedges have been left in the osteotomy cuts. These, of course, can move. If the operation is terminated after the anterior approach because of, for example, significant blood loss, the patient should be maintained on a kinetic bed to eliminate the need for turning, etc., until the second operation.

The second part of the procedure is performed prone on an imaging table. The posterior incision should either be a midline incision if radiation is not contemplated, or a transverse elliptical one if it is, as described earlier (Fig. 10–10F). The surgeon performs a careful subperiosteal dissection from L2 or L3 to the terminal sacrum, being careful not to disrupt any cortical bone of the sacrum. A laminectomy of L5 is performed to identify the dural sac; it is carried caudally and laterally to expose the S1 and S2 nerve roots (Fig. 10–10G). The gluteus maximus muscles are taken off the iliac crest and incised lateral to the sacrum. The gluteal arteries and veins are ligated; however, the gluteal nerves should be maintained if possible.

The dural sac is ligated distal to the S2 nerve roots, if possible, transected, and elevated to allow the surgeon to visualize the anterior sacrum (Fig. 10–10H). The longitudinal ligament is incised at L5–S1 and the disc space identified. The sacrum is now divided either at the superior horizontal cut made earlier by the osteotomes or at the disc space: using soft finger dissection, the sacrum is elevated.

Instability results from high sacral section. Although some place instrumentation at a later time, we find little justification in subjecting the patient to prolonged hospitalization and multiple operations. Therefore, stabilization is recommended during posterior sacrectomy using the Galveston technique; as an alternative, transpedicular fixation and Jackson screws into the ileum may be employed. Again, particularly in the patient who will be irradiated, closure with myocutaneous or vascularized flaps is strongly recommended.

Conclusions

The management of primary spinal tumors is challenging and requires great discretion on the part of the spine surgeon. Ensuring accurate diagnosis and monitoring spinal stability is typically all that is necessary in plasma cell lesions. However, for most other lesions discussed in this chapter, efforts to be "conservative" in surgical planning often lead to treatment failure. Alternatively, technically demanding surgical procedures that consider the biomechanics of the region can be associated with gratifying short- and long-term outcomes.

REFERENCES

1. Adapon BD, Legada BD Jr, Lime VA, et al: CT guided closed biopsy of the spine. J Comput Assist Tomogr 5:73–78, 1981.

2. Alexanian R: Localized and indolent myeloma. Blood 56: 521–525, 1980. J Bone Joint Surg 77A:405–411, 1995.

3. Ayala AG, Zornosa J: Primary bone tumors: Pathologic study of 222 biopsies. Radiology 149:675–679, 1983.

4. Azzarelli A, Quagliuolo V, Cerasoli S, et al: Chordoma: Natural history and treatment: Results in 33 cases. J Surg Oncol 37:185–191, 1988.

5. Babu NV, Titus VTK, Chittaranjan S, et al: Computed tomographically guided biopsy of the spine. Spine 19:2436–2442, 1994.

6. Baker ND, Dorfman DM: Ewing's sarcoma of the sacrum. Skeletal Radiol 25:302–304, 1996.

7. Ballance WA, Mendelsohn G, Carter JR, et al: Osteogenic sarcoma: Malignant fibrous histiocytoma subtype. Cancer 62:763–771, 1988.

8. Barlogie B, Hall R, Zander A, et al: High-dose melphalan with autologous bone marrow transplantation for multiple myeloma. Blood 67:1298–1301, 1986.

9. Barlogie B, Smith L, Alexanian R: Effective treatment of advanced multiple myeloma refractory to ankylating agents. N Engl J Med 310:1353–1356, 1984.

10. Barwick KW, Huvos AG, Smith J: Primary osteogenic sarcoma of the vertebral column: A clinicopathologic correlation of ten patients. Cancer 46:595–604, 1980.

11. Bataille R, Sany J: Solitary myeloma: Clinical and prognostic features of a review of 114 cases. Cancer 48:845–851, 1981.

12. Beltran J, Noto AM, Chakeres DW, et al: Tumors of the osseous spine: Staging with MR imaging versus CT. Radiology 162:565–569, 1987.

13. Belza MG, Urich H: Chordoma and malignant fibrous histiocytoma: Evidence for transformation. Cancer 58:1082–1087, 1986.

14. Benson H, Scarffe J, Todd ID, et al: Spinal cord compression in myeloma. Br Med J 1:1541–1544, 1979.

15. Bentzen SM, Poulsen HS, Kaae S, et al: Prognostic factors in osteosarcomas: A regression analysis. Cancer 62:194–202, 1988.

16. Bergsagel D, Dailey A, Langley G, et al: The chemotheraphy of plasma cell myeloma and the incidence of acute leukemia. N Engl J Med 301:743–748, 1979.

17. Bethke KP, Neifeld JP, Lawrence W Jr: Diagnosis and management of sacrococcygeal chordoma. J Surg Oncol 48:232–238, 1991.

18. Bjornsson J, Wold LE, Ebersold MJ, et al: Chordoma of the mobile spine. A clinicopathologic analysis of 40 patients. Cancer 71:735–740, 1993.

19. Black P: Spinal metastasis: Current status and recommended guidelines for management. Neurosurgery 5:726–746, 1979.

20. Boriani S, Biagini R, De Iure F, et al: Primary bone tumors of the spine: A survey of the evaluation and treatment at the Istituto Ortopedico Rizzoli. Orthopedics 18:993–1000, 1995.

21. Boriani S, Chevalley F, Weinstein JN, et al: Chordoma of the spine above the sacrum: Treatment and outcome in 21 cases. Spine 21:1569–1577, 1996.

22. Brenner B, Carter A, Tatarsky I, et al: Incidence, prognostic significance, and therapeutic modalities of central nervous system involvement in multiple myeloma. Acta Haematol 68:77–83, 1982.

23. Breslau J, Eskridge JM: Preoperative embolization of spinal tumors. J Vasc Interv Radiol 6:871–875, 1995

24. Brien EW, Mirra JM, Kessler S, et al: Benign giant cell tumor of bone with osteosarcomatous transformation ("dedifferentiated" primary malignant GCT): Report of two. Skeletal Radiol 26:246–255, 1997.

25. Broaddus WC, Grady MS, Delashaw JB Jr, et al: Preoperative superselective arteriolar embolization: A new approach to enhance resectability of spinal tumors. Neurosurgery 27:755–759, 1990.

26. Brown AP, Fixsen JA, Plowman PN: Local control of Ewing's sarcoma: An analysis of 67 patients. J Radiol 60:261–268, 1987.

27. Brugieres P, Revel MP, Dumas JL: CT-directed vertebral biopsy: A report of 89 cases. J Neuroradiol 18:351–359, 1991.

28. Burger EL, Lindeque BG: Sacral and non-spinal tumors presenting as backache. A retrospective study of 17 patients. Acta Orthop Scand 65:344–346, 1994.

29. Camins MB, Duncan AW, Smith J, et al: Chondrosarcoma of the spine. Spine 3:202–209, 1978.

30. Cammisa F, Glasser D, Lane J, et al: Chondrosarcoma of the spine and sacrum. Orthop Trans 11:578, 1987.
31. Catton C, O'Sullivan B, Bell R, et al: Chordoma: Long-term follow-up after radical photon irradiation. Radiother Oncol 41:67–72, 1996.
32. Cervoni L, Celli P, Salvati M, et al: Solitary plasmacytoma of the spine: Relationship of IgM to tumour progression and recurrence. Acta Neurochir 135:122–125, 1995.
33. Chak LY, Cox RS, Bostwick DG, et al: Solitary plasmacytoma of bone: Treatment, progression and survival. J Clin Oncol 5:1811–1815, 1987.
34. Chambers PW, Schwinn CP: Chordoma: A clinicopathologic study of metastasis. Am J Clin Pathol 72:765–776, 1979.
35. Congdon CC: Proliferative lesions resembling chordomas following puncture of the nucleus pulposus in rabbits. J Natl Cancer Inst 12:893–906, 1951.
36. Coombs RJ, Coiner L: Sacral chordoma with unusual posterior radiographic presentation. Skeletal Radiol 25:679–81, 1996.
37. Cortet B, Cotten A, Boutry N, et al: Percutaneous vertebroplasty in patients with osteolytic metastases or multiple myeloma. Revue Du Rhumatisme, English Edition. 64:177–183, 1997.
38. Corwin FK, Lindberg RD: Solitary plasmacytoma of bone versus extramedullary plasmacytoma and their relationship to multiple myeloma. Cancer 43:1007–1013, 1979.
39. Craig FS: Vertebral body biopsy. J Bone Joint Surg 38:93–102, 1956.
40. Daffner RH, Lupetin AR, Dash N, et al: MRI in the detection of malignant infiltration of bone marrow. Am J Radiol 146:353–358, 1986.
41. De Bruine FT, Kroon HM: Spinal chordoma: Radiologic features in 14 cases. Am J Radiol 150:861–863, 1988.
42. Delamarter RB, Sachs BL, Thompson GH, et al: Primary neoplasms of the thoracic and lumbar spine. Clin Orthop 256:87–100, 1990.
43. Delauche-Cavallier MC, Laredo JD, Wybier M, et al: Solitary plasmacytoma of the spine. Long-term clinical course. Cancer 61:1707–1714, 1988.
44. DeSantos LA, Murray JA, Ayala AG: The value of percutaneous needle biopsy in the management of primary bone tumors. Cancer 43:735–739, 1979.
45. Dreghorn CR, Newman RJ, Hardy GJ, et al: Primary tumors of the axial skeleton: Experience of the Leeds Regional Bone Tumor Registry. Spine 15:137–140, 1990.
46. Erikkson B, Guntegurg B, Kindblom LG: Chordoma: A clinicopathologic and prognostic study of a Swedish national series. Acta Orthop Scand 52:49–58, 1981.
47. Evans RG, Nesbit ME, Gehan EA, et al: Multimodal therapy for the management of localized Ewing's sarcoma of pelvic and sacral bones: A report from the second intergroup study. J Clin Oncol 9:1173–1180, 1991.
48. Faccioli F, Luna J, Bricolo A: One-stage decompression and stabilization in the treatment of spinal tumors. J Neurosurg Sci 29:199–205, 1985.
49. Feldenzer JA, McGauley JL, McGillicuddy JE: Sacral and presacral tumors: Problems in detection and management. Neurosurgery 25:884–891, 1989.
50. Firooznia H, Golimbu C, Rafii M, et al: Computed tomography of spinal chordomas. J Comput Tomogr 10:45–50, 1986.
51. Fruehwald FX, Tscholakoff D, Schwaighofer B: Magnetic resonance imaging of the lower vertebral column in patients with multiple myeloma. Invest Radiol 23:194–199, 1988.
52. Fuller DB, Bloom JG: Radiotherapy for chordoma. Int J Radiat Oncol Biol Phys 15: 331–339, 1988.
53. Fyfe IS, Henry APJ, Mulholland RC: Closed vertebral biopsy. J Bone Joint Surg 65B:140–143, 1983.
54. Gahrton G, Tura S, Flesch M: Bone marrow transplantation in multiple myeloma: Report from the European Cooperative Group for Bone Marrow Transplantation. Blood 69:1262–1264, 1987.
55. Gennari L, Azzarelli A, Quagliuolo V: A posterior approach for the excision of sacral chordoma. J Bone Joint Surg 69:565–568, 1987.
56. Ghelman B, Lospinuso MF, Levine DB, et al: Percutaneous computed tomography guided biopsy of the thoracic and lumbar spine. Spine 16:736–739, 1991.
57. Gitsch G, Jensen DN, Hacker NF: A combined abdominoperineal approach for the resection of a large giant cell tumor of the sacrum. Gynecol Oncol 57:113–116, 1995.
58. Gokaslan ZL, Romsdahl MM, Kroll SS, et al: Total sacrectomy and Galveston L-rod reconstruction for malignant neoplasms: Technical note. J Neurosurg 87:781–787, 1997.
59. Gosselin M, Benk V, Charron F, et al. Postoperative radiotherapy for chondrosarcoma of the L1 vertebral body: A case report. Med Dosim 19:217–222, 1994.
60. Han JS, Kaufman B, El Yousel SJ, et al: NMR imaging of the spine. Am J Roentgenol 141:1137–1145, 1983.
61. Heffelfinger MJ, Dahlin DC, MacCarty CS, et al: Chordomas and cartilaginous tumors of the skull base. Cancer 32:410–420, 1973.
62. Helms CA, Vogler JB III, Genant HK: Characteristic

CT manifestations of uncommon spinal disorders. Orthop Clin North Am 16:445–459, 1985.

63. Hermann G, Sacher M, Lanzieri CF, et al: Chondrosarcoma of the spine: An unusual radiographic presentation. Skeletal Radiol 14:178–183, 1985.

64. Hershey A, Bos GD, Stevens K: Successful treatment of spinal osteosarcoma with radiation and chemotherapy. Orthopedics 19:617–618, 1996.

65. Hirsh LF, Thanki A, Spector HB: Primary spinal chondrosarcoma with eighteen year follow-up: Case report and literature review. Neurosurgery 14:747–749, 1984.

66. Hruban RH, May M, Marcove RC, et al: Lumbosacral chordoma with high-grade malignant cartilaginous and spindle-cell components. Am J Surg Pathol 14:384–389, 1990.

67. Huang TL, Cohen NJ, Sahgal S, et al: Osteosarcoma complicating Paget's disease of the spine with neurologic complications. Clin Orthop 141:260–265, 1979.

68. Ikeda H, Honjo J, Sakurai H, et al: Dedifferentiated chordoma arising in irradiated sacral chordoma. Radiat Med 15:109–111, 1997.

69. Karakousis CP: Sacral resection with preservation of continence. Surg Gynecol Obstet 163(3):270–273, 1986.

70. Kattapuram SV, Khurana JS, Rosenthal DI: Percutaneous needle biopsy of the spine. Spine 17:561–564, 1992.

71. Kawahara N, Tomita K, Fujita T, et al: Osteosarcoma of the thoracolumbar spine: Total en bloc spondylectomy. A case report. J Bone Joint Surg 79:453–458, 1997.

72. Kim RY: High energy irradiation in the management of chondrosarcoma. South Med J 76:729, 1983.

73. Kornblum MB, Wesolowski DP, Fischgrund JS, et al: Computed tomography guided biopsy of the spine: A review of 103 patients. Spine 23:81–85, 1998.

74. Korovessis P, Repanti M, Stamatakis M: Primary osteosarcoma of the L2 lamina presenting as "silent" paraplegia: Case report and review of the literature. Eur Spine J 4:375–378, 1995.

75. Kozlowski K, Barylak A, Campbell J, et al: Primary sacral bone tumors in children. Australas Radiol 34:142–149, 1990.

76. Kreicbergs A, Boquist L, Borssen B et al: Prognostic factors in chondrosarcoma: A comparative study of cellular DNA content and clinicopathologic features. Cancer 50:577–583, 1982.

77. Krol G, Sundaresan N, Deck M: Computed tomography of axial chordomas. J Comput Assist Tomogr 7:286–289, 1985.

78. Kumar PP, Good RR, Skultety FM, et al: Local control of recurrent clival and sacral chordoma after interstitial irradiation with iodine-125: New techniques for treatment of recurrent or unresectable chordomas. Neurosurgery 22:479–483, 1988.

79. Le Pointe H, Brugieres P, Chevalier X, et al: Imaging of chordomas of the mobile spine. J Neuroradiol 18:267–276, 1991.

80. Lee BJ, Sahakian G, Clarkson BD, et al: Combination chemotherapy of multiple myeloma with alkeran, cytoxan, vincristine, prednisone, and BCNU. Cancer 33:533–538, 1974.

81. Leis AA, Fratkin J: Chondrosarcoma of the spine and thyroid carcinoma following radiation therapy for Hodgkin's lymphoma. Neurology 48:1710–1712, 1997.

82. Loftus CM, Michelson CB, Rapoport F, et al: Management of plasmacytoma of the spine. Neurosurgery 13:30–36, 1983.

83. Ludwig H, Tscholakoff D, Neuhold A, et al: Magnetic resonance of the spine in multiple myeloma. Lancet 1987:364–366.

84. Luken MG, Michelsen WJ, Whelan MA, et al: The diagnosis of sacral lesions. Surg Neurol 15:377–383, 1981.

85. MacCarty CS, Waugh JM, Mayo CW, et al: The surgical treatment of sacral and presacral tumors other than sacrococcygeal chordoma. J Neurosurg 22:458–464, 1965.

86. Matsukuma S, Kawabata M, Takemoto T, et al: Paget sarcoma of the cervical vertebrae: An autopsy case report and review of the literature. Pathol Intern 45:885–889, 1995.

87. Meis JM, Butler JJ, Osborne BM, et al: Solitary plasmacytomas of bone and extramedullary plasmacytomas: A clinicopathologic and immunohistochemical study. Cancer 59:1474–1485, 1987.

88. Meyer JE, Lepke RA, Lindfors KK, et al: Chordomas: Their CT appearance in the cervical, thoracic, and lumbar spine. Radiology 153:693–696, 1984.

89. Mill WB, Griffith R: The role of radiation therapy in the management of plasma cell tumors. Cancer 45:647–652, 1980.

90. Moulopoulos LA, Dimopoulos MA, Smith TL, et al: Prognostic significance of magnetic resonance imaging in patients with asymptomatic multiple myeloma. J Clin Oncol 13:251–256, 1995.

91. Moulopoulos LA, Dimopoulos MA, Weber D, et al: Magnetic resonance imaging in the staging of solitary plasmacytoma of bone. J Clin Oncol 11:1311–1315, 1993.

92. Murphy WA: Radiologically guided percutaneous musculoskeletal biopsy. Orthop Clin North Am 14:223–241, 1983.

93. Nelson PK, Setton A, Berenstein A: Vertebrospinal angiography in the evaluation of vertebral and spi-

nal cord disease. Neuroimaging Clin North Am 6:589–605, 1996.
94. Ozaki T, Hillmann A, Winkelmann W: Surgical treatment of sacrococcygeal chordoma. J Surg Oncol 64:274–279, 1997.
95. Patel DV, Hammer RA, Levin B, et al: Primary osteogenic sarcoma of the spine. Skeletal Radiol 12:276–279, 1984.
96. Person S, Kindbolm LG, Angervall L: Classical and chondroid chordomas: A light microscopic, histochemical, ultrastructural and immunohistochemical analysis of various t cell types. Pathol Res Pract 187:828–838, 1991.
97. Poor MM, Hitchon PW, Riggs CE: Solitary spinal plasmacytomas: Management and outcome. J Spinal Disord 1:295–300, 1989.
98. Rahmouni A, Divine M, Mathieu D, et al: MR appearance of multiple myeloma of the spine before and after treatment. Am J Radiol 160:1053–1057, 1993.
99. Rahmouni A, Divine M, Mathieu D, et al: Detection of multiple myeloma involving the spine: Efficacy of fat-suppression and contrast-enhanced MR imaging. Am J Radiol 160:1049, 1993.
100. Ribbert H: Ueber die experimentelle Erzeugung einer ecchondrosis physalifora. Ver Deutsch Kong Inn Med 13:455–464, 1895.
101. Rich TA, Schiller A, Suit HD, et al: Clinical and pathologic review of 48 cases of chordoma. Cancer 56:182–187, 1985.
102. Rosenthal DI, Scott JA, Mankin HJ, et al: Sacrococcygeal chordoma: Magnetic resonance imaging and computed tomography. Am J Radiol 145:143–147, 1985.
103. Rubins J, Quazi R, Woll JE: Massive bleeding after biopsy of plasmacytoma: Report of two cases. J Bone Joint Surg 62A:138–140, 1980.
104. Saltutti C, Di Cello V, Marzocco M, et al: Sacrococcygeal chordoma: Clinicoradiological study. Urol Int 45:372–375, 1990.
105. Samson IR, Springfield DS, Suit HD, et al: Operative treatment of sacrococcygeal chordoma: A review of twenty-one cases. J Bone Joint Surgery 75A:1476–1484, 1993.
106. Saunders WM, Castro JR, Chen GT, et al: Early results of ion beam radiation therapy for sacral chordoma: A Northern Oncology Group study. J Neurosurg 64:243–247, 1986.
107. Seifert RS, Arkin AM: Trephine biopsy of bone with special reference to the lumbar vertebral bodies. J Bone Joint Surg 31:146–149, 1949.
108. Settle WJ, Ebraheim NA, Saunders RC, et al: CT guided biopsy of metastatic sacral tumors. Orthopedics 137:753–758, 1990.
109. Shikata J, Yamamuro T, Kotoura Y, et al: Total sacrectomy and reconstruction for primary tumors. J Bone Joint Surg 70A:122–125, 1988.
110. Shikata J, Yamamuro T, Mikaway, et al: Instrumentation surgery for primary tumors of the spine. Arch Orthop Trauma Surg 108:144–149, 1989.
111. Shives TC, Dahlin DC, Sim FH, et al: Osteosarcoma of the spine. J Bone Joint Surg 68A:660–668, 1986.
112. Siegal T, Siegal T: Spinal epidural involvement in hematological tumors: Clinical features and therapeutic options. Leuk Lymphoma 5:101–110, 1991.
113. Simpson AH, Porter A, Davis, et al: Cephalad sacral resection with a combined extended ilioinguinal and posterior approach. J Bone Joint Surg 77A:405–411, 1995.
114. Smith J, Ludwig RL, Marcove RC: Sacrococcygeal chordoma: A clinicoradiological study of 60 patients. Skeletal Radiol 16:37–44, 1987.
115. Smith SR, Saunders PW, Todd NV: Spinal stabilisation in plasma cell disorders. Eur J Cancer 31A:1541–1544, 1995.
116. Soo C, Wallace S, Chuang V, et al: Lumbar artery embolization in cancer patients. Radiology 145:655–659, 1982.
117. Stener B, Gunterberg B: High amputation of the sacrum for extirpation of tumors: Principles and technique. Spine 3:351–366, 1978.
118. Stener B: Complete removal of vertebrae for extirpation of tumors: A 20-year experience. Clin Orthop 245:72–82, 1989.
119. Stephens GC, Schwartz HS: Lumbosacral chordoma resection: Image integration and surgical planning. J Surg Oncol 54:226–232, 1993.
120. Suga K, Tanaka N, Nakanishi T, et al: Bone and gallium scintigraphy in sacral chordoma: Report of four cases. Clin Nucl Med 17:206–212, 1992.
121. Suit H, Goitein M, Munzenrider J, et al: Definitive radiation therapy for chordoma and chondrosarcoma of the base of the skull and spine. J Neurosurg 56:377–385, 1982.
122. Sundaresan N, DiGiacinto GV, Krol G, et al: Spondylectomy for malignant tumors of the spine. J Clin Oncol 7:1485–1491, 1989.
123. Sundaresan N, Galicich JT, Chu FC, et al: Spinal chordomas. J Neurosurg 50:312–319, 1979.
124. Sundaresan N, Huvos AG, Krol G, et al: Postradiation sarcoma involving the spine. Neurosurgery 18:721–724, 1986.
125. Sundaresan N, Huvos AG, Krol G, et al: Surgical treatment of spinal chordomas. Arch Surg 122:1479–1482, 1987.
126. Sundaresan N, Huvos AG, Rosen G, et al: Post radiation sarcoma of the spine following treatment of Hodgkin's disease. Spine 11:90–92, 1986.

127. Sundaresan N, Rosen G, Huvos AG, et al: Combined modality treatment of osteosarcoma of the spine. Neurosurgery 23:714–719, 1988.

128. Sundaresan N: Chordomas. Clin Orthop 204:135–142, 1986.

129. Sung HW, Shu WP, Wang HM, et al: Surgical treatment of primary tumors of the sacrum. Clin Orthop 215:91–98, 1987.

130. Sze G, Uichanco LS, Brant-Zawaddzki MN, et al: Chordomas: MR imaging. Radiology 166:187–191, 1988.

131. Takaishi H, Yabe H, Fujimura Y, et al: The results of surgery on primary malignant tumors of the spine. Arch Orthop Trauma Surg 115:49–52, 1996.

132. Tasdemiroglu E, Bagatur E, Ayan I, et al: Primary spinal column sarcomas. Acta Neurol 138:1261–1266, 1996.

133. Tehranzadeh J, Freiberger RH, Ghelman B: Closed skeletal needle biopsy: Review of 120 cases. Am J Radiol 140:113–115, 1983.

134. Tigani D, Pignatti G, Picci P, et al: Vertebral osteosarcoma. Ital J Orthop Traumatol 14:5–13, 1998.

135. Tomita K, Kawahara N, Baba H, et al: Total en bloc spondylectomy: A new surgical technique for primary malignant vertebral tumors. Spine 22:324–333, 1997.

136. Tomita K, Tsuchiya H: Total sacrectomy and reconstruction for huge sacral tumors. Spine 15:1223–1237, 1990.

137. Utne JR, Pugh DG: The roentgenologic aspects of chordoma. Am J Radiol 74:593–608, 1955.

138. Villas C, San Julian M: Ewing's tumor of the spine: Report on seven cases including one with a 10-year follow-up. Eur Spine J 5:412–417, 1996.

139. Waisman M, Kligman M, Roffman M: Posterior approach for radical excision of sacral chordoma. Int Orthop 21:181–184, 1997.

140. Weinstein JB, Siegel MJ, Griffith RC: Spinal Ewing sarcoma: Misleading appearances. Skeletal Radiol 11:262–265, 1984.

141. White LM, Schweitzer ME, Deely DM: Coaxial percutaneous needle biopsy of osteolytic lesions with intact cortical bone. Am J Radiol 166:143–144, 1996.

142. Wilkins RM, Pritchard DJ, Burgert EO, et al: Ewing's sarcoma of bone! Experience with 140 patients. Cancer 58:2551–2555, 1986.

143. Wojno KJ, Hruban RH, Garin-Chesa P, et al: Chondroid chordomas and low-grade chondrosarcomas of the craniospinal axis: An immunohistochemical analysis of 17 cases. Am J Surg Pathol 16:1144–1152, 1992.

144. Wollersheim HC, Holdrinet RS, Haanen C: Clinical course and survival in 16 patients with localized plasmacytoma. Scand J Hematol 32:423–428, 1984.

145. Wu RK, Trumble TE, Ruwe PA: Familial incidence of Paget's disease and secondary osteogenic sarcoma: A report of three cases from a single family. Clin Orthop 265:306–309, 1991.

146. Wuisman P, Harle A, Matthiass HH, et al: Two-stage therapy in the treatment of sacral disorders. Arch Orthop Trauma Surg 108:255–260, 1989.

147. Yalniz E, Er T, Ozyilmaz F: Fibrous dysplasia of the spine with sarcomatous transformation: A case report and review of the literature. Eur Spine J 4:372–374, 1995.

148. Yang RS, Eckardt JJ, Eilber FR, et al: Surgical indications for Ewing's sarcoma of the pelvis. Cancer 76:1388–1397, 1995.

CHAPTER 11

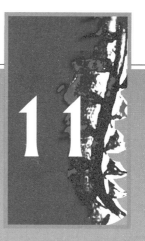

Metastatic Tumors of the Lumbar Spine

Epidemiology

Pathophysiology

Clinical Presentation

Radiography in Evaluation and Diagnosis

Diagnostic Biopsy

Factors Affecting Treatment Outcomes

Management

Conclusions

Metastatic Tumors of the Lumbar Spine

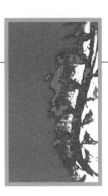

For an area perceived as being so important to the spine surgeon, this is a surprisingly brief chapter. Several reasons exist for this: first, management principles are similar for many types of lesions; and second, improvements in diagnosis and nonsurgical treatment appear to have decreased the number of patients undergoing surgery.[125,134]

In a retrospective series by Leviov et al,[100] 70 patients with metastatic tumors of varying radiosensitivity underwent radiotherapy (30–45 Gy) and steroid treatment; only 5 ultimately came to surgery. Most ambulatory patients remained so; one-third of the nonambulatory patients, including 16% who were paraplegic, had motor recovery. These results have been repeated many times in many series over many years: although outcomes in individual patient series may be altered by one treatment versus another, the aggregate results often seem the same.[28,170]

Epidemiology

Eighty percent of all skeletal metastases are produced by four primary malignancies: breast, lung, prostate, and renal cell. Spinal metastases represent approximately one-third of these, of which 6% produce spinal cord compression. Typically, such metastases are initially asymptomatic but eventually grow to cause invasion of intraspinal spaces or produce increased paravertebral soft tissue. In addition, pathologic fractures are commonly a cause of neurological deficit.[74]

Skeletal metastases are seen in over 20% of those with cancer, and they occur most commonly in the spine: studies have shown that the incidence of metastases is 5 to 7%, with two-thirds secondary to breast, lung, or prostate carcinoma, myeloma, or lymphoma.[144,175] The incidence of spinal cord compression is approximately 20%. Spinal cord compression is the initial symptom in 8% of patients with cancer; in another 9%, the primary tumor cannot be identified.[17,23,130,136]

Metastasis can also be the initial presentation of cancer. Schiff et al performed a retrospective review of 337 patients seen at Mayo Clinic with a radiographically verified diagnosis of spinal metastasis over an 8 year period. In 20%, these metastases were the initial presentation of the cancer. Carcinoma of the lung, cancer of unknown primary, multiple myeloma, and non-Hodgkin's lymphoma accounted for 78% of this group. Only 27% of patients with a first diagnosis of cancer had nonspecific symptoms suggesting malignancy, and in only 24% did the history or physical examination suggest the primary site of malignancy. Percutaneous needle biopsy of the vertebral lesion was diagnostic of malignancy in 18 of 19 patients.[136] Black observed that metastasis was the first manifestation of cancer in 8% of victims.[25]

Pathophysiology

The predilection of cancer to attack the spine and the vertebral body has been studied extensively. The lumbar arteries are closely applied to the vertebral body. Networks on the anterior and lateral body surfaces and arterioles run throughout the cortex and ramify within the marrow. End arteries also penetrate the end plate.[43] Arguello performed elegant experimental studies in mice demonstrating that marked tumor cells injected into the arteries grew into the bone marrow of the vertebra, where bone remodeling is maximal.[11] The products of bone resorption are chemotactic for the cancer cells that are known to form bone metastases.[122]

The venous drainage, which also contributes to the dissemination of cancer, includes the well-known Batson's plexus lining the vertebral canal as well as sinusoids within the bone marrow itself. The walls of these sinusoids lack a basement membrane, and thus growths can readily traverse the endothelial gaps.[19] The relevance of Batson's plexus in cancer spread was recently reappraised by Geldof.[64] He reviewed animal studies involving transplanted prostate cancer cells and bone involvement. Prostate tumor cells reaching the vertebral venous plexus of the spine, especially during transient increased intra-abdominal pressure, led to metastatic tumor deposits in the vertebrae.

Analyses of pathological findings have been instrumental in further confirming tumor transmission within Batson's plexus. A retrospective radiologic review was performed by Yuh et al, who examined magnetic resonance images in 49 patients with known spinal metastases. They argued that, considering the venous anatomy of the vertebra, metastases should be first seen in the central or dorsal portion of the vertebra, whereas deposits from arterial spread would be initiated at the end plate. They divided the vertebral bodies into 27 cells and considered the metastatic deposits to be central or peripheral. Surprisingly, no pattern of deposit was determinable. They concluded that a pure venous or arterial route for dissemination is unlikely, and that spread is from multiple sources.[171]

In another histologic evaluation, 19 solitary vertebrae filled with metastatic tumor obtained by en bloc spondylectomy were analyzed to determine the mechanisms of local spread of vertebral tumors. Analysis of tumor location showed that metastatic tumors reached the vertebral column by invading the bone marrow of the dorsal region of the vertebral body. The anterior longitudinal ligament, posterior longitudinal ligament, periosteum abutting the spinal canal, ligamentum flavum, periosteum of the lamina and spinous process, interspinous ligament, supraspinous ligament, cartilaginous end plate, and annulus fibrosus served as barriers to tumor progression (belying the concept of tumor extending to adjacent vertebrae by direct vertebral extension): the pathways allowing tumor spread to adjacent vertebrae were from the edge of the vertebral body to the adjacent vertebral body beneath the longitudinal ligament and through the paravertebral muscles to the neighboring lamina. The most common path for tumor spread is through the posterior longitudinal ligament to the epidural space.[59]

Involvement of the anterior spinal canal is more predictable from anatomic considerations. Metastatic deposits typically have a bibulbar appearance with a central septum initially on magnetic resonance imaging (MRI), conforming to the inner surface of the vertebral body and posterior longitudinal ligament. The two sections grow independently and often detach from each other at a certain size.[135]

Clinical Presentation

Virtually all patients with metastatic tumor producing spinal cord–dural sac compression give histories of local pain ranging from weeks to years prior to the onset of neurological deficit.[65] Radiculopathy may also occur.[97,104] By the time most patients present, however, three-fourths demonstrate significant motor weakness, including one-fifth who are paraplegic. Approximately 50% complain of sensory loss, either due to cord compression or to radicular abnormalities. Bowel and bladder dysfunction used to be a common presentation in earlier series.[65] More recently, however, bowel and bladder abnormalities are uncommon, presumably as a result of improved and earlier noninvasive imaging.[40]

Spinal fracture following minor trauma may also be the initial presentation, especially in older people.[61,62] In one series, of 70 cases of thoracic fracture in patients over the age of 50, 15 were due to trauma, 34 to osteoporosis, and 18 to metastasis, a much higher percentage than would be expected.[24] Hence, we recommend that patients over 50 with fractures should undergo advanced imaging to exluded tumor.

Determining if fractures are pathologic is difficult, at best. Successful identification is more related to bone density and the status of supporting structures (i.e., disc) than the quality of the vertebral body itself.[10] Taneichi et al attempted to create clinically useful criteria for pathologic fractures about to collapse. They suggested that vertebral collapse is likely if the body is more than 35% occupied by tumor, or 20% with posterior element involvement. They recommended prophylactic surgery for lesions of this size to prevent neurological catastrophe due to vertebral collapse.[160] Certainly, prophylactic radiotherapy, adjunctive chemotherapy, and possible orthotic stabilization are indicated in sizable asymptomatic lesions; it is harder to justify surgical treatment in the asymptomatic patient.

Radiography in Evaluation and Diagnosis

Plain Radiography

Although plain radiography is routinely used for detecting metastatic disease, its value must often be considered questionable.[17] At least 30 to 50% of the trabecular bone must be destroyed, or deformity exist, before lesions can typically be identified on plain radiography.[49] By then most tumors have produced cord compromise and neurological deficit. Over 60% of patients with epidural lymphoma present with normal plain radiographs.[102,105,175] Indeed, plain radiography is far more likely to be of value in slow-growing tumors such as meningiomas or ependymomas, which may cause erosion of foramina and enlargement of the spinal canal, rather than actual vertebral body compromise.

Baron et al found abnormalities on plain radiographs in 80% of patients with pain due to spinal metastasis. The studies were less valuable because they were typically positive in cancers of the breast and prostate as well as myeloma, but were negative in patients with renal cell carcinoma and lung carcinoma, even in advanced lesions.[18] In a large prospective series comparing myelography and neurological function, plain radiographs were abnormal in only 85% of patients with actual spinal cord compression, of whom the vast majority had osteolytic metastases.[78] Only prostate cancer was associated primarily with osteoblastic lesions. Clearly, whether metastatic lesions are lytic or blastic matters in terms of production of deformity; however, it is unclear whether overall prognosis is altered.[63]

Breast cancer presents some unique radiographic features. Rauschning examined spines riddled with breast cancer, comparing cryosections with plain radiography and computed tomography (CT). Most lesions were located near the cortical bone of the vertebrae or end plates. Lytic lesions at the end plate were more likely to be due to disc herniation (as noted earlier, disc expansion is common in metastatic cancer) than tumor infiltration. Posterior vertebral extrusion was uncommon, even when the vertebrae were collapsed, and epidural tumor extension was seldom seen.[128]

Computed tomography is critical in differentiating collapse due to osteopenia from tumor.[72,77] Determining the extent of bony destruction is important in surgical planning and is often necessary for determining the techniques of fixation to be used.[174] Contrast enhancement is rarely of value in the evaluation of metastatic disease.

Radionuclide Studies

These are commonly used by oncologists and others for staging purposes. Unfortunately, although sensitive, they are nonspecific and have a very high false positive rate in patients with metastases outside the spine.[124]

However, radionuclide studies may identify spine metastases several months prior to radiographic (even sometimes MRI) abnormalities.[31,58] Early definition may allow radiotherapy as soon as abnormalities are identified. Even nonspecific evidence of widespread metastasis may alter treatment planning (such as electing not to perform surgery in patients with disseminated disease).

Single positron emission computed tomography (SPECT) has a better threshold for localizing metastatic lesions than general radionuclide scanning. It also often defines the sites of the lesion within a given vertebra (i.e., pedicle versus facet), which is extremely difficult on planar images.[31]

Myelography

Before the widespread use of MRI, myelography was the diagnostic procedure of choice in metastatic disease. However, there are a number of disadvantages to this procedure. First of all, the tumor process itself cannot be precisely imaged, particularly the relationship of epidural masses to the vertebral body. Second, more often than not, a block is present and multiple punctures may have to be performed; even a single puncture, however, may be associated with neurological deficit.[81,129] Third, because of the often multifocal incidence of metastatic disease, a total spine myelogram needs to be performed, a time-consuming, potentially hazardous, and most uncomfortable process. In our institution, myelography has been largely abandoned in the evaluation of the cancer patient.

Two recent series, however, successfully used myelography and postmyelogram CT to precisely define tumor extent and to predict treatment outcome. The extent of myelographic block correlated well with the preradiotherapy neurological status: complete block was commonly associated with nonambulation and vice versa. Vertebral body collapse as a cause of canal compromise was not, however.[34,36] Sensory abnormalities did not correlate with any radiographic abnormalities. Following radiotherapy, complete or almost complete epidural tumor regression occurred in almost all patients that remained or became ambulatory. Patients whose myelograms showed no improvement did not improve clinically.[78,79] In the latter series, postmyelographic CT was more accurate than MRI in defining tumor extension. So we use myelography only when MRI is not available or for follow-up in patients with instrumentation in whom MRI is unsuccessful.

Magnetic Resonance Imaging

In our institution, a paradigm has been developed for rapid MRI scanning that includes sagittal MRI images throughout the entire spine followed by careful axial images of identified pathology. Several recent studies have shown that MRI is more accurate in the diagnosis and definition of metastatic tumors of the spine than other techniques.[22,148] MRI is 93% sensitive and 97% specific for multifocal metastatic disease and epidural tumor when compared to myelography, surgical pathology, and clinical course.[102]

In addition to demonstrating multilevel disease, MRI scanning provides accurate surgical definition, with its cranial/caudal orientation. The MRI scan is also highly sensitive to the involvement of vertebral bodies.[138] Needless to say, there are disadvantages to MRI: first of all, even at the time of this writing, machines are not universally available. In addition, an occasional patient may have enough claustrophobia that MRI scanning becomes unfeasible. Because of the superior nature of MRI scanning, it is this author's preference to perform MRI under heavy sedation or anesthesia standby, rather than accept the less sensitive and more technically difficult myelography.

On occasion, we have found that the signal changes and vertebral body collapse due to metastatic disease is difficult to distinguish from infection and sometimes osteoporosis.[70] However, vertebral body collapse due to benign causes usually is at a ratio greater than 0.8 in comparison to adjacent bodies, whereas the collapse in metastatic disease is typically less than that value.[172] Also, apparent disc expansion resulting from an intact disc, in the presence of a weakened vertebra, is a common finding in cancer.[165] Actually, the intervertebral disc is rarely involved in metastasis, though it often is involved in infection.[83] Also, metastases typically demonstrate high intensity on fat saturation T1-weighted imaging, which is not the case for nonmalignant lesions.[163]

Gadolinium is rarely necessary in imaging metastatic tumors.[167] On occasion, it may be helpful in certain nonenhancing tumors, but rarely distinguishes cancer from infection. In trauma, enhancement is rarely seen.

However, it is of value in monitoring treatment. For example, gadolinium is particularly valuable in distinguishing between scar and tumor recurrence.[32,46] Following radiation therapy of metastases, the T1 signal usually increases because of replacement of bone marrow by fat. This increased T1 signal can be distinguished from changes due to metastases recurrence by gadolinium.[127,150,158,159]

One of the classical radiographic signs of metastasis is the loss of the pedicle, historically considered to be an early abnormality.[85,169] However, more recent studies incorporating MRI have very clearly indicated that the vertebral body is involved much earlier and that destruction of the pedicle is a late finding.[13] Metastasis to the pedicle alone does not occur with any frequency;[5] instead this represents direct extension from the vertebral body. The finding of pedicle destruction and normal vertebral body reflects the sensitivity of plain radiography for cortical bone, rather than any particular involvement pattern.

Metastatic disease in the spine prominently affects the bone marrow. Therefore, MRI is extraordinarily sensitive, since it provides images of marrow rather than bone.[14,16,45,84,103] Abnormalities are typically seen in both T1- and T2-weighted images, with enhancement of the T2 effect using gradient echo sequences.[126]

Sanal et al considered bone marrow changes in patients with breast cancer of varying stages. Only some patients with marrow evidence of metastasis had positive bone marrow studies for tumor. However, in the 14 of the 23 with positive MRI studies suggesting marrow involvement, half had normal bone scans at that time. Four of 5 patients with stage II or III disease with initial marrow abnormalities showed metastatic disease within 5 to 18 months at those points.[132] Thus, not only can MRI diagnose existing metastases, but sequential scanning may be of value in defining future disease and allowing expectant treatment.

Dynamic MRI may also accurately define marrow infiltration:[27] dynamic contrast-enhanced imaging was performed prior to and following therapy in patients with leukemia. Opposed-phase and in-phase dynamic imaging before and after gadolinium were compared for controls and patients with suspected vertebral involvement. In patients with higher-grade marrow involvement, signal intensity increased with out-of-phase imaging. Although technically challenging, this may have some value in the future in determining the extent of vertebral involvement.

substantially better than those reported by others, and avoided open diagnostic biopsies in several patients.[95]

Indeed, in one series,[86] 32 patients underwent transpedicular biopsy for tumor diagnosis. Of these, 26 were performed on an outpatient basis. C-arm fluoroscopy or CT was used to confirm biopsy needle placement. Only 2 patients required repeat biopsy because of inability to make the histologic diagnosis; there were no complications, and all outpatients were discharged after observation.

Needless to say, biopsy does not substitute for, and should not delay, timely and appropriate surgical treatment for spinal cord decompression or spinal stabilization. In addition, biopsy is of little value if the radiographic picture is diagnostic, as is increasingly the case with new imaging modalities, or in patients with known primary disease and typical metastasis. It may be dangerous in vascular tumors, such as hemangiomas. Furthermore, as is discussed in the section on sacral tumors, we do not recommend transrectal biopsy, since this may cause tumor spread and lead to colostomy.

Diagnostic Biopsy

In patients with unknown primary disease and multiple levels of metastases or minimal neurological deficit, CT-directed biopsy can be helpful. The advantage of biopsy, of course, is that patients who are relatively asymptomatic can avoid major surgical procedures for some time. Furthermore, needle biopsy can be used to provide tissue diagnosis in lieu of potentially damaging procedures such as laminectomy used for diagnostic purposes alone.[1,47,55,56,60,117]

By most accounts, CT-directed biopsy has a high accuracy rate.[2,15,140,161] Success rates are approximately equal for masses located in the vertebral body, in posterior elements, or in paraspinal masses. Generally, trocar needles are used for sclerotic lesions, and thin spinal needles for lytic or soft tissue masses.[3,42,92,139] Several have reported better results for osteolytic than osteosclerotic or blastic lesions.[30,166]

Kornblum et al recently reported a series of 103 successful CT biopsies of the spine; of these, 53 were lumbar and 14 sacral. Ninety of these provided enough material for pathologic evaluation, and 67 of 94 were diagnostic. These results are

Factors Affecting Treatment Outcomes

Tumor Biology

Ultimate prognosis may depend more on tumor biology than on any other single factor. Clearly, metastatic lesions are rarely totally resectable. Thus the natural history of the tumor is of extraordinary importance. Behavior determines both local growth as well as dissemination; it is related directly to the results of treatment. This biological behavior will determine local versus systemic aggresiveness and will reflect long-term survival as well as quality of life. Myelomas and breast and prostate carcinomas[142,168,173] have a better prognosis than most sarcomas and lung cancer.

Several studies have suggested that radiosensitivity can be related to a favorable prognosis; thus the tumor cell type may mean more than the type of surgery used.[37] Patients who do respond to aggressive treatment survive longer and their quality of life may be much better if treatment is judicious.[17]

Lymphomas are generally widely metastasized before spinal lesions become symptomatic. Although when isolated they carry a good prognosis, the more typical picture is rarely associated with long-term survival. On occasion, lymphoma presents as epidural tumor; far more commonly, vertebral involvement is ultimately seen (Fig. 11–1). Surgery is useful only in severe deformity or severe neurological deficit in the presence of spinal cord compression.[35,107]

Metastatic melanoma has, by and large, a dismal prognosis, except if limited to one vertebra and not disseminated elsewhere.[149] Age and tumor location do not significantly influence survival. Patients with vertebral column disease and poor prognostic factors, including paraplegia, lung or colon metastasis, or multilevel disease, have a short life expectancy, and therefore radical surgery is not recommended.

Prostate cancer causes spinal cord compression in 7% of men affected with the disease, and spinal metastasis in about 20%. Back pain is the most common initial presentation, and typically responds to radiotherapy. Surgery is indicated only in selected cases of neurological deficit or severe compression with deformity.[123]

Approximately 140,000 new cases of breast cancer are diagnosed annually; one-half eventually demonstrate systemic involvement.[12,99] Most include spinal metastasis (60% of deaths), and a substantial percentage of spinal metastases originate from the breast. Most patients with metastatic breast cancer complain of back pain and radicular abnormalities.[66] Since the majority of lesions are lytic, plain radiographs will be abnormal, often with multilevel involvement (Fig. 11–2). MRI is critical; myelography suffers from the difficulties associated with imaging the entire spine, which is necessary before treatment of suspect local disease. Interestingly, most end plate failures are due to disc expansion rather than tumor ingrowth. Most canal compromise is caused by a fractured or collapsed vertebral body; rarely is there intrusion of epidural tumor.[12] Posterior element abnormalities are a consequence of tumor spread or bony changes, presumably due, in part, to instability.[88,89]

Neurological Status Prior to Treatment

There is a clear correlation between pretreatment motor status and functional outcome.[26] Two-thirds of patients walking at the time of diagnosis will do

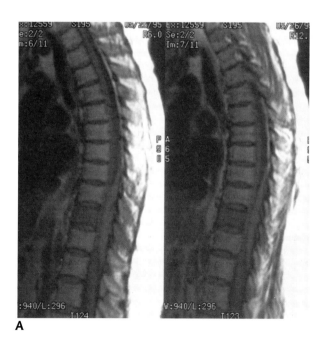
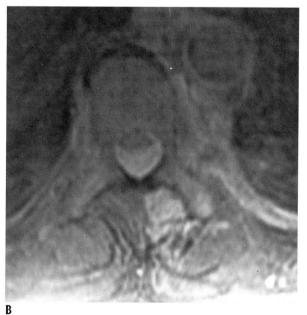

A B

FIGURE 11–1 Seventy-year-old female with lymphoma and increasing neurological deficit. **A** Sagittal MR image demonstrating vertebral body involvement and extensive posterior epidural mass. **B** Axial image showing large paravertebral mass on left, extending into spinal canal via the foramen. The patient underwent laminectomy (radiographs unavailable) and developed a deformity.

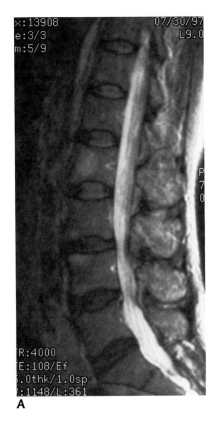
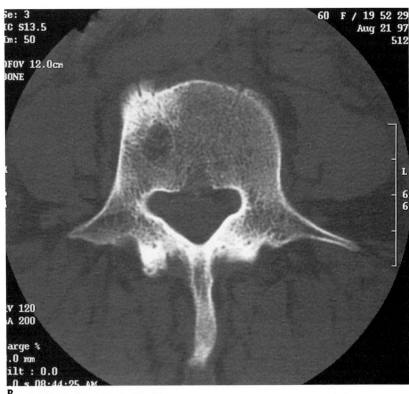
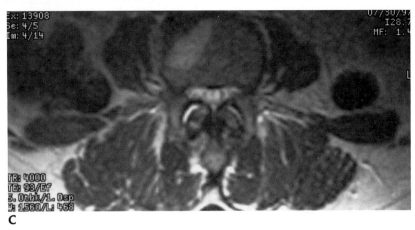

FIGURE 11–2 Sixty-year-old female with back pain and history of breast cancer and back pain. **A** Sagittal MRI with lesion at L2, questionable lesion at L4. **B** Mixed blastic/lytic lesion in vertebra. **C** Axial MRI of same lesion. Symptoms resolved with radiotherapy.

so after treatment; 35% who are paraparetic improve to the point of being somewhat ambulatory, but only 5% will regain the ability to walk.[54,56,78,145,146] There seems to be no difference between simple decompression (laminectomy[67]) and radiation therapy in that regard.

Definitive treatment prior to rapid deterioration is imperative. In almost all instances, patients present with spinal pain several weeks to months before they develop neurological deficit. Similarly, radicular pain may occur months prior to the development of myelopathy. Therefore, it is appropriate to definitively image patients with spinal pain who have known cancer. MRI is the diagnostic procedure of choice, since epidural tumor is defined quite early.

In one study considering tumor biology versus preadmission neurological status, Sioutos et al attempted to determine criteria by which clinicians could predict outcomes following treatment. In their series, lung, prostate, and breast were the most common primaries. Patients walking prior to admission survived statistically longer than nonambulatory patients or those with bowel and bladder dysfunction. Patients with renal cell carcinoma survived the longest, followed by those with breast, prostate, lung, and colon cancer.[147]

The real question is whether patients presenting with even recent-onset complete paraplegia benefit from surgical treatment. Siegal and Siegal found that only 2% of patients treated following onset of complete paraplegia demonstrated useful motor recovery.[144,145] Our experience with radical decompression is slightly better. Furthermore, a significant question exists as to whether neurological function in patients with rapidly progressive neurological deficit can be salvaged. Unfortunately, many of the retrospective series available are difficult to interpret: again, the value of surgical approaches is uncertain, in part because of poor standardization of procedures.

Tumor Location

The location of the tumor within the spinal canal should affect the choice of therapy, and also determines outcome. Several studies have shown that most epidural tumors do not arise in the venous plexus but rather in the vertebral body and invade the epidural space secondarily. Indeed, 85% of tumors thought to be epidural actually arise in the body or pedicle.[18,66,137] Thus they are primarily located anterior to the spinal cord.

Some tumors enter the canal via the neural foramina either from paravertebral lymph nodes or through direct growth (Fig. 11–3). Epidural tumors without any of the above come from direct hematogenous spread from the vascular supply of the primary tumor.[19] In our unpublished series of 329 metastatic tumors, only 9 solid tumors—as opposed, for example, to lymphoma [33,130]—failed to show bone involvement on pretreatment or subsequent imaging, or at surgery.

Lung cancer tends to metastasize into the bone marrow sinuses, extending first into the bone marrow and then causing osteolytic lesions. Pure epidural metastases, therefore, are extremely unusual.[68,90]

Several studies[17,20,50,51,56,94,101,153,162] have indicated that dorsal epidural masses are more successfully treated than those anterior to the cord. This observation does not reflect different biologic characteristics of posterior masses; rather laminectomy was used in many of these procedures and is likely only to be helpful in patients with dorsal metastatic disease. Ultimately, it may actually make the neurological situation worse in others, since vertebral body collapse can be expected when the posterior elements are radically resected. When anterior and anterolateral approaches are used, over 70% of incomplete patients will maintain ambulation.[9,29,74,75,93,114,116,121,141,156]

Management

Specifics of the management of metastatic disease have changed significantly in recent years. Earlier diagnosis because of improved imaging techniques, more focal radiation therapy, and advances in chemotherapy have altered our thinking. They have also altered surgical indications: although some have reported an increasing incidence of spinal metastasis, we are seeing fewer surgical cases, reflecting the success of earlier and more aggressive nonoperative treatment.

For this reason, specific indications remain controversial. Certainly, the last two decades have witnessed changes in therapeutic approaches, ranging from the old and now largely disfavored isolated laminectomy to nonoperative treatment, to radical surgical decompression and stabilization (which has been advocated by the senior author since at least 1970). Unfortunately, there have been few appropriately controlled trials to provide consensus on surgical management. Similarly, there is little evidence that overall prognosis, particularly in terms of ambulation and bowel and bladder function, has improved for most patients treated for spinal metastases, although selected patients have benefited dramatically. Indeed, one fundamental fact of management has remained the same for decades: the primary determinant of ultimate functional prognosis is pretreatment neurological status followed by tumor biology and radiosensitivity.[144]

Drug Therapy

Current opinion is that the use of high-dose dexamethasone decreases venous or vasogenic edema

FIGURE 11–3

Fifty-six-year-old male with history of renal cell carcinoma who developed an acute L5 radiculopathy. **A and B** Lateral MR image with involvement of L5 vertebra (note preservation of the intervertebral discs) and epidural mass. The intraoperative pathology was lymphoma. Because of the radiosensitivity of the tumor, it was elected not to resect the vertebra, and to perform a simple fixation followed by radiotherapy. **C and D** Anteroposterior and lateral radiographs 7 months later; symptoms have resolved.

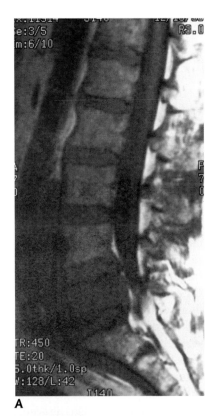
A

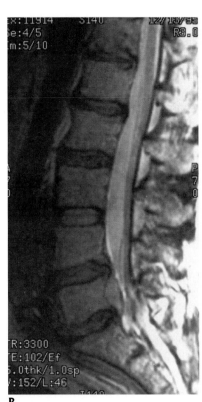
B

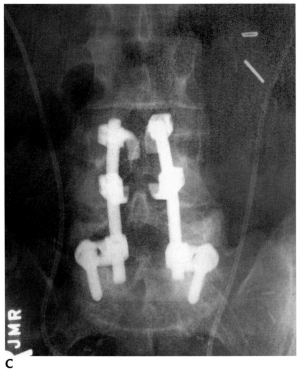
C

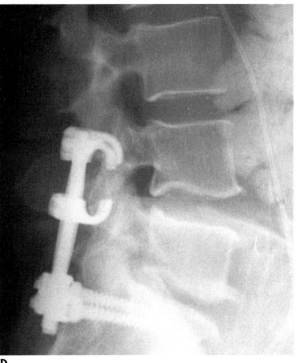
D

and slows neurological deterioration. However, experimental studies have shown that the edema of spinal cord compression is primarily due to prostaglandin production. Methylprednisolone does indeed reduce cord edema and tumor mass, particularly in blood-borne tumors.[19,115,143] Thus dexamethasone may not be the drug of choice in tumors, and methylprednisolone may be actually more effective.

It remains to be shown that reduction of edema will improve neurological status or at least delay devastating changes. Although steriods are universally used, we question the reliance on steriods to "buy time." Rather, definitive treatment should be provided with appropriate speed in a patient with progressive neurological deficit.

Surgical Treatment

Throughout this section, an emphasis is made on the appropriate decompression of masses. That is, anterior masses should be decompressed through approaches that allow vertebral resection.[116] The use of laminectomy as a decompressive technique for other than dorsal epidural tumor has marginal results. It has long been argued that patients with metastatic cancer are systemically incapable of undergoing aggressive anterior surgical procedures and therefore laminectomy is appropriate as a temporizing procedure. However, the morbidity of anterolateral approaches, especially the extracavitary approach, in our hands has not been significantly greater than laminectomy and instrumentation. Furthermore, the performance of a procedure that will not decompress the spinal cord, even if theoretically less morbid, would appear to be largely useless and often dangerous.[56] Therefore, surgeons are encouraged to consider all the components of successful spine surgery (appropriate decompression, stabilization, fusion) in patients with metastatic disease, as they do with other conditions of the spine.[96]

Indications

Siegal and Siegal emphasize that spinal instability and minor deformity are not necessarily a surgical indication.[144] For example, pathologic vertebral body fracture in the absence of progressive neurological deficit or increasing deformity may respond well to external immobilization and radiotherapy. This is commonly used in radiosensitive tumors such as myeloma and even breast cancer,[12] in which vertebral collapse is quite common.

On occasion, patients may require surgery for histological diagnosis. Commonly, newer radiologic techniques will provide significant information about tumor type; biopsies are more likely to delay definitive treatment in the patient with increasing deficit and therefore should be reserved for those with stable conditions and unknown tumor type.

Therefore, surgical treatment should be considered primarily in patients with progressive neurological deficit and resectable lesions. Aggressive surgical treatment is often appropriate for those with intractable pain or early disease and/or deformity. Again, the choice of the procedure must be based primarily on the location of the tumor and treatment needs, including decompression as well as stabilization. Furthermore, other metastatic disease, general health and survivability, and prognosis for the tumor type need to be considered. DeWald et al recommend prophylactic surgical stabilization of metastasis, even in the absence of deficit or pain;[48] however, many of these individuals respond to radiotherapy and orthotic use.

Prognosis

An important issue in the management of metastatic tumor to the spine is prognosis. Certainly, it is important from the standpoint of advising patients and families as to appropriate and realistic treatment, as well as choosing therapeutic options.

Bauer and Weddin[21] presented a detailed report on 88 patients treated for spinal metastases since 1990. Of the total, 28 were in the lumbar spine, and surgical indication was usually neurological compromise. Most patients underwent posterior decompression and stabilization. Prostate, breast, kidney, myeloma, and lung were the five most common sources of known disease. Over 10% had unknown primaries.

Approximately one-third of the population survived a year. This survival rate seemed to be most related to the metastatic load elsewhere in the spine. For example, survival rates were highest in those with isolated spinal metastasis and lowest for those with brain or visceral metastases; the question is whether surgical treatment of spinal metastasis is indicated in patients with these other lesions. Age was not related to outcome in any of the studies presented in this section.

Patients with myeloma, lymphomas, and renal cell carcinomas were more likely to survive a year than those with bronchogenic carcinoma, all else being equal. Patients with sarcomas typically did most poorly.[21] Perhaps diffuse metastatic load reflects tumor biology, rather than the length of time that the patient has had the disease.[112]

So do we tell our patients that it is tumor biology or extent of disease that ultimately predicts outcome? Bauer and Wedin argue that the type of tumor has great impact on prognosis, particularly myeloma and renal cell carcinoma, as well as breast cancer confined to the skeleton.[21] In Harrington's report, over two-thirds of the patients survived 1 year, but patients were treated with anterior decompression, which precluded those in poor general health.[75]

Our own unpublished data indicate that the morbidity of anterior and anterolateral surgery is no higher than that for laminectomy and that the surgeon's bias makes the decision, rather than any other conditions. Furthermore, for metastatic carcinoma, it appears to be tumor load or extent of soft tissue disease that is the major prognostic determinant.[147]

Techniques

Vertebroplasty Vertebroplasty has recently become popular in selected patients with metastatic disease. Weill et al reported a series of patients undergoing percutaneous vertebroplasty purely for analgesic purposes. Most achieved significant and long-term (6 months) pain relief.[164] In Cortet et al's series, 37 patients with myeloma or metastases underwent vertebroplasty under fluoroscopic control under local anesthesia. Most had very good or excellent pain relief for 6 months or longer, and only two patients suffered complications: leakage of cement causing nerve root compression.[41] These results are equivalent to surgical stabilization, as reported below, with much lower complication rates.

Laminectomy Do we really need to emphasize the limitations of laminectomy again? Overall, post-treatment ambulation rates of 40 to 50% are achieved by either radiotherapy or laminectomy. Furthermore, patients with anterior masses are as likely to deteriorate from laminectomy as improve. Nicholls and Jarecky presented a 20-year experience of laminectomy for metastatic disease: the vast majority of patients were not helped, the few who enjoyed only very short-term benefit, and complications, including infection, increased deficit, and deformity, were not trivial.[118]

The use of laminectomy for "emergent decompression" as a temporizing measure should also be discouraged. If surgery is to be performed, it should be a definitive procedure with appropriate decompression, stabilization, and fusion. Performance of laminectomy because the surgeon has little experience or success in anterior approaches and fears the morbidity is often unwise. Rather, referral to a center where such procedures are commonly carried out would be in the patient's best interests.

Transpedicular Approaches Alternatives to laminectomy have long been used, for tumor resection, with varying degrees of success. Transpedicular decompression via dorsal approaches can allow partial removal of anterior masses, especially soft, necrotic tumors (Fig. 11–4). However, even when approached bilaterally, the most central aspect of the vertebra may be difficult to reach without manipulating the cord, although Akeyson et al recommend it for patients who cannot tolerate what they perceive as larger procedures, such as the extracavitary approach.[4]

Several groups have described their experience with a modification of transpedicular decompression and partial vertebral resection in association with posterior fixation, but rarely anterior bone fusion, with good results with neurological recovery.[50,89,141] Magerl and Coscia even presented success with total vertebrectomy via posterior exposures, arguing that the ability to provide posterior multilevel fixation justifies the technical difficulties of their procedure;[106] the lateral extracavitary approach offers better exposure, maximal safe decompression, and the ability to perform stabilization. The latter, in our opinion, represents a critical advantage of posterior approaches: the ability to perform multilevel fixation, which is a critical element in the integrity of the spine affected with cancer.

The major attractiveness of transpedicular decompression is its relative ease, the somewhat effective, if incomplete, removal of anterior masses, and low morbidity. For patients with short anticipated survivals, it is often ideal and is used extensively. However, it is probably not the best approach for patients who may enjoy long-term survival, or those with resectable disease.

We performed a cadaveric study in an attempt

to determine the amount of vertebra safely removed through various approaches (Maiman, unpublished data). Approximately the middle third of the canal was difficult to reach with normal surgical instruments without manipulating the dura. This problem is considerably magnified in the patient with a firm or blastic tumor, or an extremely vascular tumor where hemostasis is made more laborious because of the indirect decompression.

Anterior fusion is also difficult through these approaches: although anterior strut grafts, for instance, can be placed in some instances without manipulating the thecal sac, more commonly surgeons pour hardening acrylic into the cavity.[151] Although this certainly adds some stability to the spine, it can be difficult to control, and certainly is not as useful as anterior grafting. The major advantages, then, of transpedicular decompression are its ease, the ability to perform bilateral decompression, and the ability to perform posterior instrumentation at the same operative approach. However, as mentioned earlier, these limited procedures are inadequate for a significant percentage of patients with thoracolumbar metastases.[29]

Anterior Lumbar Approaches Sundaresan and associates have published several clinical series that examine operative approaches and results. In the early 1980s, they analyzed results in a group of patients with metastatic lung cancer—largely involving the spine via direct extension—and myelopathy, most of whom were ambulatory.[151,155] Patients underwent radical vertebrectomy via anterolateral approaches, with stabilization using methylmethacrylate and subsequent local brachytherapy in most. Two-thirds were able to ambulate for at least 6 months, and pain was significantly improved with minimal morbidity. In light of these excellent results, the authors advocated aggressive surgical treatment.

Unfortunately, this relatively early series failed to consider the problems of spinal deformity development and extension of disease into adjacent vertebral segments. Shortly thereafter, the authors presented a small series of patients who underwent complete spondylectomy via staged approaches. In the first stage, anterior spondylectomy was accomplished; in the second, laminectomy and transpedicular removal on the opposite side and posterior fixation were performed.[154] Several patients had significant long-term survival, and morbidity was minimal.

More recently, Sundaresan and others[153,156] have advocated anterior-posterior decompression/ stabilization. In a series of 110 patients treated for both primary and metastatic tumors, approximately half were treated with anterior-posterior surgery, a third anterior decompression and fixation alone, and a smaller number posterior approaches only, or decompression without stabilization. Patients with solitary or contiguous metastases, or those who had three-column involvement, were selected for the most aggressive surgical treatment. Most patients improved neurologically, and overall median survival was 16 months. Although complications were seen in almost 50% of the entire group, the rate appeared no higher in those treated with combined anterior-posterior approaches. The technique of vertebrectomy has been modified in the MRI era. Alleyne et al have substituted titanium screws for Steinmann pins to allow for subsequent MRI.[6]

McAfee and Zdeblick also reported a series of patients undergoing anterior vertebrectomy, methylmethacrylate stabilization, anterior fixation with Harrington distraction rods, and sacral hooks.[114] Surgical indications included vertebral collapse due to metastasis with neurological compromise. In their early series, posterior fixation was not performed. More recently, they used various configurations of anterior fixation plates; in curable lesions such as primary tumors, posterior fixation is performed via a separate incision. Results are reportedly better than for other types of treatment; all in the group became ambulatory.

Lateral Extracavitary Approach Our preferred approach for the majority of patients with pathologic fractures and/or deformity and spinal cord compression is the lateral extracavitary approach. This procedure allows vertebral body, pedicle, and laminar removal through a single incision. In addition, it can be used bilaterally to perform bilateral pedicle and posterior element removal, and total vertebrectomy. Both anterior strut grafting and/or methylmethacrylate fixation can be used anteriorly, although we do not often perform the latter. Under certain circumstances, anterior plate or screw rod fixation can be performed.

Posterior stabilization, through recommended long-segment hook/rod or wire/rod fixation, is easily accomplished, as much as four-to-five levels above and below the lesion.[57] We do not use short-segment fixation using pedicle screws: although easily accomplished, adjacent pedicles are likely to become involved with tumor relatively early.[44,52]

By performing the entire anterior-posterior procedure through one incision and during one an-

244 Surgery of the Lumbar Spine

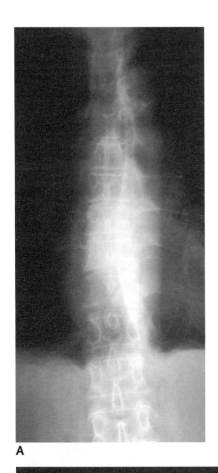

A

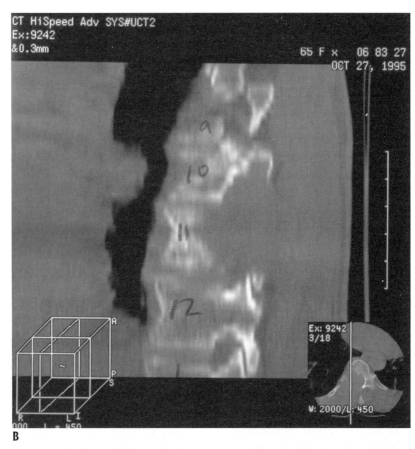

B

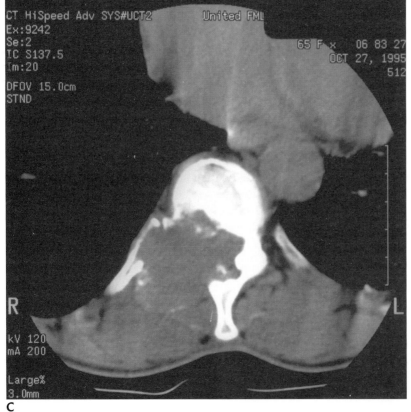

C

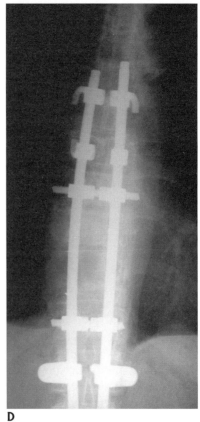

D

FIGURE 11-4

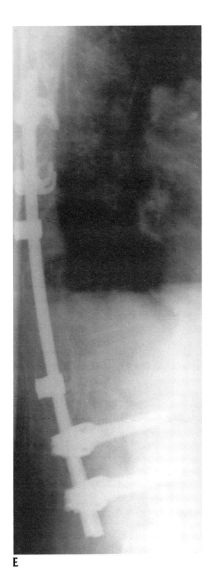
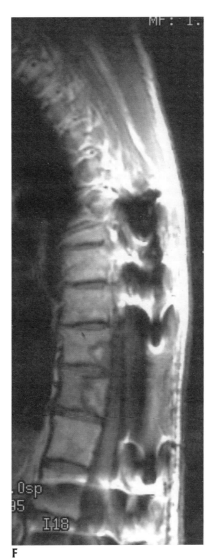
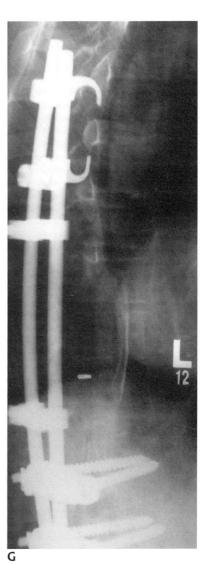

E F G

FIGURE 11–4 Seventy-year-old female with 30-lb weight loss, progressive paraparesis, and back pain. **A** Anteroposterior radiograph with pedicle loss right T11, and enlarged T12 pedicle. **B** Sagittal computed tomogram with erosion of portions of the T10 and T11 vertebrae. **C** Axial image showing massive erosion/tumor mass in right spinal canal, posterior elements, and soft tissue extension. The patient underwent emergent transpedicular decompression and posterior fixation, with moderate neurological improvement. Pathology: transitional malignant ganglioglioma. **D and E** Anteroposterior and lateral radiographs showing instrumentation. Because the lesion is potentially curable, MRI was repeated with fat suppression techniques. **F** Continued tumor present on MRI, but with good canal decompression. **G** Lateral radiograph following extracavitary approach to the spine with vertebrectomy. Note rib grafts. At 12 months, the patient was neurologically intact.

esthesia, we minimize perioperative morbidity. Patients are mobilized more quickly, and adjunctive treatment need not await two procedures. As discussed in the technique chapter, the lateral approach is difficult in lesions extending more than three levels, however.

In a yet-unpublished series from our institution, the lateral extracavitary approach to the lumbar spine was used in 83 patients with thoracolumbar spinal malignancies. Over 70% evidenced myelopathy, but only 20% were plegic. All had vertebral resection; 21 were performed bilaterally. Sixty-five patients, all treated since 1982, were stabilized posteriorly as well. Two patients died in the immediate perioperative period, 1 of myocardial infarction, and 1 of intraoperative hemorrhage and uncorrectable coagulopathy. There were nine wound infections, and 2 patients required reoperation for instrumentation removal. All ambulatory patients remained able to walk; half of the non-ambulators—including 4 patients who were thought plegic—became able to ambulate independently. Most patients succumbed to their primary disease, with a median survival of 17 months. A surprising 9 patients lived at least 5 years. Tumor type seemed to have less impact on survival than how early the metastasis was discovered. Overall, patients who underwent this more aggressive approach seemed to do better than those undergoing transpedicular decompression, although selection criteria may have biased these results.

Presurgical Planning

Embolization Emobolization is of great value in many vascular metastatic tumors, such as renal cell carcinoma. It is typically performed with minimal morbidity.[28,80,152] In one series, embolization minimized the most common complication associated with excision of these lesions. Indeed, in this series, 27 of 30 patients noted neurological improvement following embolization and excision. Median survival was 16 months. This experience has been reported by others.[80] We have been able to reduce intraoperative bleeding from an average blood loss of 6000 ml to 2000 ml.

O'Reilly et al performed embolization in four patients with renal cell carcinoma, presumably to decrease vascularity before surgical treatment. The resulting decrease in venous pooling led to substantial neurological improvement that persisted for several months.[120] Perhaps some results being attributed to surgical decompression might actually be due to embolization.[99]

Hemorrhage may also be a consequence of coagulopathy, which is common in metastatic cancer. Full coagulation studies should be obtained, and abnormalities corrected, prior to surgery. Fatal or serious intraoperative coagulopathy may be seen in as many as 5 to 8% of cancer patients undergoing spinal surgery.

Radiotherapy

Radiotherapy is the first-line treatment for most patients with metastatic disease who have stable vertebral body disease and/or epidural tumor with little or no neurological deficit.[8,52] It is not usually recommended as primary therapy in patients with pathologic fractures and deformity. However, in at least one large prospective trial of radiotherapy for breast carcinoma, there was no correlation between vertebral collapse and ambulatory outcome.[110] It may well be that collapse without deformity or spinal instability—the latter particularly in radiosensitive lesions such as myeloma—does not alter prognosis.

Does radiotherapy work? In another prospective trial, conducted in 1995, 255 of 275 patients with various cancers underwent primary radiotherapy.[108,109] Two schedules of radiotherapy plus steroids were given. Most patients (82%) reported substantial back pain relief. Three-fourths achieved excellent or good motor recoveries, and almost half had improved bowel and bladder function (Fig. 11–5). Even with late diagnosis, radiosensitive tumors such as breast, myeloma, and prostate responded well. Those with nonsensitive tumors were associated with unnecessary complications. Survival times correlated most to ambulatory status. Vertebral collapse did not affect survival or response.

Sugiyama[150] recently presented a series of 50 patients with 63 spinal metastases. Most patients presented with pain alone or pain with radiculopathy; about one-third had myelopathy. Primary tumors were, in order of occurrence, lung, breast, colon-rectal (9 cases each) and prostate (7). Rather than classifying the patients by tumor type, the researchers grouped patients by the MRI appearance of the lesion. Osteolytic lesions producing pathologic fracture or destructive masses were more likely to be associated with deformity.[133] Osteoblastic masses rarely did so, however. Radiotherapy was

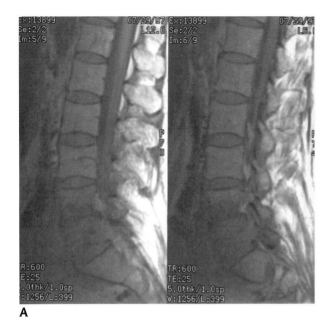
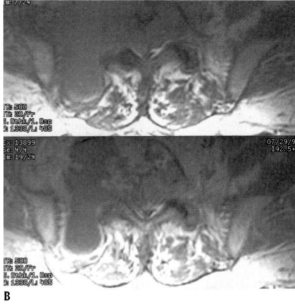
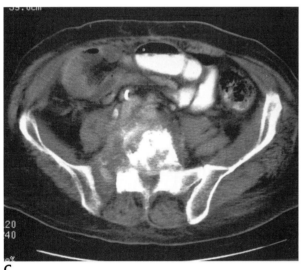

FIGURE 11-5

Sixty-two-year-old male with recent history of obstipation, increasing low back pain, and no previous history of cancer. Needle biopsy of right sacroiliac joint revealed undifferentiated adenocarcinoma.
A Sagittal MRI with destruction of L5 vertebra and involvement of L4 body; note disc preservation.
B Axial MRI showing extensive retroperitoneal mass and spinal involvement. **C** Axial computed tomogram. Because of abdominal problems, the patient underwent a bowel diversion and radiotherapy. He died 6 months later without neurological deficit.

much more likely to produce symptomatic relief in patients with blastic lesions than in those with lytic lesions. The presence or absence of epidural tumor was not related to outcome from radiation.[150]

A total of 3000 cGy over 10 to 12 treatments is typical and will arrest progress or promote resolution.[68] However, Maranzano et al have used alternative radiotherapy schemes in an effort to minimize toxicity and improve outcomes. They treated patients with metastatic spine lesions due to tumors ranging from poorly radiosensitive tumors, such as non–small cell lung, to those that are highly radiosensitive, such as prostate cancer. Short-course radiotherapy, 8 Gy repeated in one weeks by another 8 Gy, was given. Two-thirds of patients had significant pain relief, and almost all maintained ambulation if the disease was discovered early. In patients with more advanced disease, the results were not as good.[111] Indeed, the results presented in this report are quite analogous to those reported for traditional treatment using much longer courses.

Patients who have failed radiation therapy should undergo prompt surgery. Unpublished data have indicated that the risks of surgical injury to the spinal cord and surgical morbidity are lower than the neurological morbidity associated with excess radiation therapy. Many consider radiation myelopathy to be a low-risk phenomenon in patients with metastasis, since it is rarely seen at less than 18 months with conventional treatment protocols.[39,53,87,98] However, it occasionally occurs acutely, presumably as a result of cord infarction due to vasculitis.[87] There is little treatment at present.

Chemotherapy

Chemotherapy is rarely indicated as primary treatment in spinal cord compression due to metastatic disease. It may be a later adjunct in well-resected cases. For example, oncologists recommend chemotherapy to virtually every patient with spinal metastasis from breast carcinoma.[76] This ranges from cytotoxic agents to hormonal and immunotherapy and even bone transplantation,[7] and may extend survival an additional 6 to 12 months or more.

Conclusions

In spite of improved surgical techniques and earlier diagnoses, overall results of treatment are not necessarily better than in years past. However, in individual patients, definitive radiographic studies, aggressive decompression and stabilization, and appropriate radiation seem optimal for many neurologically impaired patients and will greatly improve their quality of life. We expect that in the future, advances in chemotherapy and more focused radiation may significantly improve survival, as well.

REFERENCES

1. Ackerman W: Application of the trephine for bone biopsy: Results of 635 cases. JAMA 184:11–17, 1963.
2. Adapon BD, Legada Jr BD, Lime VA, et al: CT guided closed biopsy of the spine. J Comput Assist Tomogr 5(1):73–78, 1981.
3. Adler O, Rosenberger A: Fine needle aspiration biopsy of osteolytic metastatic lesions. AJR 133:15–18, 1979.
4. Akeyson EW, McCutcheon IE: Single-stage posterior vertebrectomy and replacement combined with posterior instrumentation for spinal metastatic. J Neurosurg 85:211–220, 1996.
5. Algra PR, Heimans JJ, Valk J, et al: Do metastases in vertebrae begin in the body or the pedicles? Am J Roentgenol 158:1275–1279, 1992.
6. Alleyne CH Jr, Rodts GE Jr, Haid RW: Corpectomy and stabilization with methylmethacrylate in patients with metastatic disease of the spine: A technical note. J Spinal Disord 8:439–443, 1995.
7. Anonymous. Systemic treatment of early breast cancer by hormonal, cytotoxic, or immune therapy. One hundred thirty-three randomized trials involving 31,000 recurrences and 24,000 deaths among 75,000 women. Early Breast Cancer Trialists' Collaborative Group: Systemic treatment of early breast cancer by hormonal, cytotoxic, or immune therapy. Lancet 339:1–15, 1992.
8. Arcangeli G, Micheli A, Giannarelli D, et al: The responsiveness of bone metastases to radiotherapy: The effect of site, histology and radiation dose on pain relief. Radiother Oncol 14:95–101, 1989.
9. Arbit E, Galicich JH: Vertebral body reconstruction with a modified Harrington rod distraction system for stabilization of the spine affected with metastatic disease. J Neurosurg 83:617–620, 1995.
10. Ardran GM: Bone destruction not demonstrable by radiography. Br J Radiol 24:107–109, 1951.
11. Arguello F, Baggs RB, Duerst RE, et al: Pathogenesis of vertebral metastasis and epidural spinal cord compression. Cancer 65:98–106, 1990.
12. Asdourian PL, Mardjetko S, Rauschning W, et al: An evaluation of spinal deformity in metastatic breast cancer. J Spin Disord 3:119–134, 1990.
13. Asdourian PL, Weidenbaum M, DeWald RL, et al: The pattern of vertebral involvement in metastatic vertebral breast cancer. Clin Orthop Rel Res 250:164–170, 1990.
14. Avrahami E, Tadmor R, Dally O, et al: Early MR demonstration of spinal metastases in patients with normal radiographs and CT and radionuclide scans. J Comput Assist Tomogr 13:598–602, 1989.
15. Babu NV, Titus VTK, Chittaranjan S, et al: Computed tomographically guided biopsy of the spine. Spine 19:2436–2442, 1994.
16. Baker L, Goodman S, Perkash I, et al: Benign versus pathologic compression fractures of vertebral bodies: Assessment with conventional spin-echo, chemical shift, and STIR MR imaging. Radiology 174:495–502, 1990.
17. Barcena A, Lobato RD, Rivas JJ, et al: Spinal metastatic disease: Analysis of factors determining functional prognosis and the choice of treatment. Neurosurgery 15:820–827, 1984.
18. Barron KD, Hirano A, Araki S, et al: Experiences with metastatic neoplasms involving the spinal cord. Neurology 9:91–106, 1959.
19. Batson OV: The function of the vertebral veins and their role in the spread of metastases. Ann Surg 112:138–149, 1940.
20. Bauer HC: Posterior decompression and stabilization for spinal metastases: Analysis of sixty-seven

consecutive patients. J Bone Joint Surg 79A:514–522, 1997.
21. Bauer HCF, Wedin R: Survival after surgery for spinal and extremity metastases: Prognostication in 241 patients. Acta Orthop Scand 66:143–146, 1995.
22. Beltran J, Noto AM, Chakeres DW, et al: Tumors of the osseous spine: Staging with MR imaging versus CT. Radiology 162:565–569, 1987.
23. Bernat H, Greenberg ER, Barrett J: Suspected epidural compression of the spinal cord and cauda equina by metastatic carcinoma: Clinical diagnosis and survival. Cancer 51:1953–1957, 1983.
24. Biyani A, Ebraheim NA, Lu J: Thoracic spine fractures in patients older than 50 years. Clin Orthop 328:190–193, 1996.
25. Black P: Spinal metastases: Current status and recommended guidelines for management. Neurosurgery 5:726–746, 1985.
26. Boland P, Lane JM, Sundaresan N: Metastatic disease of the spine. Clin Orthop 169:95–102, 1982.
27. Bollow M, Knauf W, Korfel A, et al: Initial experience with dynamic MR imaging in evaluation of normal bone marrow versus malignant bone marrow infiltrations in humans. J Magn Reson Imaging 7:241–250, 1997.
28. Breslau J, Eskridge JM: Preoperative embolization of spinal tumors. J Vasc Interv Radiol 6:871–875, 1995.
29. Bridwell KH, Jenny AB, Saul T, et al: Posterior segment spinal instrumentation (PSSI) with posterolateral decompression and debulking for metastatic thoracic and lumbar spine disease: Limitations of the technique. Spine 13:1383–1394, 1988.
30. Brugieres P, Revel MP, Dumas JL: CT-directed vertebral biopsy: A report of 89 cases. J Neuroradiol 18:351–359, 1991.
31. Bushnell DL, Kahn D, Huston B, et al: Utility of SPECT scanning for determination of vertebral metastases in patients with known primary tumors. Skeletal Radiol 24:13–16, 1995.
32. Bydder GM, Brown J, Niendorf HP, et al: Enhancement of cervical intraspinal tumors in MR imaging with intravenous Gadolinium-DTPA. JCAT 9:847–851, 1985.
33. Byrne TN: Spinal cord compression from epidural metastases. N Engl J Med 327:614–619, 1992.
34. Calkins AR, Olson MA, Ellis JH: Impact of myelography on the radiotherapeutic management of malignant spinal cord compression. Neurosurgery 19:614–616, 1986.
35. Cappellani G, Giuffre F, Garusi G: Primary spinal epidural lymphomas: Report of ten cases. J Neurosurg Sci 30:147–151, 1986.
36. Carmody R, Yang P, Seeley G, et al: Spinal cord compression due to metastatic disease: Diagnosis with MR imaging versus myelography. Radiology 173:225–229, 1989.
37. Cobb CA, Leavens ME, Eckles N: Indications for non-operative treatment of spinal cord compression due to breast cancer. J Neurosurg 47:653–658, 1977.
38. Colman LK, Porter BA, Redmond J III, et al: Early diagnosis of spinal metastases by CT and MR studies. J Comput Assist Tomogr 12:423–426, 1988.
39. Combes PF, Daly N: Late progressive radiation myelopathy: A study of 27 cases. J Radiol Electrol Med Nucl 57:815–825, 1975.
40. Constans JP, de Divitiis E, Donzelli R, et al: Spinal metastases with neurological manifestations: A review of 600 cases. J Neurosurg 59:111–118, 1983.
41. Cortet B, Cotten A, Boutry N, et al: Percutaneous vertebroplasty in patients with osteolytic metastases or multiple myeloma. Revue Du Rhumatisme, English Edition. 64:177–183, 1997.
42. Craig FS: Vertebral body biopsy. J Bone Joint Surg 38A:93–102, 1956.
43. Crock HV, Yoshizawa H: The blood supply of the vertebral column. Clin Orthop 115:6–21, 1976.
44. Cybulski GR: Methods of surgical stabilization for metastatic disease of the spine. Neurosurgery 25:240–252, 1989.
45. Daffner RH, Lupetin AR, Dash N, et al: MRI in the detection of malignant infiltration of bone marrow. Am J Roentgenol 146:353–358, 1986.
46. Davis PC, Freedman NC, Fry SM: Leptomeningeal metastases: MRI imaging. Radiology 163:449–454, 1987.
47. DeSantos LA, Murray JA, Ayala AG: The value of percutaneous needle biopsy in the management of primary bone tumors. Cancer 43:735–739, 1979.
48. DeWald RL, Bridwell KH, Prodromas C, et al: Reconstructive spinal surgery as palliation for metastatic malignancies of the spine. Spine 10:21–26, 1985.
49. Edelstyn GA, Gillespie PF, Grebbell FS: The radiological demonstration of skeletal metastases. Clin Radiol 18:158–162, 1967.
50. Erickson DL, Leider LL Jr, Brown WB: One-stage decompression-stabilization for thoracolumbar fractures. Spine 2:53–56, 1977.
51. Faccioli F, Lima J, Bricolo A: One-stage decompression and stabilization in the treatment of spinal tumors. J Neurosurg Sci 29:199–205, 1985.
52. Faul CM, Flickinger JC: The use of radiation in the management of spinal metastases. J Neuroncol 23:149–161, 1995.
53. Fein DA, Marcus RB Jr: Lhermitte's sign: Incidence and treatment variables influencing risk after irra-

diation of the cervical spinal cord. Int J Radiat Oncol Biol Phys 27:1029–1033, 1993.
54. Findlay GF: The role of vertebral body collapse in the management of malignant spinal cord compression. J Neurol Neurosurg Psychiatry 50:150–154, 1987.
55. Findlay GF, Sanderman DR, Buxton P: The role of needle biopsy in the management of malignant spinal compression. Br J Neurosurg 2(4):479–484, 1988.
56. Findlay GFC: Adverse effects of the management of malignant spinal cord compression. J Neurol Neurosurg Psychiatry 47:761–768, 1984.
57. Flately TJ, Anderson MH, Anast GT: Spinal instability due to malignant disease: Treatment by segmental spinal stabilization. J Bone Joint Surg 66A:47–52, 1984.
58. Frank JA, Ling A, Patronas NJ, et al: Detection of malignant bone tumors: MR imaging vs scintigraphy. Am J Roentgenol 155:1043, 1990.
59. Fujita T, Ueda Y, Kawahara N, et al: Local spread of metastatic vertebral tumors: A histologic study. Spine 22:1905–1912, 1997.
60. Fyfe IS, Henry APJ, Mulholland RC: Closed vertebral biopsy. J Bone Joint Surg 65B:140–143, 1983.
61. Galasko CSB: Mechanisms of lytic and blastic metastatic disease of bone. Clin Orthop 169:20–27, 1982.
62. Galasko CSB: Spinal instability secondary to metastatic cancer. J Bone Joint Surg 73B:104–108, 1991
63. Galasko CSB, Doyle FH: The detection of skeletal metastases from mammary cancer. A regional comparison between radiology and scintigraphy. Clin Radiol 23:295–297, 1972.
64. Geldof AA: Models for cancer skeletal metastasis: A reappraisal of Batson's plexus. Anticancer Res 17:1535–1539, 1997.
65. Gilbert LW, Kim J-H, Posner JB: Epidural spinal cord compression from metastatic tumor: Diagnosis and treatment. Ann Neurol 3:40–51, 1978.
66. Gilbert RW, Kin JH, Posner JB: Epidural spinal cord compression from metastatic tumor: Diagnosis and treatment. Ann Neurol 3:40–51, 1978.
67. Greenberg HS, Kim JH, Posner JB: Epidural spinal cord compression from metastatic tumor: Results with a new treatment protocol. Ann Neurol 8:361–386, 1980.
68. Greenberger JS: The pathophysiology and management of spine metastasis from lung cancer. J Neurooncol 23:109–120, 1995.
69. Grem JL, Burgess J, Trump DL: Clinical features and natural history of intramedullary spinal cord metastasis. Cancer 56:2305–2314, 1985.
70. Haddad MC, Sharif HS, Aideyan OA, et al: Infection versus neoplasm in the spine: Differentiation by MRI and diagnostic pitfalls. Eur Radiol 3:439, 1993.
71. Haller J, Andre MP, Resnick D, et al: Detection of thoracolumbar vertebral body destruction with lateral spine radiography: Part I. Investigation in cadavers. Invest Radiol 25:517–522, 1990.
72. Haller J, Andre MP, Resnick D, et al: Detection of thoracolumbar vertebral body destruction with lateral spine radiography: Part II. Clinical investigation with computed tomography. Invest Radiol 25:523–532, 1990.
73. Han JS, Kaufman B, El Yousel SJ, et al: NMR imaging of the spine. Am J Roentgenol 141:1137–1145, 1983.
74. Harrington KD: Anterior cord decompression and spinal stabilization for patients with metastatic lesions of the spine. J Neurosurg 61:107–117, 1984.
75. Harrington KD: Anterior decompression and stabilization of the spine as a treatment for vertebral collapse and spinal cord compression from metastatic malignancy. Clin Orthop 233:177–197, 1988.
76. Harris JR, Lippmann ME, Veronesi U, et al: Breast cancer. N Engl J Med 327:319–328, 1992.
77. Helms CA, Vogler JB III, Genant HK: Characteristic CT manifestations of uncommon spinal disorders. Orthop Clin North Am 16:445–459, 1985.
78. Helweg-Larsen S, Johnsen A, Boesen J, et al: Radiologic features compared to clinical findings in a prospective study of 153 patients with metastatic spinal cord compression treated with radiotherapy. Acta Neurochir 139:105–111, 1997.
79. Helwig-Larsen S, Wagner A, Kjaer L, et al: Comparison of myelography combined with post-myelographic spinal CT and MRI in suspected metastatic disease of the spinal canal. J Neurooncol 13:231–237, 1992.
80. Hess T, Kramann B, Schmidt E, et al: Use of preoperative vascular embolisation in spinal metastasis resection. Arch Orthop Trauma Surg 116:279–282, 1997.
81. Hollis PM, Malis LI, Zappula RA: Neurological deterioration after lumbar puncture below complete subarachnoid block. J Neurosurg 64:253–256, 1986.
82. Holtas SL, Kido DK, Simon JH: MR imaging of spinal lymphoma. J Comput Assist Tomogr 10:111–115, 1986.
83. Hovi I, Lamminen O, Raininko R: MR imaging of the lower spine: Differentiation between infectious and malignant disease. Acta Radiol 35:532–540, 1994.
84. Hyman RA, Gorey MT: Imaging strategies for MR of the spine. Radiol Clin North Am 26:505–533, 1988.
85. Jacobson HG, Poppel MH, Shapiro JH, et al: The vertebral pedicle sign. Am J Roentgenol 80:817–821, 1958.

86. Jelenik JS, Kransdorf MJ, Gray R, et al: Percutaneous transpedicular biopsy of vertebral body lesions. Spine 21:2035–2040, 1996.
87. Jeremic B, Djuric L: Incidence of radiation myelitis of the spinal cord at doses of 5500 cGy or greater. Cancer 68:2138–2141, 1991.
88. Jonsson B, Petren-Mallmin M, Jonsson H Jr, et al: Pathoanatomical and radiographic findings in metastatic breast cancer. J Spinal Disord 8:26–38, 1995.
89. Jonsson B, Sjostrom L, Olerud C, et al: Outcome after limited posterior surgery for thoracic and lumbar spine metastases. Eur Spine J 5:36–44, 1996.
90. Kamby C, Vejborg I, Daugaard S, et al: Clinical and radiologic characteristics of bone metastases in breast cancer. Cancer 60:2524–2531, 1987.
91. Kato M, Ushio Y, Hayakawa T, et al: Circulatory disturbance of the spinal cord with epidural neoplasm in rats. J Neurosurg 63:260–265, 1985.
92. Kattapuram SV, Khurana JS, Rosenthal DI: Percutaneous needle biopsy of the spine. Spine 17:561–564, 1992.
93. King GJ, Kostuik JP, McBroom RJ, et al: Surgical treatment of metastatic renal carcinoma of the spine. Spine 16:265–271, 1991.
94. Kocialkowski A, Webb J: Metastatic spine tumors: Survival after surgery. Eur Spine J 1:43–48, 1992.
95. Kornblum MB, Wesolowski DP, Fischgrund JS, et al: Computed tomography guided biopsy of the spine: A review of 103 patients. Spine 23:81–85, 1998.
96. Kostuik JP, Errico TJ, Gleason TF, et al: Spinal stabilization of vertebral column tumors. Spine 13:250–256, 1988.
97. Ku A, Henry A, Tunkel R, et al: Lumbosacral radiculopathy secondary to L5 metastatic melanoma of unknown primary. Arch Phys Med Rehabil 77:307–309, 1996.
98. Lambert PW, Davis RL: Delayed effects of radiation on the human central nervous system. Neurology 14:912–917, 1964.
99. Landreneau FE, Landreneau RJ, Keenan RJ, et al: Diagnosis and management of spinal metastases from breast cancer. J Neurooncol 23:121–134, 1995.
100. Leviov M, Dale J, Stein M, et al: The management of metastatic spinal cord compression: A radiotherapeutic success ceiling. Int J Radiat Oncol Biol Phys 27:231–234, 1993.
101. Levy WJ, Latchawa JP, Hardy RW, et al: Encouraging surgical results in walking patients with epidural metastases. Neurosurgery 11:229–233, 1982.
102. Li MH, Holtas S, Larsson EM: MR imaging of spinal lymphoma. Acta Radiol 33:338–342, 1992.
103. Linden A, Zankovich R, Theissen P, et al: Malignant lymphoma: Bone marrow imaging versus biopsy. Radiology 173:335–339, 1989.
104. Livingston KE, Perrin RG: The neurosurgical management of spinal metastases causing cord and cauda equina compression. J Neurosurg 49:839–843, 1978.
105. Love JC, Miller RH, Kerghan JW: Lymphomas of the spinal epidural space. Arch Surg 69:66–76, 1954.
106. Magerl F, Coscia MF: Total posterior vertebrectomy of the thoracic or lumbar spine. Clin Orthop 232:62–69, 1988.
107. Maiuri F, Gangemi M, Giamundo A, et al: Primary spinal epidural lymphomas. Acta Neurol 10:213–219, 1988.
108. Maranzano E, Latini P: Effectiveness of radiation therapy without surgery in metastatic spinal cord compression: Final results from a prospective trial. Int J Radiat Oncol Biol Phys 32:959–967, 1995.
109. Maranzano E, Latini P, Checcaglini F, et al: Radiation therapy in metastatic spinal cord compression: A prospective analysis of 105 consecutive patients. Cancer 67:1311–1317, 1991.
110. Maranzano E, Latini P, Checcaglini F, et al: Radiation therapy of spinal cord compression caused by breast cancer: Report of a prospective trial. Int J Radiat Oncol Biol Phys 24:301–306, 1992.
111. Maranzano E, Latini P, Perrucci E, et al: Short-course radiotherapy (8 Gy × 2) in metastatic spinal cord compression: An effective and feasible treatment. Int J Radiat Oncol Biol Phys 38:1037–1044, 1997.
112. Martenson JA, Evans RG Jr, Lie MR, et al: Treatment outcome and complications in patients treated for malignant epidural spinal cord compression. J Neurooncol 3:77–84, 1985.
113. Masaryk TJ: Neoplastic diseases of the spine. Radiol Clin North Am 29:829–845, 1991.
114. McAfee PC, Zdeblick TA: Tumors of the thoracic and lumbar spine: Surgical treatment via the anterior approach. J Spinal Dis 2:145–154, 1989.
115. Mones RJ, Dozier D, Berrett A: Analysis of medical treatment of malignant extradural spinal cord tumors. Cancer 19:1842–1853, 1996.
116. Moore AJ, Uttley D: Anterior decompression and stabilization of the spine in malignant disease. Neurosurgery 24:713–717, 1989.
117. Murphy WA: Radiologically guided percutaneous musculoskeletal biopsy. Orthop Clin North Am 14:223–241, 1983.
118. Nicholls PJ, Jarecky TW: The value of posterior decompression by laminectomy for malignant tumors of the spine. Clin Orthop 201:210–213, 1985.
119. O'Connor MI, Currier BL: Metastatic disease of the spine. Orthopedics 15:611–620, 1992.

120. O'Reilly GV, Kleefield J, Klein LA, et al: Embolization of solitary spinal metastases from renal cell carcinoma: Alternative therapy for spinal cord or nerve root compression. Surg Neurol 31:268–271, 1989.

121. Olerud C, Jonsson B: Surgical palliation of symptomatic spinal metastases. Acta Orthop Scand 67:513–522, 1996.

122. Orr W, Varani J, Gondek MD, et al: Chemotactic responses of tumor cells to products of resorbing bone. Science 203:176–179, 1979.

123. Osborn JL, Getzenberg RH, Trump DL: Spinal cord compression in prostate cancer. J Neurooncol 23:135–147, 1995.

124. Pagani JJ, Libshitz HI: Imaging bone metastases. Radiol Clin North Am 20:545–560, 1982.

125. Poulson HS, Nielsen OS, Klee M: Palliative irradiation of bone metastases. Cancer Treat Rev 16:41–48, 1989.

126. Rahmouni A, Divine M, Mathieu D, et al: Detection of multiple myeloma involving the spine: Efficacy of fat-suppression and contrast-enhanced MR imaging. Am J Roentgenol 160:1049, 1993.

127. Ramsey RG, Zacharias CE: MR imaging of the spine after radiation therapy: Easily recognizable effects. Am J Roentgenol 144:1131–1135, 1985.

128. Rauschning W: Pathoanatomical and radiographic findings in spinal breast cancer metastases. J Spinal Dis 8:26–38, 1995.

129. Rodichok LD, Ruckdeschel JC, Harper GR, et al: Early detection and treatment of spinal epidural metastases: The role of myelography. Ann Neurol 20:696–702, 1986.

130. Rodriguez M, Dinapoli RP: Spinal cord compression with special reference to metastatic epidural tumors. Mayo Clin Proc 55:442–448, 1980.

131. Sacks EL, Goris ML, Glatstein E, et al: Bone marrow regeneration following large field radiation: Influence of volume, age, dose and time. Cancer 42:1057–1065, 1978.

132. Sanal SM, Flickinger FW, Caudell MJ, et al: Detection of bone marrow involvement in breast cancer with magnetic resonance imaging. J Clin Oncol 2:1415–1421, 1994.

133. Sartoris DJ, Clopton P, Nemcek A, et al: Vertebral-body collapse in focal and diffuse disease: Patterns of pathologic processes. Radiology 160:479–483, 1986.

134. Schaberg J, Gainor BJ: A profile of metastatic carcinoma of the spine. Spine 10:19–20, 1985.

135. Schellinger D: Patterns of anterior spinal canal involvement by neoplasms and infections. Am J Neuroradiol 17:953–959, 1996.

136. Schiff D, O'Neill BP, Suman VJ: Spinal epidural metastasis as the initial manifestation of malignancy: Clinical features and diagnostic approach. Neurology 49:452–456, 1997.

137. Schimandle JH, Levine AM: An isolated nonosseous metastasis to the epidural space from an osteogenic sarcoma. Cancer 69:103–107, 1992.

138. Scotti G, Scialfa G, Colombo N, et al: Magnetic resonance diagnosis of intramedullary tumors of the spinal cord. Neuroradiology 29:130–135, 1987.

139. Seifert RS, Arkin AM: Trephine biopsy of bone with special reference to the lumbar vertebral bodies. J Bone Joint Surg 31A:146–149, 1949.

140. Settle WJ, Ebraheim NA, Saunders RC, et al: CT guided biopsy of metastatic sacral tumors. Orthopedics 137:753–758, 1990.

141. Shaw B, Mansfield FL, Borges L: One-stage posterolateral decompression and stabilization for primary and metastatic vertebral tumors in the thoracic and lumbar spine. J Neurosurg 70:405–410, 1989.

142. Sherry MM, Greco FA, Johnson DH: Metastatic breast cancer confined to the skeletal system: An indolent disease. Am J Med 81:381–386, 1986.

143. Siegal T, Shohami E, Shapira Y, et al: Indomethacin and dexamethasone treatment in experimental neoplastic spinal compression: Effect on edema and prostaglandin synthesis. Neurosurgery 22:334–339, 1988.

144. Siegal T, Siegal TZ: Current considerations in the management of neoplastic spinal cord compression. Spine 14:223–228, 1989.

145. Siegal TZ, Siegal T: Vertebral body resection for epidural compression by malignant tumors: Results of 27 consecutive operative procedures. J Bone Joint Surg 67A:375–282, 1985.

146. Siegal T, Tiqva P, Siegal TZ: Vertebral body resection for epidural compression by malignant tumors: Results of 47 consecutive procedures. J Bone Joint Surg 67A:375–382, 1985.

147. Sioutos PJ, Arbit E, Meshulam CF, et al: Spinal metastases from solid tumors. Analysis of factors affecting survival. Cancer 76:1453–1459, 1995.

148. Smoker WRK, Godersky JC, Knutzon RK, et al: The role of MR imaging in evaluating metastatic spinal disease. Am J Roentgenol 149:1241–1248, 1987.

149. Spiegel DA, Sampson JH, Richardson WJ, et al: Metastatic melanoma to the spine: Demographics, risk factors, and prognosis in 114 patients. Spine 20:2141–2146, 1995.

150. Sugiyama A: Radiotherapy for vertebral metastases: Analysis of symptoms and clinical effects by MR imaging. Nippon Igaku Hoshasen Gakkai Zasshi 54:1368–1379, 1994.

151. Sundaresan N, Bains, McCormack P: Surgical treatment of spinal cord compression in patients with lung cancer. Neurosurgery 16:350–356, 1985.

152. Sundaresan N, Choi IS, Hughes JE, et al: Treatment of spinal metastases from kidney cancer by presurgical embolization and resection. J Neurosurg 73:548–554, 1990.
153. Sundaresan N, Digiacinto GV, Hughes JE: Treatment of neoplastic spinal cord compression: Results of a prospective study. Neurosurgery 29:645–650, 1991.
154. Sundaresan N, DiGiacinto GV, Krol G, et al: Spondylectomy for malignant tumors of the spine. J Clin Oncol 7:1485–1491, 1989.
155. Sundaresan N, Galicich JH, Bain MS, et al: Vertebral body resection in the treatment of cancer involving the spine. Cancer 53:1393–1396, 1984.
156. Sundaresan N, Steinberger AA, Moore F, et al: Indications and results of combined anterior-posterior approaches for spine tumor surgery. J Neurosurg 85:438–446, 1996.
157. Sykes MP, Chu FCH, Wilkerson WG: Local bone marrow changes secondary to therapeutic irradiation. Radiology 74:919–924, 1960.
158. Sze G: Magnetic resonance imaging in the evaluation of spinal tumors. Cancer 67:S1129–1141, 1991.
159. Sze G, Krol G, Zimmerman RD, et al: Intramedullary disease of the spine: Diagnosis using gadolinium-DTPA-enhanced MR imaging. Am J Roentgenol 151:1193–1204, 1988.
160. Taneichi H, Kaneda K, Takeda N, et al: Risk factors and probability of vertebral body collapse in metastases of the thoracic and lumbar spine. Spine 22:239–245, 1997.
161. Tehranzadeh J, Freiberger RH, Ghelman B: Closed skeletal needle biopsy: Review of 120 cases. Am J Roentgenol 140:113–115, 1983.
162. Turner PL, Prince HG, Webb JK, et al: Surgery for malignant extradural tumors of the spine. J Bone Joint Surg 70B:451–456, 1988.
163. Uchida N, Sugimura K, Kajitani A, et al: MR imaging of vertebral metastases: Evaluation of fat saturation imaging. Eur J Radiol 17:91–94, 1993.
164. Weill A, Chiras J, Simon JM, et al: Spinal metastases: Indications for and results of percutaneous injection of acrylic surgical cement. Radiology 199:241–247, 1996.
165. White MJ, Jinkins JR: Pathologic vertebral compression in spinal malignancy secondary to intervertebral disc expansion. Comput Med Imaging Graph 15:373–377, 1991.
166. White LM, Schweitzer ME, Deely DM: Coaxial percutaneous needle biopsy of osteolytic lesions with intact cortical bone. Am J Roentgenol 166:143–144, 1996.
167. Williams MP, Cherryman GR, Husband JE: Magnetic resonance imaging in suspected metastic spinal cord compression. Clin Radiol 40:286, 1989.
168. Yamashita K, Denno K, Ueda T, et al: Prognostic significance of bone metastases in patients with metastatic prostate cancer. Cancer 71:1297–1302, 1993.
169. Young JM, Funk FJ: Incidence of tumor metastasis to the lumbar spine: A comparative study of roentgenographic changes and gross lesions. J Bone Joint Surg 35A:55–64, 1953.
170. Young RF, Post EM, King GA: Treatment of spinal epidural metastases: Randomized prospective comparison of laminectomy and radiotherapy. J Neurosurg 53:741–748, 1980.
171. Yuh WT, Quets JP, Lee HJ, et al: Anatomic distribution of metastases in the vertebral body and modes of hematogenous spread. Spine 21:2243–2250, 1996.
172. Yuh WTC, Zachar CK, Barloon TJ, et al: Vertebral compression fractures: Distinction between benign and malignant causes with MR imaging. Radiology 172:215–218, 1989.
173. Zelefsky MJ, Scher HI, Krol G, et al: Spinal epidural tumor in patients with prostate cancer: Clinical and radiographic prediction of response to radiation therapy. Cancer 70:2319–2325, 1992.
174. Zimmer WD, Berquist TH, McLeod RA, et al: Bone tumors: Magnetic resonance imaging versus computed tomography. Radiology 155:709–718, 1985.
175. Zimmerman RA: Central nervous system lymphoma. Radiol Clin North Am 28:697–721, 1990.

CHAPTER 12

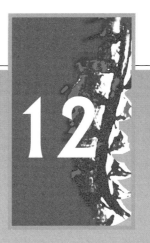

Bone Grafts and Orthoses

Bone Grafts and Fusion

Autogenous Graft Versus Allograft for Fusion Surgery

Bone Substitutes

Smoking

Enhancement of Bone Fusion

Orthoses

Bone Grafts and Orthoses

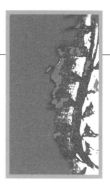

This chapter precedes the description of surgical techniques, to stress the importance of many of the principles presented here. Older (defined as pre-universal instrumentation) spine surgeons often bemoan the lack of concern on the part of younger surgeons for osteogenesis. Needless to say, as this chapter shows, that is not the case. Tremendous effort is being expended in this area, and there is little doubt that fusions will be performed differently, and better, in years to come.

Bone Grafts and Fusion

Probably no topic is more likely to lead to fisticuffs in any gathering of spine surgeons than that of the principles of taking and placing bone grafts. In spite of the arguments and controversies, the fundamental fact remains that in order for fusion to occur, grafting of bone occurs across a space; true fusion requires cessation of active motion across that space.[40] Three components must come together: osteogenic, osteoinductive, and osteoconductive forces must work in concert. These depend on the quality of the local fusion host site, including blood supply and immunological status, the graft material to be used, and local motion.[17,31–33]

Cell Types and Bone Growth

Osteogenic cells are either determined or inducible. The determined cells differentiate and replicate in a predictable manner. These are found in the marrow as well as on bone surfaces.[24] Inductive cells, on the other hand, require an osteoinductive agent such as bone morphogenetic protein to produce bone.[17] These can be recovered from connective tissue and bone marrow.[19,32,33,80,91,92]

The primary function of bone graft is to accelerate the regenerative capacity of bone. Ideally, this graft material will promote osteogenesis as well as provide inductive and conductive activities. Certainly, autogenous bone does this effectively. Allograft, although not osteogenic, is osteoinductive. Artificial materials such as ceramics are only osteoconductive in nature.

The use of vascularized autologous grafts has been occasionally reported. Fusion rates seem to be higher.[13,94,95] Sources include vascularized iliac crest, rib, and fibula. Minami et al used vascularized fibula in patients undergoing anterior spinal fusion for kyphosis. Vascular anastomosis could not be obtained in almost 20% of the patients; the bone graft dislodged in another. Fusion occurred in the rest at an average of 5.5 months.[64] Unfortunately, the length of time required to harvest these grafts and to perform the vascular anastomosis is significant. In light of the high fusion rate for nonvascularized grafts, we suggest that vascularized bone grafts be reserved for exceptionally high-risk fusions, such as selected cancer patients who are to undergo radiation therapy.

Surgical Considerations

The most critical single factor in the achievement of successful fusion is the preparation of the graft site. Since few of the osteocytes in autogenous bone survive transplantation, optimal tissue preparation facilitates the healing process.[33,35,80] During surgical procedures, traumatized, avascular, and other soft tissues should be carefully removed.

Host bone serves as the primary source of osteogenic cells and inductive proteins, as well as a conductive surface for graft incorporation; therefore, meticulous decortication of host bone surfaces is important. During transverse process fusion, injury to the vessels lateral to the transverse process should be avoided.

There is evidence that increasing the decorticated surface area available for grafting does improve fusion rates.[54] This increases the number of exposed osteogenic cells and provides better blood supply, as well as better chemotactic surface between the osteogenic host bone and graft material.[19,80] Maintaining blood supply to the decorticated surfaces is important. Furthermore, active decortication stimulates an inflammatory reaction with production of hemotactic agents that mediate local blood flow. This may explain why nonsteroidal drugs such as indomethacin, which inhibit prostaglandin synthesis, may delay mineralization when given shortly after fusion.[73]

Anecdotal evidence suggests that the use of high-speed drills to remove cortical bone creates thermal necrosis which decreases fusion, and therefore they should not be used for decortication. If we use a diamond drill to decorticate, we then use a curette to further roughen the bone surface.

Autogenous Graft Versus Allograft for Fusion Surgery

Most investigators have suggested that anterior grafts are more likely to fuse than those placed via posterior and lateral approaches. Therefore, for anterior lumbar surgery, we often use bank bone. When surgery is being performed for trauma or nonunion, the cancellous bone from the resected vertebra will be packed into the hollowed donor fibula or tibia and then impacted into place. Although there is no conclusive evidence that this improves fusion rates, several anecdotal reports have suggested so. Since 1988, our radiographic fusion rate for anterior lumbar fusion using allograft packed with cancellous autogenous bone has been better than 97%.

In high-risk patients, including smokers and those with trauma and diabetes, we attempt to use autogenous bone. However, harvest of iliac crest strut grafts of adequate length can be difficult. We currently do not perform autogenous fibular fusions because of the considerable morbidity and pain associated with obtaining the graft. We have no preference as to whether the bone has been freeze-dried or irradiated, although some have suggested that the former has a lower fusion rate.[24,34,41,52,55,75,77] There is little evidence that this decrease in mechanical strength is of any significance.

Just as biomechanical differences do not help in the decision making as to type of allograft, they do not help in making the decision to use autograft versus allograft. Studies have shown that fibular autograft has higher compressive strength than iliac crest; sterilization has no effect on strength.[97]

Allografts in Posterior Fusion

Allograft is not ideal for posterior fusion unless there is a paucity of iliac crest graft available.[61] Interestingly enough, it is the very patients who have the least autogenous bone available who are at most risk of nonunion. Using allograft on these individuals who are, for example, osteoporotic or who have undergone previous fusions, is therefore unwise. Therefore, a concerted effort is made to obtain adequate autogenous bone, supplementing this with allograft croutons.

There are alternatives for harvesting autogenous bone other than from the iliac crest.[62] The latter may be unavailable, as in the patient with multiple previous surgeries whose iliac crest has been violated on several previous occasions. These other alternatives can sometimes be used to avoid complications associated with iliac crest harvest, including bleeding, operative time, and infection rates. For example, local bone such as spinous process and lamina, carefully cleaned and chopped into fragments, is an ideal posterior fusion substrate. Ribs may be available.[62] Fusion rates for these will be similar to those for cancellous iliac crest.[50]

That posterior fusion rates are higher with autogenous bone has long been reported.[51] An et al performed a prospective clinical study comparing freeze-dried or frozen allograft, autograft, and combinations of the two in transverse process fusions in conjunction with transpedicular fixation. Allograft was placed on one side, and autograft on the other. Autograft had a better than 80% fusion rate. Freeze-dried allograft reabsorbed in all cases, and frozen bone led to solid fusion in only two of five patients. A mixture of allograft and autograft was somewhat better in producing fusion, but clearly autograft was much better than the other options.[2]

However, the experience of Stricker and Sher would suggest otherwise. They employed freeze-dried allograft in 32 patients undergoing posterior fusions for scoliosis. All patients demonstrated radiographic evidence of fusion at follow-ups averaging 34 months.[88] Yazici and Asher reported a similar experience in 40 patients in whom freeze-dried allograft was used for posterior fusion: solid fusion occurred in 95%.[99]

In a small prospective study, Bridwell et al studied bone incorporation and maintenance of alignment in patients undergoing anterior reconstruction and posterior instrumentation. Allograft was equal to autogenous bone for both incorporation and alignment if rigid posterior instrumentation was employed.[14] However, the authors recommended that autogenous bone be employed in conjunction with allograft; this is our practice when forced to use allograft in the posterior spine because of inadequate autogenous bone.

Tumor Surgery

In surgery performed for malignancy, we commonly use allograft for both anterior and posterior fusion, although most recommend methylmethacrylate for bone replacement.[49,80] For primary tumors that do not metastasize and are at early stages, iliac crest can be used judiciously. In the case of metastatic tumor or more malignant lesions, the possibility of local metastasis makes autograft undesirable.

Particularly in the lumbar spine, our experience is that fusion rates may not be lower for allograft even when radiation therapy is initiated 2 to 3 weeks after the surgical procedure. In this population, spinal instrumentation improves fusion rates.

Emery et al argue to the contrary.[28] Four of 25 patients undergoing anterior vertebrectomy and anterior fusion with allograft had nonunions on radiography. All 4 had undergone postoperative radiotherapy. In contradistinction to our experience, lumbar lesions were at higher risk of nonunion. However, this group of patients was not stabilized posteriorly, which the authors admit might have altered outcomes.

Bone Substitutes

Also occasionally discussed is the use of ceramics and coral as a fusion substrate. Arguments for the use of these substances in lieu of bone include availability, avoidance of bone graft site complications, and the decreased theoretical risk of disease transmission from bank bone.[45,56,100] Bone substitutes have been unevenly successful in promoting fusion, but overall are equivalent to allograft; however, they have problems of their own. Some surgeons have found them brittle and hard to shape; they may also be associated with exophytic bone growth. Fused motion segments are biomechanically equivalent to autologous fusion.[71,78,79]

But are fusion rates equivalent? Ragni et al suggested that although hydroxyapatite (HA) blocks are similar to autogenous bone in terms of experimental fusion, HA granules impregnated with bone morphogenic protein (BMP) fuse poorly. Fusion may also be a consequence of the material properties of the substance: that is, formulation of the substance in struts versus granules may be important in healing.[81]

Historically, the use of bone substitutes in posterior fusion has been considered undesirable, even more so than allograft. In recent studies, corticocancellous posterior grafts used in scoliosis were compared to posterior fusions incorporating autogenous bone and tricalcium phosphate mixture. Bone callus was equivalent at 6 months. The tricalcium resorbed at 2 years, leaving behind allograft fusion. Loss of correction was slightly higher in the latter group, but fusion rates were equivalent.[56]

Results of animal studies have been mixed: bicoral collagen composite grafts did not lead to transverse process fusion unless 300 mcg of bovine-derived osteoinductive protein was incorporated; then all animals fused. The latter is not available to clinicians at present.[12]

In spite of these acceptable results for posterior element fusion, we do not recommend bone substitutes, especially for fusions where minimal host bone surface exists: bone ingrowth is dependent on the extent of the contact between the host bone, that is, the transverse process, and the osteoinductive material. Such contact is at best limited in transverse process fusion. Thus we use artificial fusion substrates only in anterior lumbar fusion when right-sized allograft is unavailable.

Smoking

Smoking has long been known to have a deleterious effect on bone mineral content.[26] In a long-term twin study, Hopper and Seeman found reductions in bone mineral content and density in smokers; every ten-pack year history was good for at least a 3% decrease in bone mineral density.[44] This, of course, increases the risk of spinal fracture. Premature disc degeneration also occurs, probably secondary to malnutrition of the disc.[7,43]

Mechanism of Effect

There are various proposed mechanisms for this effect, many of which may occur together in a given patient.[15] Osteoblast metabolism, particularly oxygen utilization, is impaired by both nicotine and other components of cigarette smoke.[26,29,36,82] In addition, DNA and collagen synthesis are suppressed by carbon monoxide and benzene by-products. There may also be a role for toxic oxidant free radicals causing oxidation injury and inhibiting protein synthesis.[21] Smoking also promotes the development of osteoporosis through decreased production and increased metabolism of estrogens.[15,20]

Hambley and Mooney[39] and Holm and Nachemson[43] have observed metabolic changes in bone, as well as in the intervertebral disc, as a response to decreases in pH resulting from nicotine exposure. Studies from Hambley's laboratory, as well as many others, have demonstrated decreased blood supply to the entire spine; these effects are amplified by the decreased oxygen tension that results from smoke inhalation.

Decreased bone blood supply, probably the most commonly studied effect of smoking, is a consequence of injury of the vascular endothelium[84] and resultant endothlin (vasoconstrictive peptide) secretion.[39,58,98] Furthermore, the development of neovascularity, which is important in bone repair, is impaired.[25,86]

The effects of smoking on fusion are also clear. In a series of patients with failed fusions undergoing repair of pseudarthrosis, Carpenter et al[18] found smokers much less likely to heal and less likely to enjoy pain relief even if fusion did occur. Brown et al[16] and Thalgott et al[90] have both shown that smoking adversely affects even initial fusion; however, the effects begin to diminish even when smoking is stopped shortly before surgery.[42]

Fusion is most affected during the osteoconduction and osteoinduction phases.[38] Neovascularization of the graft and multiplication and differentiation of osteoblasts for the production of cartilage and bone occur during these phases. These processes are slowed, if not eliminated, in smokers. Thus, even if fusion occurs, it is mechanically weaker than fusion in nonsmokers.[1,27] For further details, see the excellent review by Hadley and Reddy.[38]

We assiduously avoid performing fusions on active smokers. As indicated above, the effects of nicotine on bone blood supply begin to reverse quickly; therefore, we insist that patients be smoke-free for several weeks prior to surgery. It is difficult to justify additional surgery (i.e., anterior as well as posterior lumbar fusion) merely to improve fusion rates in active smokers, since both costs and risks are increased. If patients decline to be smoke-free preoperatively, they are unlikely to stay so postoperatively.

In this author's series, the fusion rate for virgin transverse process fusion in nonsmokers is 96%; in smokers it drops to 66%. In patients undergoing repeat procedures—even following laminectomy—the latter figure drops below 50%. New agents, such as the antidepressant Zyban, (buproprion) have made the task of getting patients to stop smoking much simpler, at least through the postoperative period.

Enhancement of Bone Fusion

Electrical Stimulation and Magnetic Fields

There is an extensive body of basic science suggesting that direct electrical stimulation and the creation of magnetic fields can promote bone fusion.[57,72] Prospective clinical studies validating or discarding the basic science literature are in progress at the time of this writing, and therefore no absolute conclusions can be offered.[47] However, retrospective clinical data confirm the benefits of electrical stimulation demonstrated in animal studies.

In an early animal study, posterior fusions were performed on beagles, and stimulating electrodes were placed through the facets. One-half were stimulated using direct current. At 6 weeks, there were no differences between the stimulated and control fusions. However, at 12 weeks, fusion had taken place at the stimulated facets but not at the nonstimulated surfaces. This may suggest the value of electrical stimulation to promote fusion.[46] However, it does not help define when stimulation should be initiated. For example, we do not commonly employ external stimulation at surgery, but reserve this expensive adjunct for fusions that are progressing more slowly than anticipated.

Implanted Stimulation

Kane conducted a randomized study of patients who were at high risk for nonunion, including patients with high-degree spondylolisthesis, multiple previous operations, and failed fusions. There was a statistically significant improvement in fusion rates in patients undergoing direct stimulation.[48] The technique used here is straightforward: the cortical/cancellous bone is placed on the decorticated transverse processes. Wire electrodes are then placed onto each side of the bone mass, and these are further covered with bone. The battery pack is placed in the subcutaneous tissue and typically removed approximately 6 months later.[76]

Rogozinski and Rogozinski compared fusion rates with and without implanted electrical stimulation in a randomized series of patients undergoing instrumented lumbar procedures. These included high-risk patients such as smokers and those who had undergone previous surgeries. The solid fusion rate was 96% in stimulated patients and 85% in those who did not receive stimulation.[83]

Indeed, Tejano et al found that direct stimulation can improve fusion rates to levels typically seen with spinal instrumentation. Transverse process fusion was performed in 143 patients, of whom 118 were followed long-term. The overall fusion rate was 91%. Eighty-five percent returned to work, and over 90% reported good or complete relief of pain.[89]

External Stimulation

External stimulating devices have also been used. These produce magnetic fields that seem to be equivalent to direct electrical currents. Advantages include the fact that they do not require surgical implantation or removal, have lower morbidity, and are less expensive. However, their effectiveness remains to be proven. In nonrandomized studies, Simmons demonstrated and improved fusion rate for failed posterior lumbar interbody fusion (PLIF).[87] In this author's series, 37 patients with failed fusion (defined as lack of evidence of transverse process bone growth at 5 months) underwent external stimulation. Patient compliance was extremely high, aided no doubt by the ability to obtain readouts of patient utilization. The fusion rate was 85%. In a cohort population including 23 patients who did not undergo stimulation, the fusion rate at 9 months was less than 20%.

The use of pulsed electromagnetic fields (PEMF) to enhance fusion is also enjoying renewed interest. Early studies by Bassett et al clearly demonstrated improved union of long bone fractures.[56] In randomized animal studies, PEMF was associated with a better fusion rate. The fusion mass produced was significantly stiffer than autologous bone that was not stimulated. The amount of ossification within the stimulated fusion mass was also increased.[37]

Bone Morphogenetic Protein

At the time of this publication, other agents show great promise in promoting fusion.[22,67,85] Bone morphogenetic protein, isolated by Urist et al in the late 1970s,[65,82,92,93] has been used experimentally in several experimental and clinical trials.[59] Cook et al used rhBMP-7 to perform posterior fusions in dogs, comparing the time to radiographic fusion with that for traditional iliac crest grafting. The former required an average of 3 months, as opposed to 6 months or longer for iliac crest grafting.[23]

Boden et al have performed numerous investigations with these substances.[8-12] In studies comparing demineralized bone matrix with and without bovine osteoinductive protein (rhBMP-2) and autogenous iliac crest, rabbits underwent transverse process fusion. Osteoinductive protein matrix produced significantly better fusion than autogenous bone; it was dramatically superior to demineralized matrix without protein.[97] More recently, Boden's group demonstrated the effectiveness of minimally invasive video-assisted transverse process fusion in both monkeys and rabbits. In these studies, an osteoinductive growth factor in a collagen carrier was injected under video control; solid fusion was evident at 10 weeks.[9] Yet unpublished studies by this same group have shown that bone ingrowth will occur into titanium cages placed anteriorly in the lumbar spine, even without autograft.[8] Preliminary clinical trials are very promising, but little has been published in the peer-reviewed literature. This author can only contemplate with dread the specter of percutaneous fusions, without hardware, and with fusion rates paralleling the best we have to offer.

Orthoses

Next to bone graft principles, no subject is more widely debated or more controversial than the use of orthoses. In recent years, several clinical papers, anecdotal tales, and individuals speaking at conferences have suggested that the use of internal fixation can substitute for lumbosacral orthosis. Clearly, the placement of fixation devices that require surgical time, cause bleeding, increase the risk of infection and neurological deficit, and cost several thousand dollars only to obviate the need for a thermoplastic brace is somewhat ludicrous. Rather, the use of spinal instrumentation is for the purposes of providing internal fixation and promoting fusion.

Biomechanical Principles and Methods

Orthoses provide a lesser degree of immobilization, typically relying on three-point loading to prevent certain kinds of motions, such as flexion which are particularly bad for the recently fused lumbar spine. Anterior loading points are provided superiorly below the xiphoid and at the pubic symphysis, and posteriorly at the midlumbar spine. If well constructed, lumbosacral orthoses maintain or create optimal posture, and may even decrease the likelihood of "flat-back" syndrome.

Lumbosacral orthoses can rely on multiple points of contact with the skin (i.e., the Jewett hyperextension brace) or be full-contact. We use the latter almost exclusively to provide maximum control of flexion and extension (20% and 45%, respectively) and lateral bending (49%).[53] However most orthoses are relatively ineffective in reducing rotation.[60]

The most popular lumbosacral orthoses are made of a thermal polyform plastic molded individually for the patient. These function differently than corsets, which provide very little limitation of rotation or even flexion. However, neither does more than reduce gross spinal motion.

Indeed, Norton and Brown[74] placed wires in spinous processes and measured spinal motion in orthoses. They determined that increased motion occurs at L4-L5 and L5-S1 while in lumbosacral orthoses, in certain positions. Virtually no ordinary lumbar orthosis will limit translation: when control of translation is important, as in some fractures of the lumbar spine or when the lumbosacral junction is particularly at risk, it may be appropriate to use spica casts incorporating one hip; these largely eliminate hip motion.[3,4,30]

Additionally, rarely, in patients who undergo pelvic fixation, an orthosis is not provided. The use of spica casts incorporating one leg above the knee is quite common in this group.

The effectiveness of orthoses in promoting fusion and relief of back pain is not purely due to restriction of motion. There is evidence that lumbosacral orthoses cause increases in intraabdominal pressure and thereby reduce the joint reaction force at L5-S1,[66] and also cause marked decreases in intradiscal pressures in flexion.[68–70] The mechanisms for the former are poorly understood.

Indications for Use

We currently use a custom-fabricated lumbosacral orthosis on all patients undergoing surgical treatment for lumbar instability. Orthoses are used on average for 3 months after fusion, until evidence of bone bridging across the transverse processes occurs. Similarly, orthoses are used universally in patients with trauma and tumor. For the first 3 to 4 weeks, this orthosis is worn at all times when the patient is upright. After approximately 1 month, we generally allow the patient to remove the orthosis for personal hygiene, such as showering.

Orthoses are also occasionally used diagnostically: some believe that relief of pain during immobilization is evidence of spinal instability. Others use orthoses to treat low back pain.[70] These uses are controversial. Million et al failed to demonstrate significant or persistent improvement in generic low back pain with orthoses.[63] Willner, on the other hand, used them in patients with proven instability due to degenerative arthritis and spondylolisthesis; most patients obtained at least temporary pain relief, and almost 20% demonstrated actual healing of the isthmic defect.[96]

The treatment of unstable fractures of the lumbar spine requires exact sizing of the lumbosacral orthosis. Generally speaking, these orthoses should place the spine into gentle extension and should extend at least four to six levels cephalad of the injured segment, and minimally to the pelvis. Because of the need for precise fit, we rarely use prefitted bracing.

Conclusions

Unfortunately, data substantiating the use of orthoses to promote fusion following surgery do not yet exist. Presumably, decreasing spinal range of motion does improve osteogenesis. Certainly, immobilizing fractured spines improves healing. Until prospective studies suggest that immobilization is of great—or no—value we will continue to recommend their use.

REFERENCES

1. Aloia J, Cohn SH, Vaswani A, et al: Risk factors for postmenopausal osteoporosis. Am J Med 78:95–100, 1985.
2. An HS, Lynch K, Toth J: Prospective comparison of autograft versus allograft for adult posterolateral lumbar spine fusion: Differences among freeze-dried, frozen, and mixed grafts. J Spinal Disord 8:131–135, 1995.
3. Axelsson P, Johnson R, Stronqvist B: Effect of lumbar orthosis on intervertebral mobility. Spine 17:678–681, 1992.
4. Axelsson P, Johnson R, Strongqvist B: Lumbar orthosis with unilateral hip immobilization. Spine 18:876–879,1993.
5. Bassett CAL, Mitchell SN, Gaston SR: Treatment of ununited tibial diaphyseal fractures with pulsing electromagnetic fields. J Bone Joint Surg 63A:511–523, 1981.
6. Bassett C: The development and application of pulsed electromagnetic fields (PEMFs) for ununited fractures and arthrodeses. Orthop Clin North Am 15:61–87, 1984.
7. Battie MC, Videman T, Gill K, et al: 1991 Volvo award in clinical sciences: Smoking and lumbar intervertebral disc degeneration—An MRI study in identical twins. Spine 16:1015–1021, 1991.
8. Boden SD, Horton WC, Martin G, et al: Laparoscopic anterior spinal arthrodesis with rhBMP–2 in a titanium interbody threaded cage. North Am Spine Soc Annu Mtg, Oct 22–25, 1997, New York.
9. Boden SD, Moskovitz PA, Morone MA, et al: Video assisted lateral intertransverse process arthrodesis. Validation of a new minimally invasive lumbar spine fusion technique in the rabbit and non-human primate models. Spine 20:1410–1418, 1995.
10. Boden SD, Schimandle JH, Hutton WC: Lumbar intertransverse-process spinal arthrodesis with use of a bovine-derived osteoinductive protein: A preliminary report. J Bone Joint Surg 77A:1404–1417, 1995.
11. Boden SD, Schimandle JH, Hutton WC: An experimental lumbar intertransverse process spinal fusion model. Spine 20:412–420, 1995.
12. Boden SD, Schimandle JH, Hutton WC, et al: In vivo evaluation of a resorbable osteoinductive composite as a graft substitute for lumbar spinal fusion. J Spinal Disord 10:1–11, 1997.
13. Bradford DS: Anterior vascular pedicle bone grafting for the treatment of kyphosis. Spine 5:318–323, 1980.
14. Bridwell KH, Lenke LG, McEnery KW, et al: Anterior fresh frozen structural allografts in the thoracic and lumbar spine: Do they work if combined with posterior fusion? Spine 20:1410–1418, 1995.
15. Broulik PD, Jarab J: The effect of chronic nicotine administration on bone mineral content in mice. Horm Metab Res 25:219–221, 1993.
16. Brown CW, Orme TJ, Richardson HD: The rate of pseudarthrosis (surgical non-union) in patients who are smokers and patients who are nonsmokers: A comparison study. Spine 11:942–943, 1986.
17. Canalis E: Effect of growth factors on bone cell replication and differentiation. Clin Orthop 193:246–263, 1985.
18. Carpenter CT, Diets JAW, Leung KY, et al: Repair of a pseudarthrosis of the lumbar spine: A functional outcome. J Bone Joint Surg 78A:712–720, 1996.
19. Chalmers J, Grey DH, Rush J: Observations on the induction of bone in soft tissues. J Bone Joint Surg 57B:36–45, 1975.
20. Cheng S, Suominen H, Heikkinen E: Bone mineral density in relation to anthropometric properties, physical activity and smoking in 75-year-old men and women. Aging (Milano) 5:55–62, 1993.
21. Church EF, Pryor WA: Free radical chemistry of cigarette smoke and its toxicological implications. Environ Health Perspect 64:111–126, 1985.

22. Connolly J, Guse R, Lippielo L, et al: Development of an osteogenic bone-marrow preparation. J Bone Joint Surg 71A:684–691, 1989.

23. Cook SD, Dalton JE, Tan EH, et al: In vivo evaluation of recombinant human osteogenic protein (rhOP) implants as a bone graft substitute for spinal fusions. Spine 19:1655–1663, 1994.

24. Cornell CN, Lane JM, Nottebaert M, et al: The effect of ethylene oxide sterilization upon the bone inductive properties of demineralized bone matrix. Orthop Trans 11:74, 1987.

25. Daftari TK, Whitesides TE Jr, Heller JG, et al: Nicotine on the revascularization of bone graft: An experimental study in rabbits. Spine 19:904–911, 1994.

26. deVernejoul MC, Biclakoff J, Herve M, et al: Evidence for defective osteoblastic function: A role for alcohol and tobacco consumption in osteoporosis in middle aged men. Clin Orthop 179:107 6115, 1983.

27. Ducker TA: Cigarette smoking and the prevalence of spinal procedures. J Spinal Disord 5:134–136, 1992.

28. Emery SE, Hughes SS, Junglas WA, et al: The fate of anterior vertebral bone grafts in patients irradiated for neoplasm. Clin Orthop 300:207–212, 1994.

29. Fang MA, Frost PJ, Lida-Klein A, et al: Effects of nicotine on cellular function in L106-01 osteoblast-like cells. Bone 12:283–286, 1991.

30. Fidler MW, Plasmans CMT: The effect of four types of support on the segmental mobility of the lumbosacral spine. J Bone Joint Surg 65A:943–947, 1983.

31. Friedenstein AJ: Precursor cells of mechanocytes. Int Rev Cytol 47:327–359, 1976.

32. Friedenstein AJ, Chailakhyan RK, Gerasimov UV. Bone marrow osteogenic stem cells: In vitro cultivation and transplantation in diffusion chambers. Cell Tissue Kinet 20:263–272, 1987.

33. Freidenstein AJ, Petrakova KV, Kurolesova Al, et al: Heterotrophic transplants of bone marrow: Analysis of precursor cells for osteogenic and hematopoietic tissues. Transplantation 6:230–247, 1968.

34. Friedlander GE, Strong DM, Sell KW: Studies in antigenicity of bone: Freeze-dried and deep frozen allografts in rabbits. J Bone Joint Surg 58A:854–858, 1976.

35. Frymoyer JW: The role of spinal fusion. Spine 6:284–290, 1981.

36. Galvin RJ, Ramp WK, Lenz LG: Smokeless tobacco contains a non-nicotine inhibitor of bone metabolism. Toxicol Appl Pharmacol 95:292–300, 1988.

37. Glazer PA, Heilmann MR, Lotz JC, et al: Use of electromagnetic fields in a spinal fusion: A rabbit model. Spine 22:2351–2356, 1997.

38. Hadley MN, Reddy SV: Smoking and the human vertebral column: A review of the impact of cigarette use on vertebral bone metabolism and spinal fusion. Neurosurgery 41:116–124, 1997.

39. Hambly MF, Mooney V: Effect of smoking and pulsed electromagnetic fields on intradiscal pH in rabbits. Spine 16:83S–85S, 1992.

40. Heliovaara M, Makela M, Knekt P, et al: Determinants of sciatica and low back pain. Spine 16:608–614, 1991.

41. Herron LD, Newman MH: The failure of ethylene oxide gas-sterilized freeze-dried bone graft for thoracic and lumbar spinal fusion. Spine 14:496–500, 1989.

42. Hollenback KA, Barrett-Connor E, Edelstein SL: Cigarette smoking and bone mineral density in older men and women. Am J Public Health 83:1265–1270, 1993.

43. Holm S, Nachemson A: Nutrition of the intervertebral disc: Acute effects of cigarette smoking—An experimental animal study. J Bone Joint Surg 8A:243–258, 1984.

44. Hopper JL, Seeman E: The bone density of female twins discordant for tobacco use. N Engl J Med 330:387–392, 1994.

45. Jorgenson SS, Lowe TG, France J, et al: A prospective analysis of autograft versus allograft in posterolateral fusion in the same patient. Spine 18:2048–2053, 1994.

46. Kahanovitz N, Arnoczky SP: The efficacy of direct current electrical stimulation to enhance canine spinal fusions. Clin Orthop 251:295–299, 1990.

47. Kahanovitz N: Spine update: The use of adjunctive electrical stimulation to enhance the healing of spine fusions. Spine 21:2523–2525, 1996.

48. Kane WJ: Direct current electrical bone growth stimulation for spinal fusion. Spine 13:363–365, 1988.

49. Kaufman HH, Jones E: The principles of bony fusion. Neurosurgery 24:264–270, 1989.

50. Keene JS, McKinley NE: Iliac crest versus spinous process grafts in posttraumatic spinal fusions. Spine 17:790–794, 1992.

51. Kirkpatrick JS, Hadley MN: Autograft vs alloimplant bone as substrate for spinal fusion. Perspect Neurosurg 4:38–48, 1993.

52. Langer F, Czitrom A, Pritzker KP, et al: The immunogenicity of fresh and frozen allograft bone. J Bone Joint Surg 57A:216–220, 1975.

53. Lantz SA, Schultz AB: Lumbar spine orthosis wearing: Restriction of gross body motions. Spine 11:834–837, 1986.

54. Lauerman WC, Bradford DS, Ogilvie JW, et al: Results of lumbar pseudarthrosis repair. J Spinal Disord 5:149–157, 1992.

55. Lee EH, Langer F, Halloran P, et al: The immunology

of osteochondral and massive allografts. Trans Orthop Res Soc 4:61, 1979.

56. Le Huec JC, Lesprit E, Delavigne C, et al: Tri-calcium phosphate ceramics and allografts as bone substitutes for spinal fusion in idiopathic scoliosis: Comparative clinical results at four yea rs. Acta Orthop Belg 63:202–211, 1997.

57. Kane WJ: Direct current electrical bone growth stimulation for spinal fusion. Spine 13:363–365, 1988.

58. LeMonier de Gouvelle AC, Lippton HL, Cavero I, et al: Endothelin: A new family of endothelium-derived peptides with widespread biological properties. Life Sci 45:1499–1513, 1989.

59. Lovell TP, Dawson EG, Nilsson OS, et al: Augmentation of spinal fusion with bone morphogenetic protein in dogs. Clin Orthop 243:266–274, 1989.

60. Lumsden RM, Morris JM: An in vivo study of axial rotation and immobilization at the lumbosacral joint. J Bone Joint Surg 50A:1591–1602, 1968.

61. Malinin TI, Brown MD: Bone allografts in spinal surgery. Clin Orthop 154:68–73, 1981.

62. McBride GG, Bradford DS: Vertebral body replacement with femoral neck allograft and vascularized rib strut graft: A technique for treating post-traumatic kyphosis with neurological deficit. Sp ine 8:406–415, 1983.

63. Million R, Nilsen KH, Jayson MIV, et al: Evaluation of low back pain and assessment of lumbar corsets with and without back supports. Ann Rheum Dis 40: 449–454, 1981.

64. Minami A, Kaneda K, Satoh S, et al: Free vascularized fibular strut graft for anterior spinal fusion. J Bone Joint Surg 79B:43–47, 1997.

65. Mizutani H, Urist MR: The nature of bone morphogenetic protein fractions derived from bovine bone matrix gelatin. Clin Orthop 171:213–223, 1982.

66. Morris JM, Lucas DB, Bresler B: Role of the trunk in the stability of the spine. J Bone Joint Surg 43A:327–351, 1961.

67. Muthukumaran N, Reddi AH: Bone matrix-induced local bone induction. Clin Orthop 200:159–164, 1985.

68. Nachemson A, Morris J: In vivo measurements of intradiscal pressure. J Bone Joint Surg 46A:1077–1092, 1964.

69. Nachemson A, Schultz AB, Anderson GB: Mechanical effectiveness studies of lumbar spine orthoses. Scand J Rehab Med 9S:139–149, 1983.

70. Nachemson A: Orthotic treatment for injuries and diseases of the spinal column. Phys Med Rehab 1:11–24, 1987.

71. Nasca RJ, Lemons JE, Deinlein DA: Synthetic biomaterials for spinal fusion. Orthopedics 12:543–548, 1989.

72. Nerubay J, Marganit B, Bubis JJ, et al: Stimulation of bone formation by electrocurrent on spinal fusion. Spine 11:167–169, 1986.

73. Nilsson OS, Bauer HCF, Brosjo O, et al: Influence of indomethacin on heterotopic bone formation in rats: Importance of length of treatment and age. Clin Orthop 207:239–245, 1986.

74. Norton PL, Brown T: The immobilizing efficiency of back braces: Their effect on the posture and motion of the lumbosacral spine. J Bone Joint Surg 39A:111–138, 1957.

75. Oikarinen J: Experimental spinal fusion with decalcified bone matrix and deep-frozen allogenic bone in rabbits. Clin Orthop 162:210–208, 1982.

76. Paterson D: Treatment of nonunion with constant direct current: A totally implantable system. Orthop Clin North Am 15:47–59, 1984.

77. Pelker RR, Friedlander GE, Markham TC: Biomechanical properties of bone allografts. Clin Orthop 174:54–57, 1983.

78. Pintar FA, Maiman DJ, Hollowell JP, et al: Fusion rate and biomechanical stiffness of hydroxyapatite versus autogenous bone grafts for anterior cervical discectomy: An in vivo animal study. Spine 19:2524–2528, 1994.

79. Pintar FA, Yoganandan N, Droese K, et al: Biomechanical stiffness of hydroxyapatite versus autogenous bone grafts in anterior spinal fusions. Adv Bioeng 26:419–421, 1993.

80. Prolo DJ, Rodrigo JJ: Contemporary bone graft physiology and surgery. Clin Orthop 200:322–342, 1985.

81. Ragni P, Ala-Mononen P, Lindholm TS: Spinal fusion induced by porous hydroxyapatite blocks (HA): Experimental comparative study with HA, demineralized bone matrix and autogenous bone marrow. Ital J Orthop Traumatol 19:133–144, 1993.

82. Ramp WK, Leng LG, Galvin RJ: Nicotine inhibits collagen synthesis and alkaline phosphatase activity, but stimulates DNA synthesis in osteoblast-like cells. Proc Soc Exp Biol Med 197:36–43, 1991.

83. Rogozinski A, Rogozinski C: Efficacy of implanted bone growth stimulation in instrumented lumbosacral spinal fusion. Spine 21:2479–2483, 1996.

84. Rubenstein I, Yang T, Rennard SI, et al: Cigarette smoke extract attenuates endothelium-dependent arteriolar dilatation in vivo. Am J Physiol 261:H1913–H1918, 1991.

85. Sato K, Urist MR: Induced regeneration of calvaria by bone morphogenetic protein (BMP) in dogs. Clin Orthop 197:301–311, 1985.

86. Silcox DH III, Daftari T, Boden SD, et al: The effects of nicotine on spinal fusion. Spine 20:1549–1553, 1995.

87. Simmons JW: Treatment of failed posterior lumbar interbody fusion (PLIF) of the spine with pulsing electromagnetic fields. Clin Orthop 193:127–132, 1985.
88. Stricker SJ, Sher JS: Freeze-dried cortical allograft in posterior spinal arthrodesis: Use with segmental instrumentation for idiopathic adolescent scoliosis. Orthopedics 20:1039–1043, 1 997.
89. Tejano NA, Puno R, Ignacio JM: The use of implantable direct current stimulation in multilevel spinal fusion without instrumentation: A prospective clinical and radiographic evaluation with long-term follow-up. Spine 21:1904–1908, 1996.
90. Thalgott J, LaRocca, H, Gardner V, et al: Reconstruction of failed lumbar surgery with narrow AO DCP plates for spinal arthrodesis. Spine 16:S170–S175, 1991.
91. Urist MR: Bone: Formation by autoinduction. Science 150:893–899, 1965.
92. Urist MR: Bone transplants and implants. In Urist MR (ed.): Fundamental and Clinical Bone Physiology. Lippincott, Philadelphia, pp. 331–368, 1980.
93. Urist MR, Lietze A, Mizutani H, et al: A bovine low molecular weight bone morphogenetic protein (BMP) fraction. Clin Orthop 162:219–232, 1982.
94. Weiland AJ, Moore JR, Daniel RK: Vascularized bone autografts: Experience with 41 cases. Clin Orthop 174:87–95, 1983.
95. Weiland AJ, Phillips TW, Randolph MA: Bone grafts: A radiologic, histologic, and biomechanical model comparing autografts, allografts, and free vascularized bone grafts. Plast Reconstr Surg 74:368–379, 1984.
96. Willner S: Effect of a rigid brace on back pain. Acta Orthop Scand 56:40–42, 1985.
97. Wittenberg RH, Moeller J, Shea M, et al: Compressive strength of autologous and allogenous bone grafts for thoracolumbar and cervical spine fusion. Spine 15:1073–1078, 1990.
98. Yanagusawa M, Kurihara H, Kimura S, et al: A novel potent vasoconstrictor peptide produced by vascular endothelial cells. Nature 332:411–415, 1988.
99. Yazici M, Asher MA: Freeze-dried allograft for posterior spinal fusion in patients with neuromuscular spinal deformities. Spine 22:1467–1471, 1997.
100. Younger EM, Chapman MW: Morbidity at bone graft donor sites. J Orthop Trauma 3:192–195, 1989.

CHAPTER 13

Surgical Approaches

Laminectomy-Based Approaches

Posterior Intertransverse Lumbar Fusion

Transpedicular Fixation

Sublaminar Wiring

Galveston (Pelvic) Fixation

Universal (Hook-Rod) Fixation

Posterior Lumbar Interbody Fusion (PLIF)

Extracavitary Approach

Anterior Lumbar Fusion

Endoscopic Lumbar Fusion

Surgical Approaches

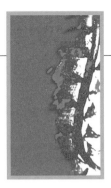

Historically, laminectomy was the favored approach to lumbar spine lesions of all types: *"When all you have is a hammer, every problem is a nail."* as the old Yiddish saying goes.

The literature is filled with retrospective studies of trauma, tumors, and other pathology of the vertebral body and disc that have been unsuccessfully treated through posterior approaches. Since patients rarely improved as the result of these inappropriate procedures, many argued that surgical treatment en toto is not beneficial in promoting neurological recovery.

In the last two decades, there has been increasing emphasis on anterior and anterolateral approaches for lumbar spine decompression. These procedures are associated with their own problems, including the technical challenges, issues of instrumentation, and indications. Because the spinal cord terminates near the thoracolumbar junction, the neurological indications for anterior decompression are somewhat different than for the cervical or thoracic spine. Furthermore, because of the unique biomechanics of the lumbar spine, including its lordosis, the importance of the facets and lamina on loading, and its massive musculoligamentous component, indications for instrumentation and types available are different as well.

In recent years, then, the pendulum seems to have gone in the other direction: that is, anterior decompression and fusion-including instrumentation are being used for indications where less extensive procedures might suffice. In addition, staged circumferential procedures are commonly used in situations where either anterior or posterior approaches would be adequate.

In this section, we describe some of the most common procedures used in lumbar spine decompression and stabilization. This discussion is not meant to be exhaustive, but rather reflects our current practice.

Laminectomy-Based Approaches

Because laminectomy is such a common procedure (and indeed the most common one performed on the lumbar spine), there are as many surgical options as there are surgeons performing them. However, there are certain common features. Needless to say, prior to making the incision, the surgeon should determine that laminectomy is the appropriate choice. Indications may include disc herniation, foraminal narrowing, dorsal tumor, and canal stenosis.

Anterior masses other than intervertebral disc herniation should rarely be approached through a pure laminectomy. Variations of laminectomy, such as transpedicular decompression, are often appropriate for certain anterior masses. However, except for very soft tumors or lateral fracture fragments, for example, the authors prefer anterior approaches for anterior problems.

Lumbar Discectomy

Standard anesthetic/preoperative techniques are used: legs are wrapped to minimize venous congestion, and patients are positioned prone. Chest rolls, Wilson frame, or Jackson table are used to minimize intraabdominal venous pressure and decrease epidural bleeding. We do not use the knee-chest or other nonanatomic positions, except in cases of deformity. Marking x-rays are obtained to ensure the appropriate level of the incision.

The authors currently use incisions that provide maximum exposure. This surgeon has abandoned microdiscectomy, finding it to be relatively unpleasant because of the increased risks of operating at the wrong level, difficulties in performing foraminotomy, and occasional difficulties in retraction. We recognize, of course, that microdiscectomy is extremely popular mostly because of the minimal dissection required and subsequent brief hospitalization. However, most people currently treated with standard single-level discectomy are also outpatients.

Following incision, the thoracolumbar fascia is opened using a knife or cutting electrocautery. Subperiosteal dissection is carefully performed, elevating the muscles and periosteum off of the lamina (Fig. 13–1A). Prior to hemilaminectomy or laminotomy as described, we obtain a confirming marking radiograph.

Laminotomy is then performed. First the ligamentum flavum is freed from the lamina using a curette, and the bone is removed using a Kerrison rongeur or high-speed drill (Fig. 13–1B). This is done layer by layer to prevent injury to the nerve roots. Following exposure of the disc to be removed, the nerve root is generally retracted laterally and the pathology identified. Bipolar electrocautery is used to coagulate the epidural vessels. A rectangular opening is incised in the annulus with a scalpel, and the disc is removed using rongeurs (Fig. 13–1C). We prefer to remove all loose fragments of degenerated disc; we do not routinely use ring curettes to scrape the end plate, unless fusion is to be performed. The wound is closed in layers, and patients should be ambulatory from the recovery room.

This author has found that using a surgical drain for several hours, if there is any venous bleeding, minimizes postoperative pain. In addition, we routinely inject half-percent Marcaine into the muscle and fascia, which certainly speeds ambulation following surgery.

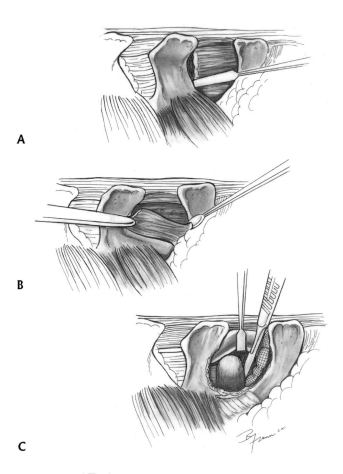

FIGURE 13–1 Technique for lumbar disc excision: see text for details. **A** Subperiosteal dissection; the laminar edge is dissected. **B** Laminatomy and removal of ligamentum flavum. **C** Incision of disc annulus and removal.

Lumbar Laminectomy

For laminectomy, a bilateral subperiosteal dissection is accomplished. The laminectomy itself may be performed in several ways: recently, we have often used a high-speed drill to thin the lamina laterally; we then lift it and cut the ligamentous attachment. Alternatively, the lamina can be removed piecemeal using Kerrison and Leksell rongeurs. However, the use of the Kerrison rongeur can be hazardous, since it may rip the dura if used to remove thickened bone.

One of the most important principles in laminectomy is adequate exposure. We strongly discourage the use of unilateral hemilaminectomies or laminotomies to treat central disc herniations. This requires a great deal of retraction of the thecal sac and may result in cauda equina syndrome. Rather, a full laminectomy and bilateral disc excision are safer.

As is discussed in the chapter on degenerative spine disease (Chapter 5), probably the leading reason for failure of surgeries performed for stenosis and foraminal narrowing is inadequate decompression. Performance of central laminectomy without foraminotomy is associated with a high degree of failure. However, facetectomy, which is often required to enlarge the narrowed foramen, is associated with a recognized incidence of instability.

To the extent possible, the degree of decompression needed should be determined preoperatively, so that fusion can be planned if necessary. Partial facetectomy, which is not as destabilizing, may be accomplished through the judicious use of osteotomes. The advantage of performing partial facetectomy this way is that the surgeon can accurately measure how much of the joint is to be removed; if partial facetectomy is accomplished with rongeurs, more joint may be removed than is necessary or desirable, leading to instability.

Transpedicular Approaches

In certain instances of tumor, infection, or fracture with relatively minor—or very lateral—canal compromise, transpedicular approaches can be safely used to decompress the spinal canal. Because a pedicle as well as a disc is removed, stabilization is frequently required.

Transpedicular approaches are often associated with an unacceptable rate of neurological injury: we suspect that the most common reason for this is inadequate lateral bone removal, thus necessitating excessive retraction on the dural sac. It is better to remove more bone to protect neural structures: instability can be dealt with much more easily than cauda equina syndrome.

Following hemi- or full-laminectomy, wide bone removal is accomplished at the pedicle to be approached. Usually, we recommend that this include the facet joint and both the superior- and inferior-articulating facets. The nerve root at the affected levels should be followed out some distance beyond the pedicle to soft tissue: this ensures its safety to some extent. The pedicle is then available adjacent to the nerve root. This can be safely drilled with a high-speed drill, or carefully rongeured and curetted.

Through this exposure anterolateral to the dural sac, lateral or very soft masses can be pushed away from the dural sac and excised. Under certain circumstances, two-level transpedicular decompression can be accomplished with partial vertebrectomy. In cases of tumor, methyl-methacrylate can be pushed into the empty space anteriorly, although this is not our preference. Again, we prefer to deal with such masses through an anterolateral approach, using the extracavitary approach whenever possible. Rarely, if ever, should transpedicular decompression be used for central masses.

Posterior Intertransverse Lumbar Fusion

Transverse process fusion was first used in the late 1940s to treat pseudoarthrosis following posterior (laminar) lumbar fusion. Since the latter procedure has been abandoned, it will not be discussed. The former was used more commonly in the late 1950s and was refined into the posterior-lateral approach by those who described the importance of exposure of the pars and full length of the transverse process as well as the posterior joints.[9]

The technique of transverse process fusion, although it may appear straightforward, requires careful knowledge of the anatomy of the spine and its blood supply to maximize fusion potential. There are few spine surgery techniques where meticulous preparation of bone surfaces is of more benefit. Although spinal instrumentation, particularly transpedicular fixation, has improved fusion rates following lumbar fusion, it cannot substitute for thoughtful technique.

Technique

The patient is positioned prone on an operating room table with chest rolls or Wilson frame. Recently, we have begun using the OSI Jackson frame for even routine lumbar fusions, and have found it to decrease blood loss and aid in positioning (Fig. 13–2A). Furthermore, it enhances intraoperative radiography. The Jackson frame tends to exaggerate lumbar lordosis; this is of value in some patients, but can decrease the ability to reduce spondylolistheses for surgeons so inclined.[36]

In patients with thin or moderate habitus, the arms are placed carefully at the sides with pressure points padded. However, in larger patients, it may be necessary to place the arms up toward the anesthesiologist in order to obtain adequate radiographs. If such is elected, positioning must be meticulous to avoid the development of brachial plexopathy. Pneumatic compression stockings are used routinely as well as Foley catheterization. Intravenous antibiotics are given, although there is no compelling evidence that prophylaxis is of any benefit. Auto-transfusion (cell saver) use is routine. Although many clinicians prefer biplanar fluoroscopy, we are more inclined to use traditional radiographs during the procedure, finding the fluoroscopic equipment annoying and the required lead vests punishing. Marking x-rays are obtained to aid in localization. We recommend a positioning film early so that the surgeon can be assured of satisfactory sagittal alignment.

Our current practice is to use a single vertical incision extending approximately one level above the desired level of fusion. In larger people, two levels are often necessary. There is little advantage to fighting the large paravertebral muscle mass, or being forced to resect muscle, rather than making the incision longer. Indeed, an important principle is the need to expose the entire transverse process for fusion, and therefore longer incisions may be useful.

The iliac crest is palpated through the fascia and an incision made through it to the thicker, more medial portion of the crest. This allows harvesting of the greatest amount of cancellous bone and typically avoids injury to the cluneal nerves. These nerves penetrate the lumbodorsal fascia over the iliac crest 6 to 10 cm lateral to the posterior superior iliac spine. Needless to say, the surgeon should avoid violating the sacroiliac joint, which can cause long-term pain.

A full-thickness iliac crest graft need not be taken. There is some risk to injuring the viscera on the ventral surface of the iliac crest. For transverse process fusion, the amount of cortical bone used is of little relevance. Therefore, we typically use a trap-door approach where the cortical bone is incised (Fig. 13–2B), cancellous bone is removed, and most of the cortical bone is allowed to fall back into place (Fig. 13–2C). Once the bone has been taken, meticulous hemostasis is performed using Gelfoam powder or thrombin and bone (Fig. 13–2D), and the fascia is closed with large absorbable sutures. We rarely drain the graft site separately from the main incision.

A meticulous subperiosteal dissection is then performed to the lateral tips of the transverse processes, where much of the blood supply is.[65] The use of cautery to minimize blood loss is critical; however, one must be careful to use only bipolar electrocautery around the pars and transverse process to avoid nerve root injury (Fig. 13–2E). Although dissection of the soft tissues off the pars may be associated with blood loss, the additional fusion surface is of value, and therefore should be done carefully with curette and blunt dissection (see Fig. 13–2F). The facet joint capsules are carefully cleared (Fig. 13–2G). Many surgeons use osteotomes to violate the facet joints, later filling them with bone graft.

The sacral ala is meticulously cleansed of soft tissue and decorticated using a sharp Cobb dissector. Intertransverse ligaments should be removed, since these will push the loose bone graft dorsally. Care is taken to avoid aggressive dissection over the sacral foramina and the medial vessels of the ala, because of the bleeding that might result.

The transverse processes and the pars are decorticated using a high-speed drill and/or curettage. Several clinicians have reported anecdotally that the failure to manually decorticate the "burned bone" leads to decreased fusion rates. Although the evidence for this is inconsistent, we carefully roughen the ala, pars, and transverse processes to their tips with a curette (Fig. 13–2H). The facet joints are then packed with small pieces of cancellous bone, and the remainder of the cortical and cancellous bone is placed on the decorticated transverse processes (Fig. 13–2I). We recommend against placing bone over the lamina, since this may lead to hypertrophied laminae and cephalad extension of the fusion.

The wound is then closed in layers, with meticulous fascial closure. This author routinely uses surgical drains.

Postoperative Care

Patients are mobilized in a full-contact TLSO on the day of surgery; currently, average patient length of stay is 3 to 4 days. Patients are advised to avoid heavy lifting or bending and the orthosis is maintained for an average of 3 months. Patients can typically resume light-duty employment within 6 weeks. Following evidence of acceptable fusion, the orthosis is removed, and patients undergo an intensive rehabilitation program. The importance of this cannot be overemphasized: several yet unpublished reports have shown such rehabilitation to be valuable in promoting long-term successful outcomes.

Complications of transverse process fusion are few. Anesthetic complications, infection, and hemorrhage may occur, as is the case for any type of operation. Persistent pain from the iliac crest graft site is very common.

The determination of successful fusion can be difficult. We routinely obtain lateral and antero-

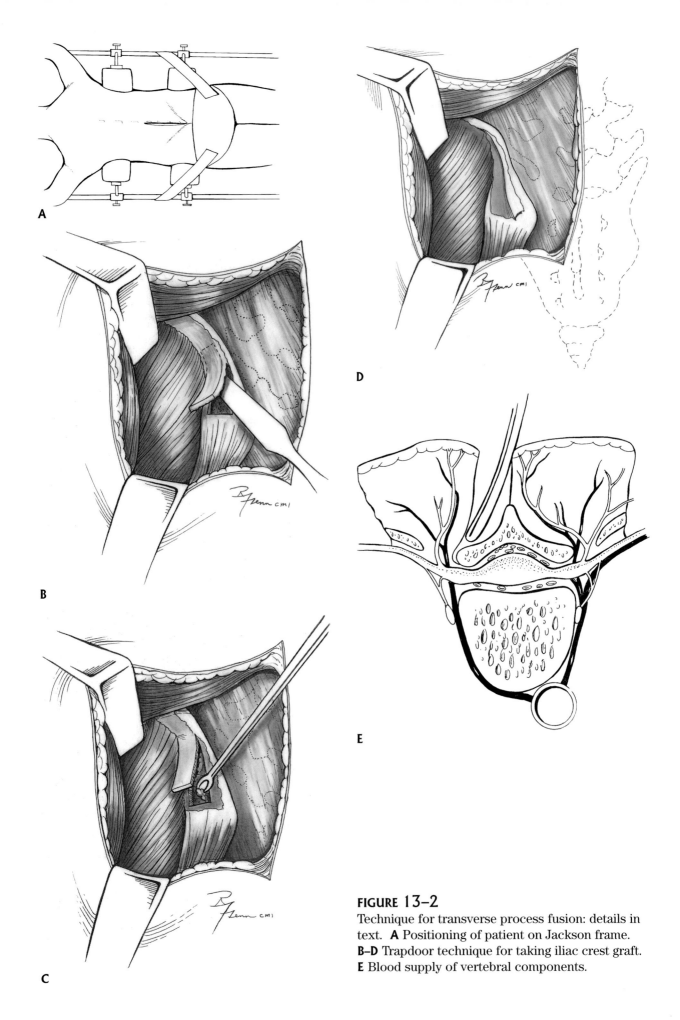

FIGURE 13-2
Technique for transverse process fusion: details in text. **A** Positioning of patient on Jackson frame. **B–D** Trapdoor technique for taking iliac crest graft. **E** Blood supply of vertebral components.

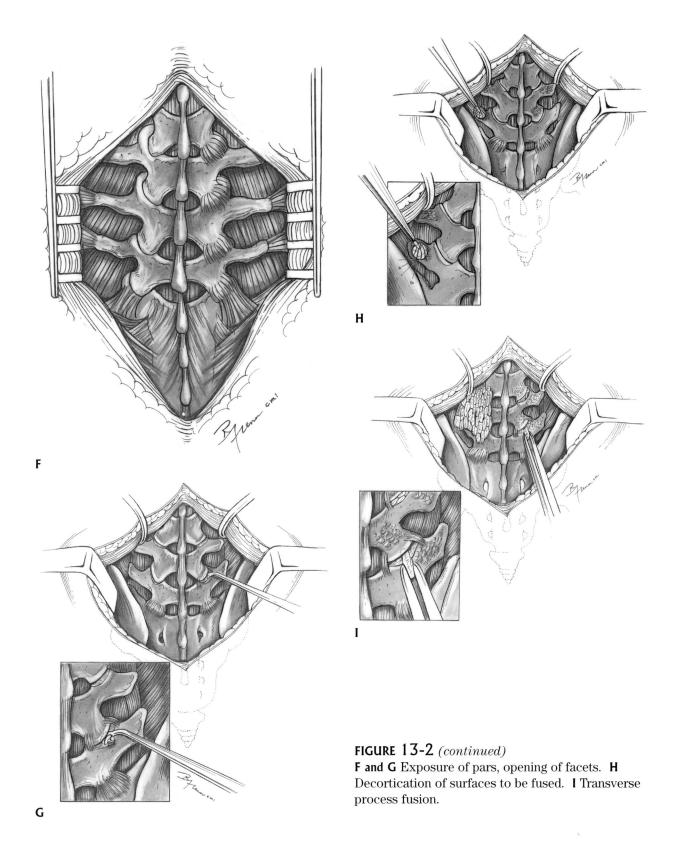

FIGURE 13-2 *(continued)*
F and G Exposure of pars, opening of facets. **H** Decortication of surfaces to be fused. **I** Transverse process fusion.

posterior radiographs at intervals, typically monthly. As do most surgeons, we assume that fusion has occurred when bone bridges the transverse processes. On occasion, we have been surprised when patients thought to have solid fusions presented with, for example, fractured pedicle screws and were subsequently shown to have nonunions.

Bosworth's dictum, coined in 1948, states that the only way to be certain that a fusion has occurred is to explore it.[9] Brodsky et al compared radiographic studies, including plain radiography and computed tomography (CT), with surgical exploration. The former were about 70% accurate in determining that fusion had occurred; CT was little better.[12] In another series, Blumenthal and Gill reviewed postoperative radiographs blindly, and then assessed fusion during hardware removal in 49 patients who had undergone transverse process fusion, transpedicular fixation, and posterior lumbar interbody fusion (PLIF). The fusion rate on intraoperative observation was 90%. Overall agreement between radiography and visual assessment was 69%; however, the range between observers was 57 to 77%. The overall false-positive rate was 42%, and the false-negative 29%.[7] Thus fusion is actually underestimated in one-fourth of patients, and plain radiographs accurately determine fusion in about 70%. CT and functional films are probably of little value in improving these results. Instead, in patients with increasing back pain that appears mechanical, and in whom radiography is unhelpful, exploration is occasionally appropriate.[12]

Results

Fusion rates are marginal for transverse process fusion without instrumentation. In our series of more than 1,400 lumbar fusions, approximately 160 were done without instrumentation. Fusion rates approached 60%. Whereas some clinicians indicate that L5,S1 is more likely to fuse than other levels, in this author's experience that has not necessarily been the case. To improve fusion rates, we typically incorporate spinal fixation. Most commonly, this consists of transpedicular fixation; in the osteoporotic patient, sublaminar or spinous process wired Luque rectangles are used; and in yet others, hook and rod instrumentation is occasionally employed.

Transpedicular Fixation

At the time of this writing, the use of pedicle fixation to promote lumbar fusion is considered almost essential by spine surgeons for many patients[86,102] but is not yet accepted by the FDA for some indications. To stay out of the fray, and hopefully out of the clutches of thousands of attorneys, we will not discuss the legal controversies. Rather, the focus is on indications and technical issues.

Internal fixation in association with transverse process and interbody fusion was first reported in 1889 by Hadra,[39] who used spinous process wiring. Spinous process plates were used by Straub, and hooks subsequently were used by Knodt.[59,91] Hook/rod constructs were employed early by Harrington and others.[40] The use of sublaminar wires for segmental fixation of the spine was popularized by Luque and still is used in selected patients, as described elsewhere in this chapter.[63]

The most dramatic advance in internal fixation of the lumbar spine has been the use of transpedicular fixation.[102] The pedicle represents the ideal point of attachment to the lumbar spine. It is the strongest component of the vertebra, consisting primarily of cortical bone. The entrance point, dimensions, and endpoint are consistent and radiographically determinable, and the pedicle is rarely affected in degenerative disease.[34] When the pedicle has been violated by trauma or tumor, the determination is easily made radiographically. Thus much of the uncertainty associated with fixation constructs is eliminated with preoperative imaging.

Although it is uncertain who first used the transpedicular screw, Roy-Camille et al were among the first to demonstrate the effectiveness of pedicle-based instrumentation.[88] Steffee was one of the earliest developers of a system that allowed the rigid anchor of a screw to the plate and variable placement.[97,98]

Since then, at least 17 transpedicular screw fixation systems have been developed. These vary from screw-and-plate to screw-and-rod systems, and often incorporate various types of transverse fixation, connectors, variable angle screws, and different profiles. The bewildering array has made the surgeon's decision more complicated. Suffice it so say that most of these systems share relatively common biomechanics and common insertion principles. Thus no effort is made in this chapter to advocate one system over another; rather the emphasis is on common features of all instrumentation systems. The clinician is urged to become familiar with one or two systems and use these regularly to understand their nuances and best compensate for their weaknesses.

Regardless of the system employed, overall improvement in fusion rates has ranged from 20% to 30%, although this has not necessarily translated into improved clinical outcomes. As is true for so many other surgical techniques, complication and morbidity rates decrease with experience.

Patient Selection and Preparation

Patients being considered for transpedicular fixation and fusion should have clinical and radiographic evidence for instability. Furthermore, to be recommended for surgery, most patients should have undergone a rehabilitation program emphasizing lumbar stabilization and strengthening of spinal musculature. A thoughtful discussion of the risks and potential benefits of transpedicular fixation as well as the FDA status (at the time of this writing) is imperative. We do not knowingly operate on smokers, as discussed elsewhere: there is considerable evidence that smoking decreases fusion rates in lumbar fusion. Since fusions are rarely emergent, patients should be expected to quit prior to the operative procedure. If they are unwilling to do so, then alternative treatments are often best considered.

Other relative contraindications include osteoporosis; we do not routinely attempts to anchor pedicle screws in osteoporotic bone using methylmethacrylate or other techniques. However, if it is felt necessary to use pedicle fixation in the osteoporotic spine, the surgeon should strongly consider simultaneous PLIF. In a study by Bennett et al, interbody fusion increased stiffness of the fixated spine even with lower bone densities.[4]

Morbid obesity is a relative contraindication, in part because of problems with intraoperative radiography: image-directed screw placement may be of benefit in this population, but the preoperative planning which incorporates CT in such individuals may be inaccurate.

Preoperative radiographic requirements include a spinal canal study, such as magnetic resonance imaging (MRI), as well as bone imaging. Plain radiographs are important for overall anatomy and for defining the preoperative sagittal alignment. CT is used to define pedicle diameter as well as projected screw length. Generally, we do not use screws that are more than 65% of the diameter of the pedicle. We do not use, recommend, or condone discography. Although some have knowingly placed screws through fractured pedicles, we strongly discourage this practice, since it is biomechanically unsound.

We prefer that patients donate autologous blood for the procedure. Two to three units are generally recommended, in addition to intraoperative cell salvage.

The preparation for transpedicular fixation is much as was discussed previously for transverse process fusion. If transpedicular fixation is to be used, the incision is generally carried caudally over the sacrum to allow exposure some distance beyond the first sacral foramen.

Surgeons often like to debate the advantages of rod versus plate systems. Currently, the former are commonly used by the authors. They allow appropriate contouring to carefully maintain sagittal alignment, which has been our practice for several years. Three-dimensional alignment can be much more capably performed. Less injury to adjacent levels (i.e., facet disruption) is required, and more surface for bone grafting is available. Unfortunately, rod-based systems often require multiple connections, which can make placement more complicated and result in a higher profile.

The technical description provided below is not adequate for even an accomplished surgeon to acquire the skills for transpedicular fixation. Rather, cadaver study in courses that are readily available to most surgeons, as well as proctored practice, is important. The hazards of transpedicular fixation, including nerve root and dural sac injury, cerebral spinal fluid leak, hemorrhage, pedicle fracture, and injury to major vessels anteriorly cannot be overstressed. They can be minimized, however, by experience.

Technical Considerations

The pedicle is ideal as a fixation point not only because of its bony composition but also because of its geometry. A screw in the pedicle resists loads circumferentially; pull-out strength is directly related to length and is often predictable: increasing screw length by one-third will improve pull-out strength by one-third.[51,52] Zindrick et al, however, have suggested that bone density is more important in pull-out strength than screw length. They have found further that penetrating the anterior vertebral cortex improves fixation, eliminating screw toggling within the pedicle and vertebra.[116] This has not been popular clinically because of the risks of injury to visceral structures, particularly the aorta, anterior to the spine. Rather, the use of larger-diameter screws engaging the pedicle circumferentially improves fixation strength.

However, placement of larger screws is not without risk.[77] Sjostrom et al performed CT in 21 patients in whom they removed pedicle screws one year postoperatively. In some patients, medial or lateral defects in the cortical bone of the pedicle were seen. If the screw diameter was greater than 65% of the outer diameter of the pedicle, the pedicle was likely to be expanded.[96] This has the potential for decreasing stability or compressing neural structures, especially lumbar nerve roots.[33]

Unfortunately, fracture of the medial wall of the pedicle may be radiographically indeterminable. In a cadaver study, Weinstein et al inserted screws under fluoroscopy through the thoracolumbar spine. Over 20% of the screws violated the medial cortex of the pedicle, in spite of apparent satisfactory position on radiography.[106] But when all is said and done, does it really matter? No reports have documented significant deficit resulting from the typically minor violation of the canal seen with most pedicle fixation.[26,27,55,61,88]

Other means of increasing strength have also been studied. The injection of methylmethacrylate into oversized pedicle holes has been suggested to augment fixation. We have found this not to be the case, and do not generally recommend this technique. There is no compelling evidence that one type of pedicle screw thread has significantly better pull-out strength than another, although shallow threads may perform better under certain forces.

Numerous studies have been done on the ideal placement of transpedicular screws in the sacrum.[13,76,83] It is our preference to insert the screw laterally into the ala, taking advantage of maximum screw length. Bicortical purchase is often appropriate to enhance the stiffness of the construct at the lumbosacral junction. However, the screw should not penetrate the sacrum by more than 2 to 3 mm, since injury to lumbar nerve roots may occur.

Other considerable risks of transpedicular fixation exist as well, which will be discussed later. The surgeon needs to weigh the complications associated with fixation against improved fusion rates. Ultimate stiffness of internal fixation is not the terminal goal; fusion is. No matter how rigid the construct, if fusion does not occur, instrumentation will ultimately fail. If the anterior load path is inadequate to reduce loads, both the fusion and the hardware are doomed. Transpedicular fixation does not substitute for meticulous attention to fusion biomechanics and techniques.[47]

Technique

Prior to performing transpedicular fixation, we generally perform the full lateral dissection including wide exposure of the transverse processes, as discussed above. In addition, we perform neural decompression (when indicated). Some would argue that it is better to do the laminectomy after fixation, but we have found this to be technically cumbersome. In addition, laminectomy allows direct visualization of the pedicle entry point.

Prior to this point, a lateral lumbar spine film should have been performed to ensure appropriate sagittal alignment. Radiographs are also obtained liberally throughout pin and screw placement. This author does not typically use fluoroscopy because of the radiation exposure and the cumbersome nature of the technique. We have not found it to save time, either. Although some surgeons have all but abandoned intraoperative x-ray to save time and money, we prefer to have some intraoperative degree of comfort that the screws are where we want them to be. This may require only lateral radiography, according to some.[79]

Clearly, the most important part of the procedure is the identification of the pedicle. We prefer to place the screw entry point at the junction of the true facet and transverse process (Fig. 13–3A). This typically requires removal of overgrown facet joints, which are a normal consequence of instability, particularly at the lumbosacral junction, where the sacral foramen can actually be covered by hypertrophic facet joint.[43] Using an overgrown facet joint as the anatomic marker is a leading cause for misplaced pins. In addition, inadequate facet removal may lead the surgeon to put the pin and screw through a joint, which may be associated with increased risk of nonunion.

The junction of the facet joint and transverse process is then decorticated with a rongeur or power drill. Typically, the safest entry point is at the junction of the top and middle third of the transverse process (Fig. 13–3B).

We use a Steinman pin attached to a chuck to make the initial hole in the pedicle (Fig. 13–3C). Our preference is to insert the pin 50 mm if the computed tomogram indicates that the vertebra will allow this, to provide optimal identification of future screw length. The pin should pass smoothly, without jolting: jolting is often associated with violation of the cortical wall of the pedicle or vertebral body.

There are several opinions regarding medial angulation of the screws to be placed. We try to angle the screws within the limitations of the surgical exposure. At L2, the screws are angulated 0 to 5 degrees; this is increased to 5 to 10 degrees below that, and to 15 degrees in the sacrum, if possible. Similarly, the cranial-caudal angulation is increased to ensure placement of the screw in the middle of the pedicle, and to ensure that the screw is at least several millimeters away from the disc end plate.[53]

At the sacrum, the first sacral foramen is identified clearly. We decorticate the sacrum one cm cephalad to that point (Fig. 13–3B). Although there have been numerous discussion about where optimal sacral fixation occurs, our current practice is to try to keep the sacral screws more or less in line with the others, one cm cephalad to the sacral foramen, and angled quite medially (many others will direct the screws laterally). A markedly caudal direction is necessary to prevent the screw from entering the L5–S1 disc space. Although placing a screw across a disc space to be fused is not in and of itself a disaster, it may compromise the strength of fixation at the ends of the construct.

The Steinman pins are removed, and a thin awl is used to further define the holes. We carefully probe the walls and bottom of each hole down to at least 35 to 40 mm to ensure that it is well within bone. Blunt marker pins (the left pins different from the right-sided pins) are placed in each of the holes that have been made. Careful anteroposterior and lateral radiographs are performed.

Following confirmation of placement within the pedicle, the pins are sequentially removed and the screw holes tapped. We generally prefer to undertap both diameter and length; the tap should go in easily, using two fingers, without resistance. The hole should be reprobed after tapping.

We generally try to put in the longest screws that are reasonable within the holes available, and prefer larger-diameter screws (again, about 65% of the pedicle diameter), without placing a screw that will cause the pedicle to expand. Sacral bicortical purchase is reserved for cases of higher-grade spondylolisthesis, severe abnormal motion, and mild osteoporosis.

We routinely perform radiographs following screw placement, before the rods are inserted. Although it is often difficult to ascertain appropriate screw placement on plain radiography, we feel that this offers the optimal opportunity to avoid violation of the pedicle.

Rods are carefully contoured for optimal alignment. No effort is made to "overcorrect"; indeed, we rarely attempt reduction with fixation alone. Overcontouring will often place unacceptable biomechanical stresses on the screw/pedicle interface and lead to hardware failure and loss of stabilization. After all, stabilization is the primary purpose of fixation.

Connectors and rods are placed and carefully tightened (see Fig. 13–3D). In systems that do not use torque wrenches for tightening, all connections should be tightened sequentially and repeatedly, since they do loosen. Cross-linking in transpedicular fixation for degenerative disease is not usually necessary unless more than four segments are fixated. Rotational instability as a cause of fusion failure is extremely uncommon. This is not the case in trauma or tumor, however, where cross-linking is routinely employed.

Transverse process fusion is performed as discussed above. Following drain placement, wounds are closed as for lumbar fusion. Patients are ambulated on the day of surgery in a TLSO; the average length of stay is 3 days in uncomplicated cases.

Complications

Most complications are the same as those for any spinal surgery: infection, bleeding, and dural tears. Deep infection rate requiring instrumentation removal is less than 0.1%. Skin infection rate is less than 1%. Unrecognized spinal fluid leaks are seen in less than 0.5%.[29]

Nerve root injuries due to marginal screw placement or pedicle fracture are uncommon. Although some have reported nerve root injury rates of 2.5 to 7.5%,[27,107,117] we have seen only three cases: two probably due to initial hole creation, and one due to explosion of the pedicle. Most nerve root injuries can be prevented through meticulous attention to technique. Violation of the medial wall of the pedicle will rarely cause nerve root injury, and these screws need not be removed. However, screws going through the foramen generally should be.

Abdominal injury occurs rarely. Some have discussed damage to retroperitoneal structures due to violation of the anterior vertebral cortex; there is little biomechanical advantage to screws of this

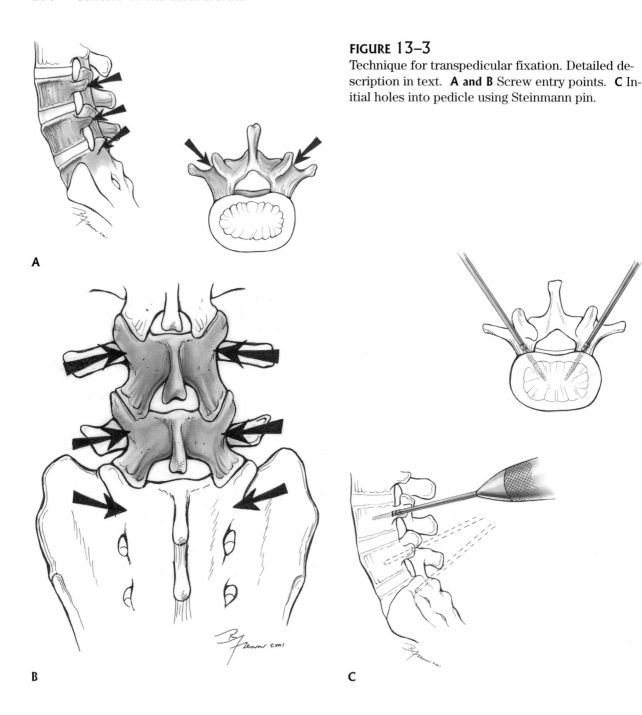

FIGURE 13-3
Technique for transpedicular fixation. Detailed description in text. **A** and **B** Screw entry points. **C** Initial holes into pedicle using Steinmann pin.

length. We have had one case of a self-tapping screw fracturing the pedicle and going into the peritoneal cavity; we again emphasize that no force should be used to tap the pedicle hole.

Screw fractures or loosening will be seen in 1 to 4% of cases: many of these are related to nonunion, since fracture of metal due to fatigue is common. However, screw failure often occurs in patients with solid fusions, reflecting the ability of even mature fusions to deform, whereas metal cannot.[111]

Nonunion is uncommon in nonsmoking individuals undergoing first operative procedures (<5%). In smokers, the failure rate increases to over 20%, and even further in those who have been operated upon previously. In managing nonunion, this author prefers anterior lumbar fusion,[49] discussed later, rather than redoing posterior fusion, although the senior author has had good results with repeat transverse process fusion. A recent clinical study has suggested superior results with anterior lumbar fusion overall.[35]

Although not really a complication of the procedure, development of instability at adjacent segments is well recognized. First of all, during insertion of the most superior screw, some violation of

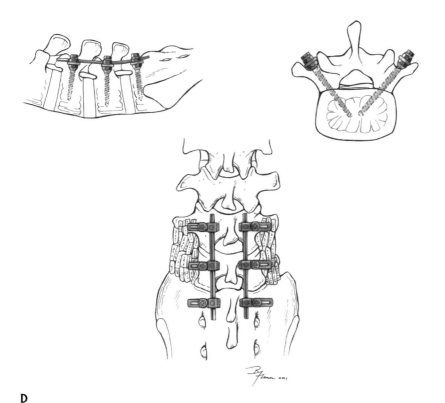

FIGURE 13–3 *(continued)*
D Completed construct.

the cephalad facet is usually necessary. In addition, stresses are increased above the fixation, as we have observed in biomechanical studies.[69,113] Degeneration of even minimally altered segments may occur rapidly,[8] and the question as to whether adjacent, asymptomatic but degenerated segments should be incorporated into the initial fusion is a real one: the number of patients requiring cephalad extension of lumbar fusions over time has not been inconsequential.

Pain due solely to instrumentation is uncommon. Certain thin patients find the hardware annoying and may benefit from its removal. In patients with trigger point pain following lumbar fusion, radiography performed with skin markers may confirm that the screws are possibly related to the pain; removal is a reasonable option. Needless to say, patients should understand that significant improvement is unlikely.

Results

A local series of over 800 instrumented lumbar fusions by the senior author of this book, Sanford Larson, was reviewed. Of the total, minimum follow-up of 1 year (and average follow-up of 4.5 years) was available in 695 patients that underwent various types of instrumentation, including the Luque loop, Knodt rod, Luque and Steffee plates, CD, or Artifex pedicle fixation with or without concomitant neural decompression and with transverse process fusion using iliac autograft. For all systems, and all cases combined, the overall fusion rate was 90% with no motion on dynamic spine films as the criterion for fusion. Older fixation systems had notably lower rates of fusion. Luque loop fixation had a failure rate of 18%, Knodt rods 27%, Steffee plates 9%, and Luque plates 20%. All pedicle fixations combined had a fusion rate of 93%. Of currently used pedicle systems (CD and Artifex), the fusion rate for all cases was 95%. CD pedicle fixation had an overall fusion failure rate of 6.1%, and Artifex pedicle fixation 2.0%. Fusion failure occurred at the L4–5–S1 level in 8.7% of cases for all types of pedicle fixation combined.

Complication rates were minimal: 0.7% deep wound infections requiring hardware removal, and 1.2% (9 patients) with superficial infections resolving on antibiotics. In the placement of over 2,900 pedicle screws no vascular injuries occurred, and only two nerve root injuries occurred, with complete recovery after screw removal.

Overall, these data emphasize the value of transpedicular fixation in selected patients for the purpose of promoting fusion. Complication rates increase with the demands placed on fixation and are decreased by experience. Functional results, of course, are more difficult to measure, and the value of fusion overall remains to be proven. Indeed, Pihlajamaki recently reported on patients followed for over 4 years after transpedicular fixation to promote fusion.[82] There appeared to be no correlation between fusion and clinical outcome, whether measured as pain or return to work, except in patients with spondylolisthesis.

Sublaminar Wiring

In spite of new developments in fixation, there remains a role for sublaminar wiring in the lumbar spine.[14] We tend to use this technique in tumors where we are uncertain of the extent of the disease in the pedicles, and in patients with osteoporosis who are not candidates for other fixation techniques.[20] Biomechanical studies have shown sublaminar wiring with Luque rods to be quite effective for segmental stabilization.[70] In addition, Luque fixation with wiring can be accomplished quickly in the compromised patient.[63]

Some have reported rates of neurological deficit from sublaminar wiring approximating 4%. In our series, we have never seen a patient with spinal cord injury due to sublaminar wiring. There was one instance of thoracic radiculopathy, which resolved. In a long-term series of patients who underwent sublaminar wiring for fracture and tumor, over 6% had one or more broken wires at 2 years. However, deformity or significant loss of correction was seen in less than 1%.[20,21,24]

Generally speaking, sublaminar wiring is most suitable when the posterior elements are intact. However, we have used it when a laminectomy is performed, extending the fixation two to three levels above and below the laminar defect. Some surgeons have drilled holes in the facets laterally in the spine for wire placement in the laminectomized spine. This may offer some stability, although there is little biomechanical data indicating that it is of the quality of laminar fixation.

Several types of wire are available. The surgical drawings used here incorporate traditional prebent stainless steel or titanium wire. However, more recently, we have used titanium cable in many instances.

Technique

Subperiosteal dissection is performed in the usual manner. Laminotomies for wire placement are next performed. Using a curette, the edge of the lamina is carefully dissected, and a Kerrison rongeur is used to make a sizable window in the lamina. We prefer to remove the ligament so that the dura can be directly visualized and therefore protected. Others prefer to dissect and preserve the ligament; there is very little biomechanical advantage to this, and there is the potential for compression of neural structures.

Following exposure of the dura, the carefully bent wire is placed underneath the lamina. The edge should be in contact with the inferior surface of the lamina; this will protect the dura. The diagram in Figure 13–4A shows the rounded edge of the wire loop as the leading edge. This allows a nerve hook to be used to pull the wire through.

On occasion, it becomes necessary to expedite wiring for reasons of rapid blood loss or in an unstable patient. Under those circumstances, midline laminotomy can be performed with a Leksell rongeur. The bone is removed in the midline, and the ligament dissected and excised. If wide enough, this hole can be used to safely pass double wires to both sides of the spine.

When the wires are placed, it is important to bend one set of (half of the) wires laterally, and one set medially to make sure that they are wound properly (Figure 13–4B). Alternatively, they can be dotted with ink for the same purpose. When tightening the wires, grab them about 2 cm above the rod.

We typically use prebent Luque loops or L-rods. For pelvic fixation, we use prebent titanium Galveston rods as much as possible. However, they often require recontouring.

Sublaminar wiring and Luque rodding should generally be considered neutral fixation.[63,64] Whereas minor changes in sagittal alignment can be created by underbending or overbending the rods, we recommend that reconstruction of the spine be done through decompression rather than through the wiring technique. Certainly, tightening the wires down sequentially contributes to realignment to some extent. Rod length should approximate the number of segments to be fixated. If L-rods are used, wires should be secured at each corner.

We often supplement sublaminar wiring with spinous process wiring. In this instance, two holes are placed through the spinous processes and stain-

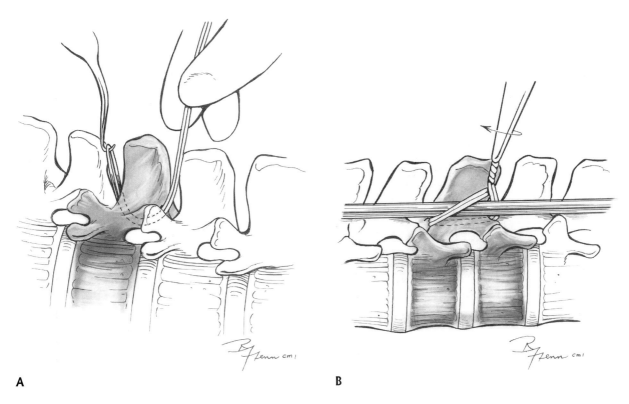

FIGURE 13-4 Sublaminar wiring technique: see details in text. **A** Wire loop being passed through laminotomies. **B** Wires are twisted snugly onto the rod.

less steel or titanium buttons are placed. The wires are then passed through the spinous processes and twisted around alternating rods. This contributes somewhat to lateral stability and limits rotation as well.

Decortication of the transverse processes follows, and bone for fusion is placed. The wound is closed in layers over a drain. Orthoses are used routinely.

Galveston (Pelvic) Fixation

Extension of transpedicular fixation or sublaminar wiring to the pelvis can be very helpful in the management of severe trauma of the lower lumbar spine, tumors and the occasional patient with deformity.[21] We occasionally use pelvic fixation when the sacrum is either osteoporotic or otherwise unsuitable for placement of pedicle screws.

Two constructs exist: the prebent Luque rod that is preconfigured to extend into the pelvis as indicated in the subsequent drawings, or a specifically designed pelvic fixation screw, which is available in many pedicle fixation sets. In recent years, we have generally used iliac screws whenever possible, since they are easier to place and attach to a rod. Pull-out strength is greater than with the nonthreaded Galveston rod. However, if the rod is properly placed within the margins of the cortical bone of ilium, the difference is relatively trivial.

Technique

Only the Galveston technique is presented here, since the principal issue is the orientation of the hole in the ilium.

First, the gluteal muscle is stripped from the ilium for maximum exposure, to allow easy palpation of the greater ischial foramen. This is critical for appropriate orientation of the drill, which should be directed approximately 1 cm above the foramen within the cortical bone. A hole is initially made through the posterior superior iliac spine, often started with a power drill (Fig. 13-5A). It is important that the initial hole be made within the

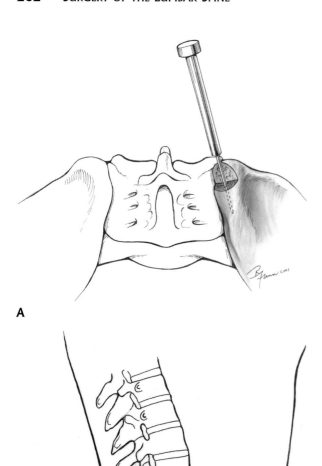
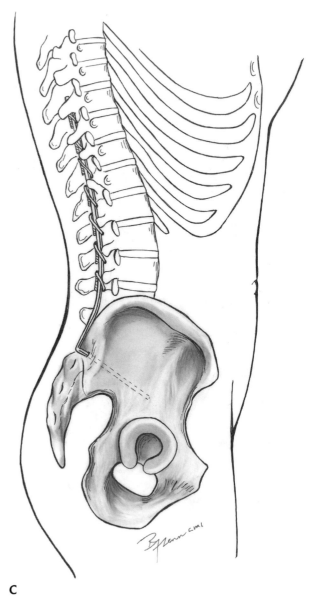

FIGURE 13-5
Extension of lumbosacral fixation into pelvis. **A** Initial hole in posterior superior iliac spine. **B** Track of hole placed within the ilium. **C** Following placement of the contoured rod into the ilium, wires are fastened sequentially.

margins of the cortical bone. We generally start with a Steinman pin and pass it carefully through the ilium, again with a finger on the greater ischial foramen, until it appears to be above the foramen, approximately 50 or 60 mm. It is then removed and the hole probed to make sure that there is good cortical bone on each side (Fig. 13–5B). The Steinman pin is then replaced and then both anteroposterior and lateral radiography are obtained.

When the position of the pin has been confirmed, the screw or rod is inserted. If prebent rods are to be used, they are contoured based on a trial using a malleable rod. This should be carefully accomplished to minimize the need for any in situ bending. If sublaminar wiring is to be used, wires should be placed as discussed earlier. If pedicle fixation is to be used, these screws should be placed as discussed earlier. The rods are then placed following appropriate contouring.

The iliac fixation should be inserted first, and the rod tightened down or wired in a cephalad direction (Fig. 13–5C). Bone grafting is accomplished as for other posterior fusions. When pelvic fixation is used, we recommend using a Spica cast, rather than TLSO.

Results

We have used the Galveston technique for tumor, trauma (Figs. 13–6 and 13–7), and degenerative disease. Before the widespread use of pedicle fixation, the Galveston procedure was commonly used for lumbosacral fusions. It still is, in certain cases of osteoporosis or in lumbosacral junction trauma. In spite of the high-risk population in whom pelvic fixation is used, our fusion rate has been close to 100%. Patients seem to complain of more long-term pain, however.

The most common *complication* is gluteal hematoma.[2] Theoretically, there is a risk of nerve injury if the terminal end of the rod perforates the iliac foramen. This technical problem can be avoided by careful attention to technique.

Universal (Hook-Rod) Fixation

On occasion, universal fixation of the lumbar spine is optimal. For example, in instances of diseased (cancer) or sclerotic pedicles, hook placement is a recommended alternative to pedicle fixation.[18,37] More commonly, we use hooks in the lower thoracic or upper lumbar spine, in conjunction with pedicle screws at lower lumbar levels.

Because of the robust laminae and transverse processes, hook placement is rarely difficult. Both upgoing and downgoing hooks can be placed in either structure. Because of the orientation of the laminae, we generally prefer to use the tranverse

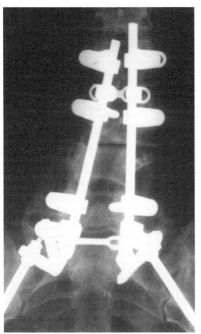
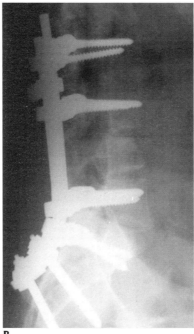

A   B

FIGURE 13–6
Thirty-four-year-old woman who had undergone three previous procedures for L4 fracture with repeated nonunions. Anteroposterior **A** and lateral **B** Radiographs demonstrating instrumentation, including iliac screw fixation.

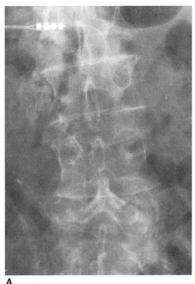
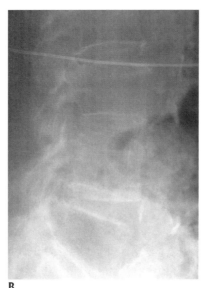

FIGURE 13-7
Sixty-year-old man with long-standing paraparesis, severe osteoporosis, new bowel and bladder dysfunction, and back pain. Anteroposterior **A** and lateral **B** radiographs and nonenhanced computed tomography through L5 **C** and through the proximal sacrum **D** Postoperative radiographs **E and F** following proximal sacral and partial L5 laminectomy and Galveston fixation, with good clinical recovery.

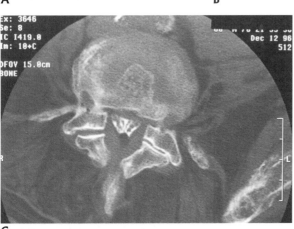
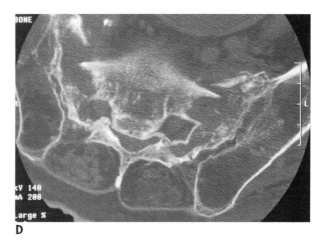
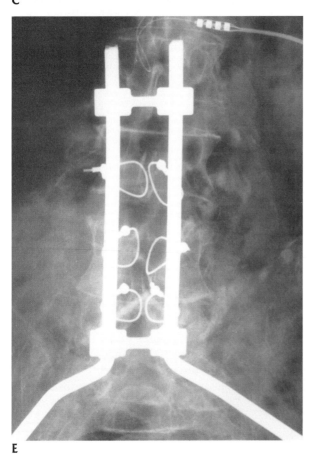
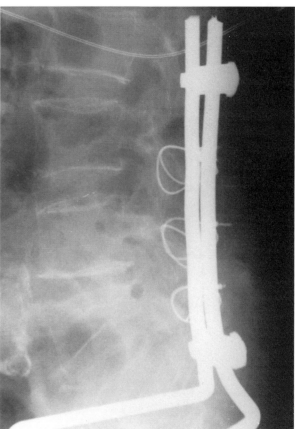

processes for downgoing hooks. In the lumbar spine, a single claw on either side (two above and two below) of the pathology to be fixated is all that is necessary. Cross-linking in instances of trauma and tumor is recommended.

Technique

The laminar hook should be placed into a squared laminotomy. A half-inch osteotome and mallet are used to develop the squared defect in the lamina. The pattern for the hook can be created manually with a curette or with a tool designed for the process; certainly the latter is easier.

Hook size selection is generally straightforward. The lumbar laminae will usually accept a wider hook. The critical issue is the length of the curved portion of the hook: the surgeon should use the shortest hook that will fit. Hooks that are longer-bodied than necessary, when tightened down, may compress the thecal sac.

A hook holder and introducer are used to place the hook into the defect (Fig. 13–8A). The opposite hook of the claw is then placed. If the transverse process is indeed being used, the cephalad surface is carefully dissected. There are several small arterial branches here that need to be coagulated. A

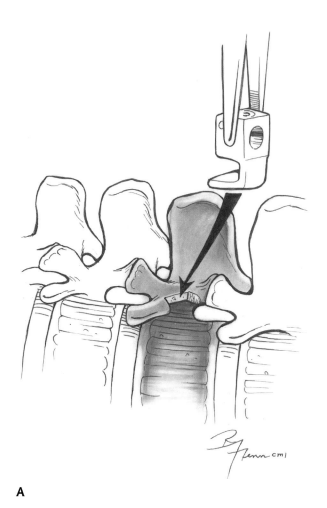

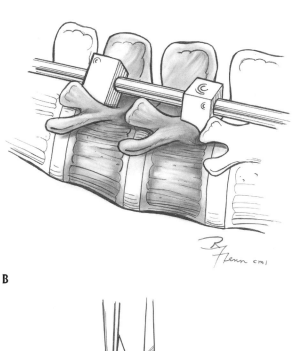

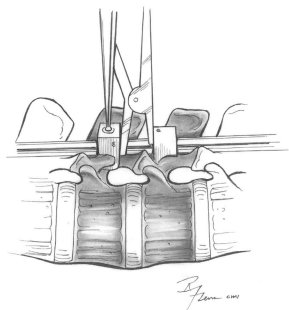

FIGURE 13-8
Universal instrumentation; details in text. **A** upgoing laminar hook placed into laminotomy. **B** Rod is inserted though transverse process and laminar hooks. **C** If third hook is incorporated, one can distract across them to improve hook fixation.

hook dissector is used, and the hook is placed. We find that transverse process hooks need to be longer than laminar hooks; during trial placement we suggest lining up the hooks to ensure that the rod will go through.

The rod is cut and contoured based on a trial with a malleable rod, such as the stylet from an endotracheal tube. Again, we do not attempt gross correction with instrumentation, and virtually never use in situ bending to attempt restoration of lordosis.

More commonly than not, we do not attempt to slide the rod through the transverse process hook at the same time as the laminar hook. Instead, we place the transverse process hook on the rod, slide the rod through the laminar hook, and then gently rotate the transverse process hook into position.

Working cephalad from the caudal claw, the rod is inserted through the lower hooks rotated 180 degrees from the spinal lordosis: this makes rod insertion much easier. When the rod approaches the upper laminar hook, it is carefully rotated and pushed through both the laminar and transverse process hooks (Fig. 13–8B). Often, two additional hooks are placed, one on each side of the pathology, in addition to the claws. Many use these additional hooks to compress an anterior graft. However, we would rather distract slightly to maintain alignment (Fig. 13–8C) and place the oversized graft later.

Some surgeons prefer to place all the hooks on the rod and sequentially position them by forcing them into the bone defects; we find this approach technically cumbersome.

If distraction or compression is contemplated, it is often useful to place one side of the instrumentation and carry out the realignment then perform insertion of the other rod since rod length and other factors may be affected. In addition, with unilateral procedures such as the extracavitary approach, more distraction may be needed on the side of the vertebrectomy to protect alignment.

Posterior Lumbar Interbody Fusion (PLIF)

For all practical purposes, the PLIF was developed by Cloward in 1943.[16] He used iliac crest grafts following radical discectomy. Others modified the procedure using the removed posterior elements for graft purposes. Early clinical reports suggested a fusion rate of approximately 90% with very good or excellent results in the same number. The complication rate, however, was reported to be in the range of 5 to 8%, with a high incidence of nerve root injury.

PLIF has recently enjoyed a dramatic resurgence. PLIF had largely fallen out of favor, in part as a result of early experience with neurological deficit occurring during decompression, as well as extrusion of bone grafts when performed without instrumentation. PLIF has been resurrected in recent years because of the observation that transverse process fusion, although biomechanically effective in stabilizing the spine, often does not eliminate micromotion at the disc.[15] This observation led to the popularity of the "360 degree approach" with a retroperitoneal or anterior approach to the spine in conjunction with posterior instrumentation. The need for two separate incisions, a general surgeon for the approach, and considerable morbidity and costs have led to increased interest in the PLIF.

PLIF has become particularly popular in recent years with the advent of preformed bone grafts and PLIF application sets, as well as titanium and carbon cages. Recent biomechanical data suggest advantages of the cages over bone; in spite of their FDA approval, the long-term implications of titanium cages in the disc space remain to be determined.[89] In the meantime, we use them routinely for PLIF, anterior lumbar interbody fusion (ALIF), and retroperitoneal fusions, even at L5–S1.

Indications

Even in patients thought to be marginal candidates for lumbar fusion (such as those with workers' compensation claims), instrumented PLIFs or 360° fusions decrease pain and increase functional activities.[41] A recent study by Hacker showed that instrumented PLIF had equal patient satisfaction, much lower costs, and faster return to work and other activities than anterior-posterior fusion.[38] Furthermore, a recent biomechanical study by Bennett et al found that PLIF doubles the spinal stiffness produced by transpedicular fixation following laminectomy and facetectomy.[4]

The indications for PLIF as opposed to other types of lumbar fusion are uncertain. Some have felt PLIF to be biomechanically superior to transverse process fusion in reducing motion within the lumbar spine. In addition, the pathophysiology of degenerative changes in the lumbar spine prominently implicates the intervertebral disc. However, one could argue that PLIF is a biomechanically inferior procedure, since the facet joints and posterior elements need to be disrupted, along with the obvious violation of the disc space. With transpedicular fixation and transverse process fusion, these concerns are eliminated.

Other theoretical advantages of PLIF are technical; a much larger area of bone surface exists for fusion, with the fusion at the center of motion and at the site of maximum compression loading. The disc space is maintained in a distracted position without the collapse often seen in transverse process fusion using transpedicular fixation. In addition, the blood supply is better at the decorticated end plate than at the transverse process.

In spite of the above, the indications for PLIF are clinical. We use PLIF in patients with broad-based herniations, totally degenerated discs with marked instability, some patients with recurrent disc herniation, and with pseudoarthrosis of transverse process fusion (as an alternative to anterior lumbar fusion) in the absence of epidural scarring. We do not recommend PLIF as a fusion technique if decompression of neural elements is not to be performed; there is little justification for exposing nerve roots to scarring or injury to achieve the spinal stability obtainable by transverse process or anterior lumbar fusion.

Technical Considerations

Before describing our preferred technique for PLIF, a discussion of other alternatives is appropriate. In Cloward's original description, following removal of the disc, osteotomes were used to remove the end plates and the articulating facets. He also recommended laminar spreaders to provide distraction for graft placement.[16] Others have altered the shape of the graft in an attempt to decrease the incidence of graft extrusion, including triangular and oversized dowels.[108] We have placed milled bone fragments anterior in the disc space, impacting the arch of the lamina into the dorsal aspect of the disc space to prevent extrusion of the small fragments.

We rarely perform noninstrumented PLIFs: because performing PLIFs in a manner that protects the neural elements introduces instability by removal of the facet joints and portions of the lamina, as well as violating the intervertebral disc, some sort of stiffening is best incorporated. This may be accomplished through the use of intervertebral cages, or through traditional posterior (transpedicular or other) fixation, or both. The decision of which to use is predicated by preoperative flexion-extension radiographs, abnormalities on nuclear imaging, back pain, and, to some extent, intraoperative impressions of the degree of instability present.

Furthermore, the amount of bone removal necessary for safe surgery participates in that determination. It is our current practice to remove the entire articulating facet joint to maximize exposure for placement of intervertebral cages or bone and to minimize dural sac retraction. This is strongly recommended; it is hard to justify injuring nerve roots or the cauda equina in order to save a few millimeters of an already compromised joint.

Technique

Once the decision has been made to perform a PLIF, the surgeon must choose between several alternative approaches. The extent of fixation desired, the type of bone, and the available variety of instrumentation techniques are almost daunting.

Surgery is performed in the prone position with chest rolls, on a Wilson frame, or using the Jackson table. Because the epidural venous structures will be disrupted almost to the midline, intraabdominal pressure should be minimized to lower venous bleeding. We typically employ cell salvage standby in these procedures. X-rays are obtained before making the skin incision.

Iliac crest bone harvest is usually not necessary. If transverse process onlay fusion is not planned—and in our practice it often is not—local bone from the laminectomy will suffice. If cages alone are to be used, local bone is always adequate. For noninstrumented PLIFs, robust spinous processes can often be trimmed to provide corticocancellous chunks. If that is not the case, a separate subfascial incision is made to obtain an iliac crest bone graft as described for transverse process fusion.

A subperiosteal dissection is performed in the usual manner, extending laterally beyond the border of the articulating facet joints and pars. The transverse processes need not be exposed, decreasing blood loss and postoperative pain. Bone removal should then take place. Following radiographic confirmation of the appropriate level, an intralaminar decompression is carried out to expose the relevant disc space. Depending on the amount of bone that needs to be removed for decompression, it is often easier to perform full laminectomy (Fig. 13–9A). However, this is not necessary for the purposes of interbody fusion. We do remove the spinous processes to make retraction safer and keep the dural sac under direct vision; their preservation is of little biomechanical value.

It is this surgeon's practice to remove the facet joints *prior to* performing laminectomy. This not only saves time, but minimizes risk to the nerve roots. Osteotomes and rongeurs are used for that purpose. Again, we strongly recommend removal of the majority—if not all—of the facet joint all the way to the pedicle to minimize compression of nerve roots as well as to minimize retraction of the thecal sac.

After gently retracting the nerve roots and thecal sac, the epidural space is identified and epidural vessels coagulated. Since the disc and end plates will be violated almost to midline, we bipolar small vessels likely to be injured.

Many surgeons attempt to minimize initial disc removal when performing PLIFs. Rather, they use osteotomes and remove the disc en bloc with the end plates and portions of the vertebral body. We do not recommend this. Instead, we remove as much disc as possible to ensure that none bunches up to the midline, compressing the dural sac, when bone grafts or cages are placed laterally. We have seen this phenomenon several times in patients treated elsewhere, with often devastating neurological results. Therefore, traditional discectomy is performed (Fig. 13–9B). Carefully retracting the nerve root at risk, a No. 15 blade is used to incise the annulus widely. A large rectangle of annulus and available disc is removed. This is done bilaterally. An up-biting biopsy forceps is used to remove disc underneath the thecal sac without manipulating it. Ring curettes are often used to further empty the disc space. Backward-angled curettes are carefully placed between the dural sac and the annulus to push down any bulging disc or osteophyte near the midline.

The PLIF procedure itself is then carried out: before beginning end plate removal, radiographs should be marked to determine how deep the osteotome cut can safely be made. A Penfield or ruler is placed into the disc space, and images obtained. The osteotome should not be placed more than 50 to 60% through the anteroposterior diameter of the vertebral body.

Osteotomes are placed parallel to the end plates both at the superior and inferior aspect of the disc space, and then medial/lateral. We have rarely been able to get osteotomes of greater than ¾ of an inch in the available space, even with maximal retraction.

Needless to say, the nerve root and dural sac should be very carefully protected with hand-held retractors that are regularly released (Fig. 13–9C, D).

After the four cuts have been made, creating a rectangle, a curette is used to push the bone and end plate into the cavity within the empty disc space. These pieces are removed with a Leksell rongeur. A bleeding cancellous bone surface should then be available on the cephalad and caudal edges of the space, and possibly laterally as well. The prepared corticocancellous grafts are then tapped into place. We generally prefer to place the more medial bone grafts first, to minimize total mobilization of the dural sac (Fig. 13–9E, F). Others place the grafts laterally, and then push them towards the midline. The superior edge of the graft should be at least 5 mm ventral to the floor of the spinal canal. Two to three pieces can safely be placed on each side of the thecal sac (Fig. 13–9G). After placing the grafts, be certain that the dural sac and nerve roots are not being compressed.

We typically place a drain for 24 hours and close the wound in layers. Patients are mobilized on the day of surgery and usually go home in an orthosis 1 or 2 days later.

Many variations in PLIF technique exist. The most prominent of these, of course, involves the use of instrumentation developed by Cloward. In this set, bone dowels are taken from the iliac crest and one placed on each side of the thecal sac. This simplifies placement of the bone graft and may well improve the safety of PLIF.

Regardless of the technique employed to place the bone, surgeons are reminded to be cautious regarding the risk of bone graft extrusion. Although this is uncommon, it may result in significant neurological deficit. Therefore, some form of fixation is desirable.

Results

In an early series of 274 PLIFs, three significant complications occurred. One was a deep infection, and two were graft extrusions. None of these patients had undergone instrumentation, although all were immobilized postoperatively in a lumbar orthosis. Most authors report fusion rates of 85 to 90% and complication rates of 2 to 5%.[11,17,60] Retropulsion rates in other series range from 2 to 9%.[95] Complication rates are lower in the hands of experienced surgeons, further defining the learning curve in this procedure.

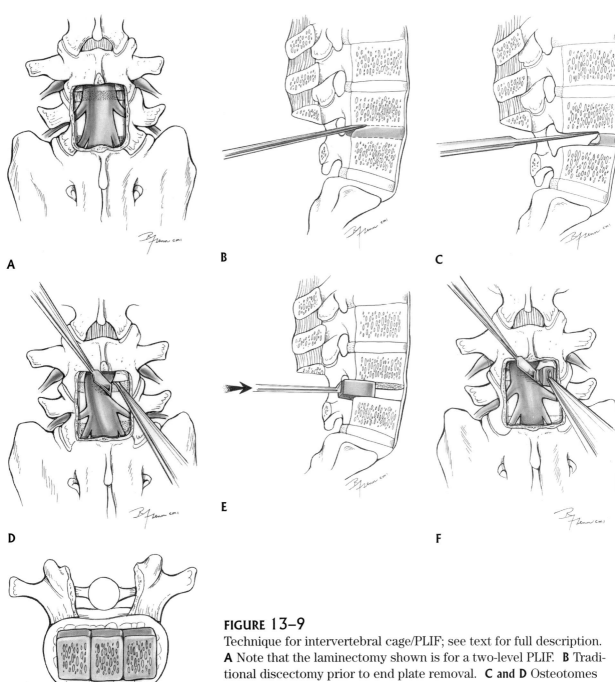

FIGURE 13–9

Technique for intervertebral cage/PLIF; see text for full description. **A** Note that the laminectomy shown is for a two-level PLIF. **B** Traditional discectomy prior to end plate removal. **C and D** Osteotomes used to cut end plates, with careful protection of neural elements. **E and F** Procedure for bone graft placement. **G** Three corticocancellous grafts can often be placed.

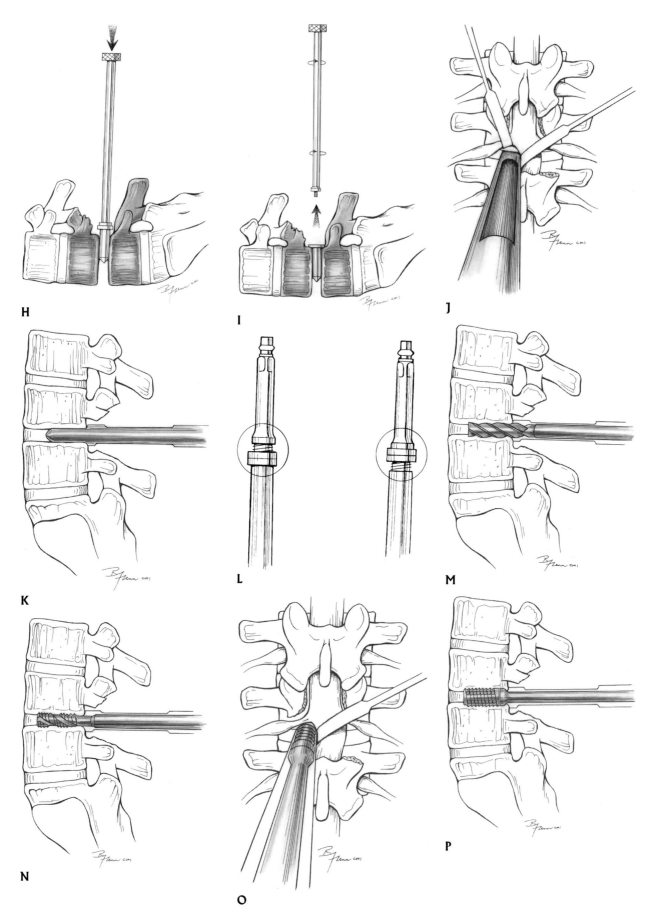

FIGURE 13-9 *(continued)* **H** Placement of distracter tip. **I** Distracter tip left in interspace. **J** Placement of tang retractor. **K** Tang and distracter blades must be against the end plates, well within the disc space. **L** Drill is set for 21 or 26 mm respectively. **M** Drilling process. **N** Tapping. **O** and **P** Cage insertion.

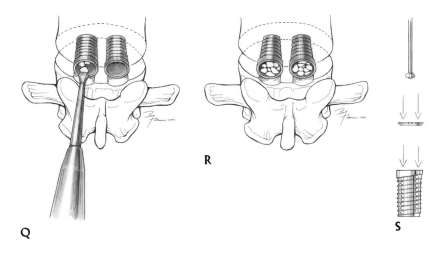

FIGURE 13-9 *(continued)*
Q and R Bone fragments are packed into the cage. **S** End cap is snapped into place.

Intervertebral Cages in PLIF

Since 1995 we have used intervertebral cages for most PLIFs. These allow distraction of the disc space,[90] grafting using cancellous bone, which is optimal for fusion but mechanically weak, optimal preparation of the host bone with excision of the end plates, and fixation that some feel approximates transpedicular fixation in a relatively safe and straightforward approach.[2,32,44,84,85,105]

Disadvantages include the morbidity of the retraction required for cage placement, the need for radiography during surgery—which is not typically necessary for bone fusion—the cost of the cages themselves, and the difficulties in visualizing the fusion radiographically.[105] To date, clinical results have been gratifying, although long-term implications remain unknown. This impression is not universally held. Many surgeons are actually hostile to cages, some on a sound biomechanical basis. For example, at least one study has shown titanium mesh implant constructs to be no stiffer than tricortical bone acutely.[44]

Described in this section is the Ray Threaded Fusion Cage, marketed by Surgical Dynamics. However, by the time this book is published, there likely will be several other systems available. Although, as for pedicle fixation, there are surgeons who adamantly insist that one company's device is vastly superior to another, differences are minimal and largely technical. The choice of systems for us is based largely on cost and ease of utilization, not graft.

The Ray cage was designed by Charles Ray as a hollow titanium alloy threaded cylinder that is fenestrated to promote bone growth into the vertebra adjacent to the cage.[85] Threads promote insertion, and have been shown to improve pull-out strength and segmental stiffness. The ultimate strength of the cage is well beyond that for vertebral bodies. Cages produce spinal stability by distracting the disc space, which stiffens the annulus. In spite of the titanium structure, the hollow nature of the cage and thread design allow more elasticity than would be expected, sharing compressive loads with the bone within the cavity of the cage.

The procedure for PLIF with intervertebral cages is the same as for bone PLIF until the point of removal of the intervertebral disc. Although some perform caged PLIFs via laminotomies with minimally cored-out facet joints, we recommend more aggressive removal, as suggested earlier. The additional time investment is minimal, and facet joint removal minimizes retraction and tension on neural structures. Furthermore, whereas many recommend preservation of the spinous processes, we recommend removal: leaving the spinous processes requires the operating surgeon to angle and toe-in the dural retractor more than we regard as being optimal. There is no evidence at present that preservation of the spinous process is of value.

Once the intervertebral disc has been partially removed, the cage size should be determined. Currently available cage systems have templates available to measure optimal cage size from the computed tomogram and/or MRI. We currently recommended that the cages be at least 6 mm shorter than the vertebral body, allowing at least 3 mm subcortical placement of the cage both anterior and posterior to be certain that there is no nerve root or dural sac compression. In addition, cage placement should be lateral enough so that the cages do not touch. Early in our experience, in a few cases insertion of the second cage pushed the first one out.

Initially, we strongly recommend that surgeons use the templates provided to measure cage size. The experienced surgeon will probably measure cage length from the blades of the tang after placement in the disc space, as discussed below.

The Ray TFC cage is available in four diameters: 12, 14, 16, and 18 mm, and two lengths: 21 and 26 mm. We believe it ideal to place the largest-diameter cage that safely fits. The limiting factors are typically not the size of the disc space; more commonly, the distance between the pedicles above and below the disc space in question determines cage diameter. Indeed, even the dural sac does not limit the diameter of the cage: the willingness of a surgeon to retract the dural sac well beyond the midline allows larger cages but may be associated with neural injury.

We prefer only minimal retraction of the thecal sac and would much rather take off more facet joint or even use a smaller cage. However, it is important that the cage selected have a wide enough diameter to cut well into the cancellous bone on both sides of the disc space. If after drilling the hole, the surgeon determines that there is not good cancellous bone on each side of the disc, a larger-diameter cage should be incorporated. If this is not possible, intervertebral fixation should be abandoned, bone alone placed into the disc space, and posterior fixation contemplated.

All distracter, tang, and cage placement should be performed under radiographic control. On the first side approached, the distracter is placed into the disc space following disc removal. Before placing the blades of the distracter into the disc space, all neural structures need to be carefully retracted using the curved retractors provided, and protected. We find that (particularly at L4–L5) both superior and inferior nerve roots need to be retracted. In addition, the thecal sac needs to be gently retracted to the opposite side. Like the skull base surgeon, we cannot emphasize enough the value of more aggressive bone removal over more aggressive retraction. Remove osteophytes or hypertrophied annulus to allow the distracter and tang to fit flush with the posterior vertebral margin.

Select the largest distracter tip that safely fits. Gently drive it into the hole in the disc space using a mallet (Fig. 13–9H). Before doing so, eyeball the angle of the disc space from the lateral radiograph and impact the distracter tip appropriately, directing the distracter slightly medially. This tip should be driven in until the flat surface of the tip is against the margin of the vertebra. Then remove the handle, leaving the distracter tip in place (Fig. 13–9I). The dural sac is allowed to fall back over the distracter.

On the contralateral side, the nerve roots and thecal sac are again carefully retracted. A tang retractor of the same diameter as the distracter is selected (Fig. 13–9J). The impacter cap is placed on the tang and the latter impacted into place between the two end plates until it is seated well. Lateral radiography or fluoroscopic images should be obtained to ensure that (a) the tang and distracter are placed well within the disc space, (b) the disc space is not wider than the tang and distracter, (c) the blades are equidistant between the edges of the disc space, and (d) the blades are perpendicular to the end plates.

The tang and distracter are the right size and appropriately placed if the blades are firmly against both end plates and are well placed within the disc space itself (Fig. 13–9K). The length of the blades of the tang allows determination of cage length as well. The blade length is 24 mm; the surgeon can use this to "eyeball" ideal cage length.

Before drilling, the surgeon should again be absolutely certain that the tang is seated flush on the vertebral body and annulus and that all neural elements are safely away from the barrel. This must be confirmed prior to drilling.

The disc space is then drilled. There are two settings on the vertebral drill, for either the 21- or the 26-mm cage (Fig. 13–9L). At the shorter drill length, a 25-mm hole will be created, and a 30-mm depth at the longer length. This overdrilling is important to prevent disc bulging back against the cage from the anterior surface (Fig. 13–9M). Following vertebral drilling, loose disc is removed with a biopsy forceps. The tang should be controlled by the assistant during this process to prevent the blades from loosening and the tang from wobbling.

The hole is then tapped: care is essential here. There are two guides on the vertebral tap: again, 21 and 26 mm (Fig. 13–9N). Carefully advance the tap clockwise to the desired depth, being certain that there is good cancellous bone on both sides. We prefer to overtap 2 to 3 mm beyond the marks to take further advantage of the overdrilling performed in the previous step.

Carelessness with tapping, such as letting the tang move, is rewarded with poorly placed threads in the cancellous bone and marginal cage placement. The tap is removed with equally careful counterclockwise unscrewing to prevent cross-threading. A nerve hook or curette is gently inserted into the tang, and the vertebral edges carefully sounded for proof of cancellous bone surfaces.

The cage on its T-handle is placed into the tang, and the cage threaded clockwise to the appropriate length, laser-etched on the handle (Fig. 13–9O, P). We then generally thread the cage another 3 mm (one complete turn) beyond what the tool indicates. The insertion handle has two small indicator pins: these identify the fenestrations in the cages that allow bone growth. These pins must be pointing directly cranial-caudal when insertion is complete. We obtain a lateral radiograph after the cages are inserted, prior to placement of the bone.

The cage is then filled with bone. A bone mill may be used to crumble the graft into small pieces. If local bone is being used, which is commonly the case, be sure that there is no soft tissue attached. A 2-cc syringe can be used to inject the amount of bone that comfortably fills a cage. As the bone is placed, it should be packed using the instrument available in the set (Fig. 13–9Q, R). Do not use a mallet to pound the bone, since this pushes out the plastic cap on the base of the cage. Bone graft placement should stop one or two screw threads below the edge of the cage to allow placement of the plastic end cap, which is gently snapped into place (Fig. 13–9S).

Following successful placement of this cage, attention is turned to the other side. Aggressive disc removal should be carried out. We have often observed disc being pushed into the midline by the first cage, under the dural sac. This central disc is easily removed after the first cage has been placed. Thus we remove the distracter and remove even more disc that had been taken out previously, extending across to the first cage. The dural retractors are again placed and a tang placed in the same position and alignment. The cage insertion procedure is then repeated. If cage PLIF is to be performed at multiple levels, which is not uncommon, distracters can be placed at multiple levels to minimize the amount of radiography required.

Recently, we have begun placing single cages in selected PLIF cases (Fig. 13–10). Typically, these are people with less preoperative evidence of instability and patients for whom removal of the contralateral facet is undesirable. The surgical procedure is identical, except that full unilateral facet removal is mandatory, and the tang is angled across the midline. Preliminary biomechanical studies suggest that a single cage with preserved contralateral facet is equal to double cage placement, and clinical results of this modification have been gratifying.

We typically use a drain and close the wound in layers using vicryl with subcuticular stitches for skin. The patients are mobilized within 3 to 4 hours of surgery and are usually able to tolerate a regular diet and ambulate freely within 24 hours in an orthosis. Orthosis is usually maintained for an average of three months.

Risks and Complications

The limitations of this technique are obvious. First of all, as is always the case, there is a learning curve for the procedure. Significant hemorrhage can be encountered with inadequate electrocoagulation of the epidural space. Nerve root and cauda equina injury through injudicious retraction is the major risk. Inadequate removal of disc under the dural sac may lead to central disc protrusion compressing the cauda equina. If the cages are not placed well below the floor of the spinal canal, they may compress and even physically injure nerve roots and the dural sac.

The determination of successful bone fusion is difficult, and requires tomography or nuclear imaging in uncertain cases. Thus we typically end up assuming fusion after a few months. To date, we have not been disappointed.

In spite of some biomechanical evidence suggesting that the stiffness provided by cages is similar to that of transpedicular fixation, we do not use cages in place of transpedicular fixation. Indeed, overconfidence in these poorly understood devices may represent their greatest risk, as is evidenced in the complication presented later. Rather, they are most useful in patients who need structural supplementation or in those who have instability that is clinically and radiographically evident but not severe. An example of effective utilization may in the individual with a badly degenerated central disc herniation and back pain but little facet arthropathy and single-level disease. Additionally, we have found them useful in patients undergoing multilevel transpedicular fixation with a single level showing much more severe motion, disc degeneration, and instability.

Although some surgeons are incorporating intervertebral cages in operations for spondylolisthesis (in lieu of or in addition to transpedicular fixation), we think this unwise for now. Although adding further stiffness to the segment is biomechanically attractive, it is difficult to adequately protect the nerve root during placement of the tang because of the vertebral step-off, and to insert the cage sym-

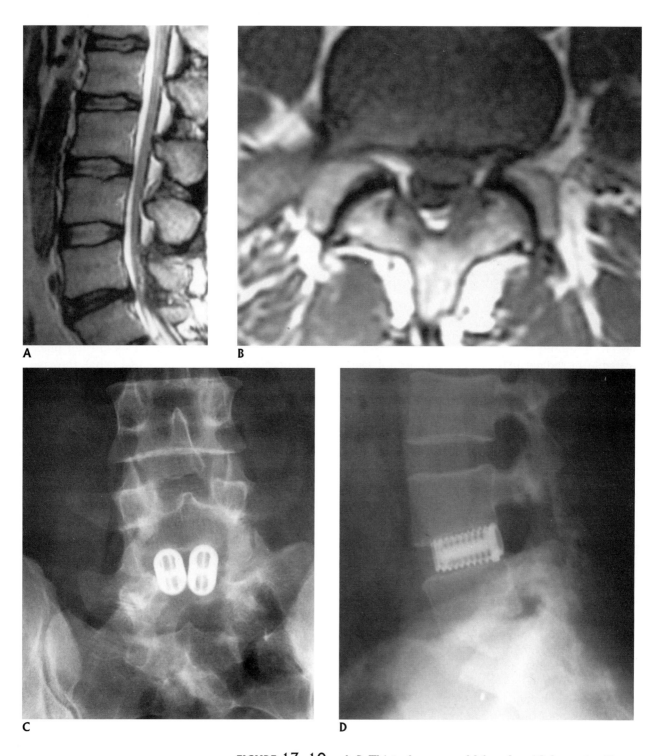

FIGURE 13–10 **A–D** Thirty-four-year-old female with long-standing mechanical back pain with known listhesis at L4–L5, severe disc degeneration, and foot drop. **A and B** Sagittal and axial MR images, demonstrating disc herniation and desiccation, and facet arthropathy. **C and D** Postoperative anteroposterior and lateral radiographs with caged PLIF. Patient returned to full-duty nursing nine weeks postoperatively.

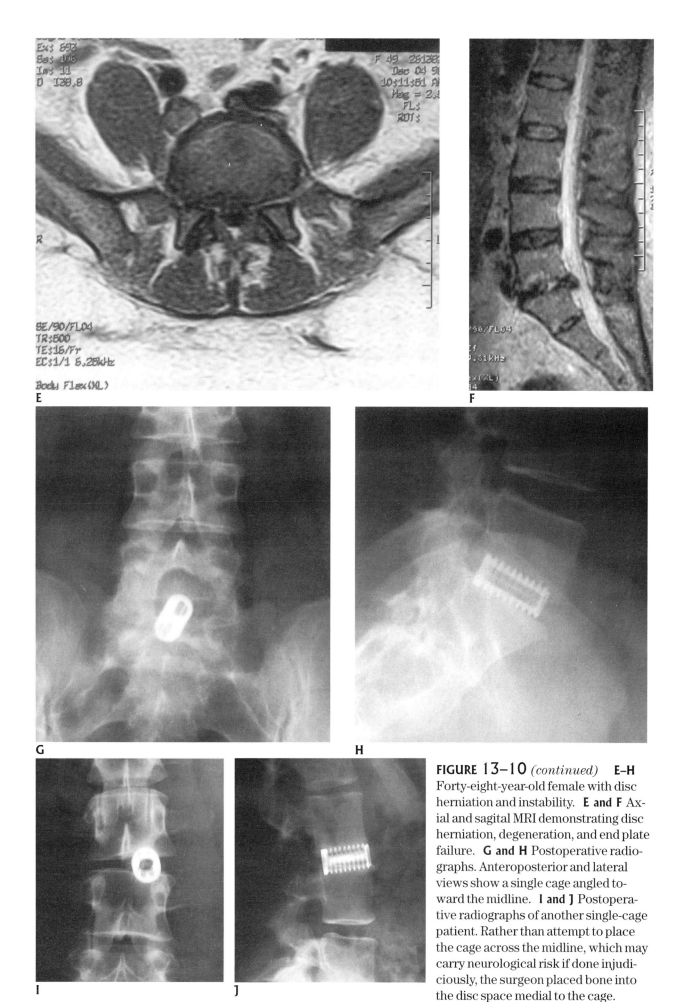

FIGURE 13–10 *(continued)* **E–H** Forty-eight-year-old female with disc herniation and instability. **E and F** Axial and sagital MRI demonstrating disc herniation, degeneration, and end plate failure. **G and H** Postoperative radiographs. Anteroposterior and lateral views show a single cage angled toward the midline. **I and J** Postoperative radiographs of another single-cage patient. Rather than attempt to place the cage across the midline, which may carry neurological risk if done injudiciously, the surgeon placed bone into the disc space medial to the cage.

metrically in all but the most minimal spondylolistheses. Rather, transpedicular fixation and, if needed, interbody fusion with bone are used. Lastly, the long-term effects of intervertebral cages remain unknown, in terms of their effects on adjacent segments and the integrity of titanium over decades. This important work remains to be done.

Results

In the last 2 years, this surgeon has performed more than 100 caged PLIFs with 12-month follow-up. One cage had to be revised because of poor location. There were two dural tears: one was incidental and related to decompression. The second was caused by inadequate dural retraction; the tang perforated a dural fold. The tear was closed without complication. There have been no wound infections. Return to previous activity, particularly employment, occurred in 74%; most patients described excellent or very good pain relief.

One case of deformity occurred (Fig. 13–11). In this particular instance, cages provided inadequate stabilization and the patient began developing an acute lateral deformity. Repeat fusion was performed with transpedicular fixation, and the patient did well. Three patients demonstrated "halos" around one cage; in all three, tomography suggested bone growth, and bone scanning showed no evidence of nonunion.

These results are similar to those reported by Ray.[84] In a series of 236 patients treated with instrumented PLIF for severe back pain in conjunction with disc herniation, end plate and osteophytes, most patients (>90%) demonstrated fusion and 65% had excellent or very good pain relief. The complication rate was less than 1%.

Extracavitary Approach

The procedure was originally developed by Capener for the treatment of Pott's disease. It had rarely been used until the modifications by Larson et al, who largely popularized the procedure.[56–58] We use this procedure from T2 to the sacrum; lower lumbar use can be difficult because of the iliac crest, although we often resect the lateral iliac wing en mass to gain exposure and then use the crest as graft.

The lateral extracavitary approach (LECA) to the spine is used extensively in our institution for the management of tumor, infection, and fracture.[5,6,56,58,66,68,109] It allows effective anterior decompression, posterior stabilization, and anterior fusion and stabilization, as necessary, in one procedure. Although technically demanding initially, its advantages make it quite useful.

The extracavitary approach is quite flexible, in that it can easily be combined with other procedures to allow maximum decompression of the spinal cord. For example, in the instance of a large midline vertebral lesion, transpedicular decompression can be used on one side, and the extracavitary approach on the other, to allow full decompression as well as anterior and posterior fusion. Similarly, in lesions such as tumors, laminectomy can be added quite easily. Of course, this is difficult to do in classic retroperitoneal or anterior approaches. In addition, a bilateral extracavitary approach can be safely accomplished with a surgeon and capable assistant, or two surgeons to allow full spondylectomy. Instead of the hockey stick incision, a lazy S incision is used. The full vertebra and both pedicles can comfortably be resected; if desired, the posterior elements can be removed as well.

This procedure is ideal for resection of one vertebral segment. However, we have used it for as many as three lumbar segments in cases of infection and tumor with excellent results. Furthermore, with recent developments in instrumentation, anterior fixation systems such as the Synthes TLSP and anterior rod screw systems can be employed when indicated. However, it must be emphasized that anterior instrumentation does not substitute for effective posterior constructs.[6,40]

Lastly, this can all be accomplished in one anesthesia, through one incision, and in a logical sequence. Anterior decompression can be performed prior to reduction of deformity, and instrumentation is placed prior to placement of anterior bone graft to eliminate the risk of loosening. In addition, posterior fusion is accomplished.

Patient Preparation

Prior to surgery, necessary spinal imaging is performed as discussed elsewhere in this book. Spinal angiography is generally recommended even for high lumbar lesions, because the radiculomedullary artery of Adamkiewicz can occur at L1 and occasionally at L2. This vessel is known to provide critical blood supply to the watershed zone of the mid to lower thoracic spinal cord. Although the increasingly popular consensus is that injury to the radiculomedullary rarely causes neurological compromise, our experience and other studies suggest that it can, and therefore we recommend angiography in lesions above L3.

Embolization is also routinely performed on vascular tumors approximately 24 hours prior to the procedure, as discussed elsewhere in this book.[10] In the past, we performed embolization immediately before the operative procedure with marginal results; in recent years, it has become evident that the 24-hour delay further decreases tumor blood supply. Complications associated with embolization are few, and dramatic decreases in blood loss often result.

Spinal stability should be determined before surgery whenever possible. If instrumentation is to be performed, the incision needs to be placed accordingly.

Antiembolism stockings and a Foley catheter are placed, as well as peripheral and central venous access. An arterial line is routinely used. Balanced anesthesia is the favorite of our anesthesiologists. We do not recommend hemodilution or hypotension during anesthesia. Cell savers are routinely used and strongly recommended for diagnoses other than cancer and infection. Although we usually do not perform intraoperative neurophysiologic monitoring, others may find it helpful.

We had historically performed this procedure on chest rolls on a standard operating table; recently we have begun using the Jackson frame and find it to be of significant utility: imaging is improved, and venous pressure in the abdomen and chest is decreased, with decreased blood loss as a result. The Jackson table also allows the table to be safely rotated 20 to 30 degrees for maximum exposure. The arms are often tucked in at the sides. This can make radiography more difficult, and in a larger individual the arms are placed above the head, carefully positioned to avoid pressure on the ulnar and radial nerves and stretch injury of the brachial plexus.

Technique

Incision Location

The skin incision should be marked after the patient is positioned. A metallic marker is placed over what is considered the level of pathology, and a radiography is performed. The incision is then marked (Fig. 13–12A). A curved hockey stick-shaped incision is typically used. Although others have used an L, the devascularized corner can become necrotic. The hockey stick is typically made to the side of the worse pathology in the instance of fracture or tumor. For disc herniation, if there is asymmetry, we prefer to operate toward that side.

If posterior decompression or fixation is not to be performed, a paramedian incision over the lateral border of the paravertebral musculature will suffice.

We avoid operating on the side of the artery of Adamkiewicz whenever possible. However, if the lesion is worse on the same side as the artery, we still approach from that side using extra caution. If there are no reasons to prefer left or right, the surgeon's personal preference is appropriate.

The vertical portion of the incision is made on the basis of the instrumentation to be used: for example, if transpedicular fixation one or two levels above and below the level of injury is to be used, the vertical incision should be two levels above and below. Similarly, if hook and rod instrumentation is to be used, the vertical incision needs to be longer. The lateral limb of the incision generally extends approximately 10 to 12 cm. In an L1 or L2 lesion, we sometimes make the curve longer to give us easier access to the iliac crest. If the lateral portion is much longer or carried more caudally, retraction later in the procedure becomes difficult. The incision is carried through the subcutaneous tissue to thoracolumbar fascia. At this point, bilateral subperiosteal dissection should be performed if spinal instrumentation is to be placed. If not, a unilateral dissection on the side of the decompression can be performed; alternatively, the surgeon can incise the thoracolumbar fascia at the lateral aspect of the paravertebral musculature.

Exposure

Following the subperiosteal dissection, the thoracolumbar fascia, subcutaneous tissue, and the skin are elevated as a flap. They are incised together along the angled portion of the incision. At the lateral aspect of the erector spinae group, a plane is defined with finger dissection; this group of muscles is then elevated and retracted medially along

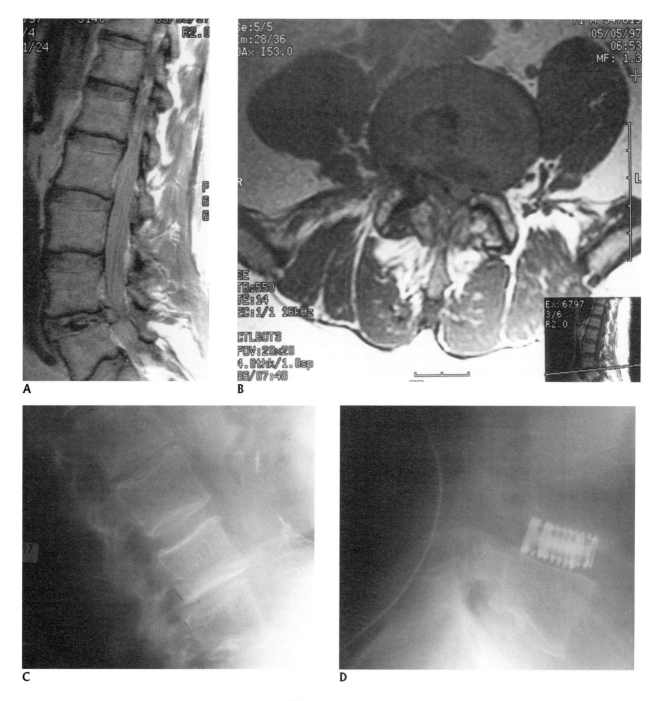

FIGURE 13–11 Sixty-eight-year-old male with eight-month history of back and leg pain and urinary frequency. **A and B** Sagittal and axial MRI demonstrating severe disc degeneration and, herniation. **C** Lateral extension radiograph demonstrating listhesis at L4–L5. Discectomy and PLIF were performed without difficulty; there was good bone purchase on cage placement. **D** Lateral radiograph two days postoperatively showing early dorsal migration of the left cage.

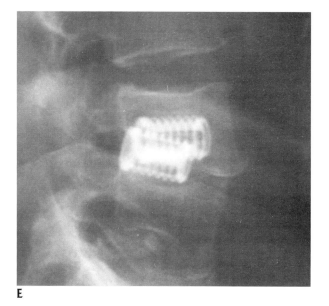
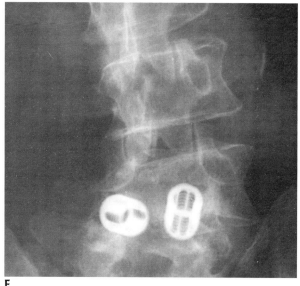
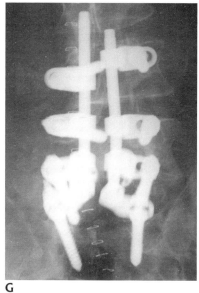
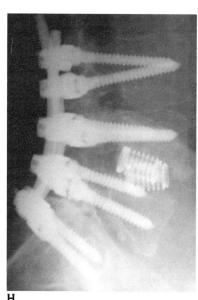

FIGURE 13-11 *(continued)*
E and **F** Three weeks later, lateral and anteroposterior radiographs demonstrate translational deformity and, significant dorsal migration of cage; patient had no neurological deficit or increased pain. **G** and **H** Following redo fixation. Cages were deep within the disc space and vertebra, and not readily retrievable. The patient enjoyed an excellent clinical outcome.

the extent of the incision. Self-retaining retractors are placed between the skin flap and the paravertebral muscles after the latter have been carefully wrapped in moistened laparotomy pads. We occasionally use a table-mounted Farley retractor; otherwise standard self-retaining retractors suffice.

For lesions at L1 or L2, removal of the 12th rib can be useful in facilitating exposure. The transverse processes of L1 and L2 typically are under the 12th rib, and thus its removal is necessary. In addition, that rib can then be used as part of the bone graft. Unlike rib removal at thoracic levels, however, the neurovascular bundle need not be identified, nor should the intercostal nerve be sacrificed.

In lesions below L3, the iliac crest typically needs to be removed for exposure. Generally speaking, this should be done after the paravertebral musculature has been elevated and after the attachments are incised off the iliac crest. This is repaired at the end of the procedure. Osteotomes are used to resect the iliac aspect of the crest, carefully protecting the sacroiliac joints. The removed bone is used as graft material.

The transverse process is visible underneath the paravertebral musculature. The processes located cephalad and caudally, as well as at the level of the lesion, are identified and dissected free of periosteum.

Frequently, the nerve roots from the level above are seen at the tip of the transverse process.

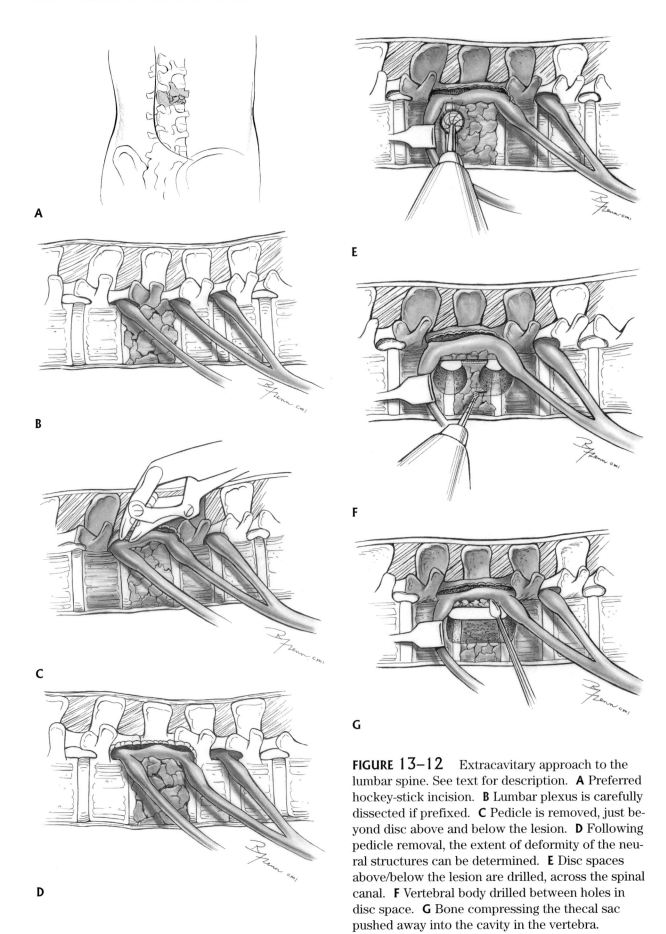

FIGURE 13–12 Extracavitary approach to the lumbar spine. See text for description. **A** Preferred hockey-stick incision. **B** Lumbar plexus is carefully dissected if prefixed. **C** Pedicle is removed, just beyond disc above and below the lesion. **D** Following pedicle removal, the extent of deformity of the neural structures can be determined. **E** Disc spaces above/below the lesion are drilled, across the spinal canal. **F** Vertebral body drilled between holes in disc space. **G** Bone compressing the thecal sac pushed away into the cavity in the vertebra.

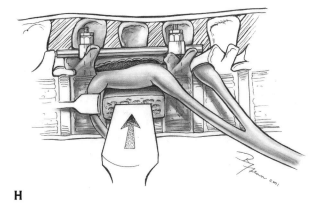

H

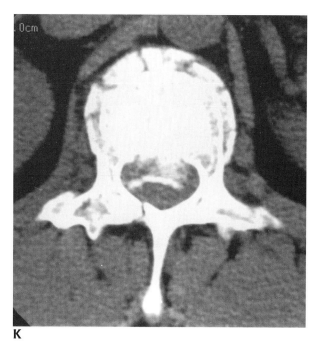

K

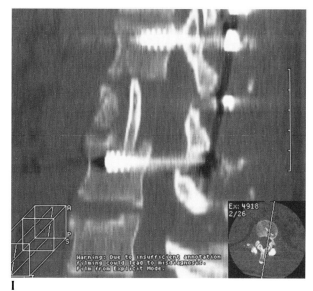

I

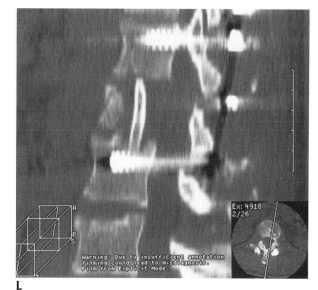

L

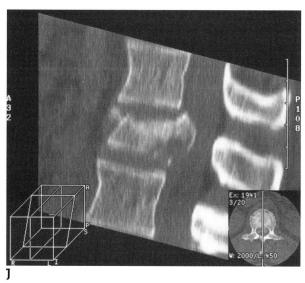

J

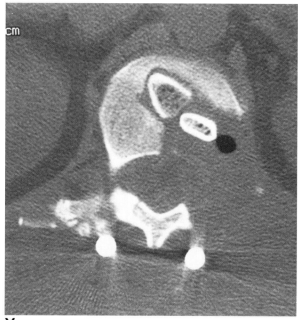

M

FIGURE 13–12 *(continued)*
H Oversized graft impacted into troughs, 1 cm anterior (**I**) of dural sac. **J–M** Thirty-year-old male with L1 fracture with paraparesis. **J and K** Sagittal and axial computed tomograms demonstrating severe canal compromise. **L and M** Postoperative computed tomography with decompression of the thecal sac.

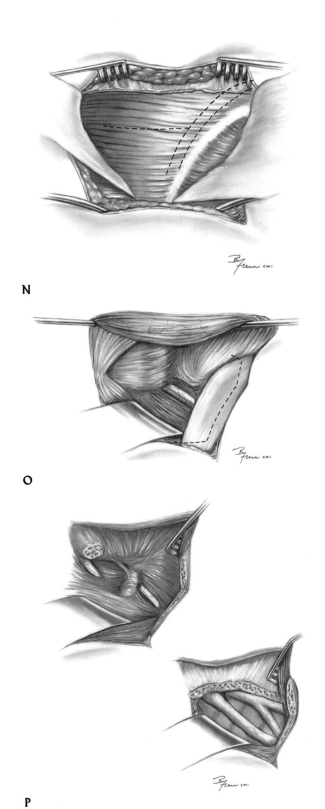

Thus it is useful to identify the nerve roots before removing the transverse processes. The transverse processes need to be removed to expose the nerve root foramina, which is critical in pedicle removal. The nerve roots between the affected vertebrae are mobilized laterally until they dive deep into the psoas. The periosteum of the vertebra at the levels of the lesion, cephalad and caudal, is bluntly dissected away from the lateral aspect of the vertebral body and pedicle. The prefixed lumbar plexus may be densely attached to the vertebral body and should be dissected carefully (Fig. 13–12B).

The amount of vertebra to be resected is directly related to the pathology. In the instance of fracture, for example, it is the dorsal half of the vertebral body that is compressing the dural sac and must be removed. For infection or tumor, however, a more radical resection is necessary. In those circumstances, the vertebral periosteum should be dissected anteriorly to the level of the anterior longitudinal ligament. Prior to this dissection, the anterior-lying segmental arteries are identified and ligated or electrocoagulated. Because injury to these vessels can cause multiliter blood loss, caution is important, regardless of how the vertebra is being approached.

Vertebral Resection

Following identification of the vertebral lesion, dissectors or blunted needles are placed into the disc spaces at the margins of the pathology and anteriorposterior or lateral radiographs obtained to ensure localization. We then rotate the table away from the surgeon, so that the patient is elevated 15 to 20 degrees vis-à-vis the surgeon.

Before incising the discs, the pedicle at the level of the injury is removed (Fig. 13–2C). This ensures visualization of the dural sac and direct definition of the pathology prior to resection of pathologic bone and disc. First, the mobilized nerve roots are followed proximally to the foramina and the margins of the foramina opened, after the venous plexus commonly surrounding the root is coagulated. The pedicle is thinned using a high-speed drill or a rongeur. The pedicle is then carefully removed to its dorsal extent using small Kerrison rongeurs and curettes. Potential for neural element injury exists here, and caution is required.

FIGURE 13–12 *(continued)* **N** Muscle entry point for L5 and S1 approach. **O** Deep muscle dissection and excision of iliac crest. **P** Transverse processes and joints are dissected free of muscle (top); transverse processes, pars, and lateral laminae are removed (bottom).

The pedicles adjacent to the affected levels may need to be at least partially removed to allow direct access to the annulus of the disc and the ligaments. It is imperative that the normal (nondeformed) dural sac be visualized both proximally and distally to the involved vertebra (Fig. 13–12D). Some epidural bleeding may occur during this step, but full removal of the pedicle makes protection of the spinal cord much simpler during vertebral decompression.

After the dissection of the periosteum, exposure of the disc spaces and localizing radiograph, and removal of the pedicle exposing the dural sac, the disc spaces above and below the lesion are ready to be incised. A scalpel is used to cut a rectangle in the annulus, and large amounts of disc are removed with biopsy forceps and curettes. The disc spaces are now drilled out using a high-speed drill or hand drill (Fig. 13–12E). The evacuation of the disc space should extend at least three-fourths of the way across the body to ensure bone removal well across the spinal canal. Failure to do so is the most common error in this procedure.

The vertebral body between the discs is then removed using a rongeur and high-speed drill. Bone removal should extend well beyond the opposite side of the spinal canal. If not, decompression will be suboptimal. Approximately 1 to 2 cm should be left at the anterior aspect of the vertebral body, unless there is tumor present, and a thin 5 mm to 1 cm shelf dorsally (Fig. 13–12F).

The last step in the decompression is the removal of the dorsal vertebral plate that is still compressing the thecal sac. Again, significant epidural bleeding may result at this step. Carefully dissect the dura away from the bony plate, breaking up adhesions as well as removing spiculae or masses stuck to the dura.

Working primarily at the junction of the disc annulus to the end plate, backward-angled Epstein ("stomper") curettes are used to push the bone plate away from the dura into the cavity created by the surgeon (Fig. 13–12G). Although it is tempting to remove the residual bone on the surgeon's side that is under direct vision, the surgeon should be careful to carry the disconnection of the residual bone process well across the spinal canal to ensure effective spinal cord decompression. By working at the margins of the pathology and by bringing this entire plate into the vertebral cavity in one piece, the surgeon does not directly manipulate bone or tumor fragments that are compressing the spinal cord at the middle of the exposure. The decompression can be verified with ultrasound, or—as we do—with dental mirrors visualizing the dural sac from its anterior aspect. Avoid palpating the dural sac as some recommend.

Anterior Graft

If spinal instrumentation is to be performed, the retractors are removed, the area carefully packed, and attention turned to the posterior elements. If fixation is not necessary, the graft is placed now: avoid the temptation to place the graft prior to spinal fixation, since the anatomic correction that often results from instrumentation may loosen the graft.[28] Troughs are cut into the adjacent bodies for the bone graft. The bone graft is prepared by cutting it 10 to 15% longer than the defect to be spanned. The ends are trimmed to 45 degree angles; the shorter is the leading edge (Fig. 13–12H). At least two or three pieces of rib and thick tri- or bicortical graft are impacted into position at least 1 cm away from the dural sac (Fig. 13–12I).[42]

If there is any question as to whether the spinal cord is adequately decompressed, it is a simple matter to perform a transpedicular decompression on the opposite side, since the exposure already exists. This is rarely necessary: in our experience, if there still is cord deformity, it is due to inadequate vertebral removal earlier in the procedure (Fig. 13–12J–M).

In the presence of spinal instability or angulation, spinal instrumentation is then performed using techniques discussed elsewhere. If the subperiosteal dissection has already been performed, the laminae are immediately available for preparation. Because the dural sac and the spinal cord have been carefully decompressed, even severe deformities can be realigned with minimal risk to the spinal cord. Posterior fusion is performed across the levels to be fused anteriorly (i.e., rod long/fuse short). Before returning anteriorly, the midline muscles are reapproximated.

Since correction of spinal deformity and stabilization have now taken place, it is appropriate to place the bone graft in neutral position. The erector spinae are again retracted medially, the dural sac visualized, and the pre-prepared bone grafts inserted into the spine. Generally, a large drain is left in the paravertebral region for one day. The wound is then closed in layers, approximating the muscles posteriorly, the thoracolumbar fascia, subcutaneous tissues, and skin.

Dumbbell and Paraspinal Lesions

The lateral extracavitary approach allows direct exposure of both the extracanal and intracanicular portions of the tumor. External masses can safely be excised without exposing the thecal or dural sac, and the pedicle is then removed and the portion of the tumor within the spinal canal visualized and removed.

McCormick et al reported on a series of dumbbell tumors operated on using the lateral extracavitary approach.[74] Histology ranged from schwanomma to sarcoma. Total resection was possible in 10 of 11 cases. Because of the nature of the procedure, anterior interbody fusion and posterior fixation were possible. The procedure was considerably more successful for these lesions than either an anterolateral approach or wide laminectomy and pedicle resection.

L5 Corpectomy

The standard approach is made as discussed above: the lateral/transverse portion of the incision is made below the wing of the iliac crest. The iliocostalis is split in the direction of its fibers; it is sometimes possible to make the dissection in the deep laminae of the lumbodorsal fascia (Fig. 13-12N). The gluteal, ileocostalis, and quadralis lumbarum are separated from the iliac wing by subperiosteal dissection. An osteotome is used to remove enough of the iliac crest to allow exposure of the lateral aspect of the lower L4 vertebra, the entire L5 vertebra, and superior sacrum, as well as to provide bone for the subsequent anterior fusion (Fig. 13-12O).

The muscular dissection is carried out down the transverse processes of L3, L4, and L5. The muscles are dissected from these transverse processes, the apophyseal joints, and the laminae (Fig. 13-12P, top). The L3 root is identified from within the psoas muscle as it emerges from beneath the L4 transverse process, the L4 from beneath the L5 transverse process, and the L5 root from its foramen. To accomplish the latter, it is necessary to resect the lateral portions of the L4–L5 and L5–S1 joints, the pars, and the lateral aspect of the laminae (Fig. 13-12P, bottom). The transverse processes are removed, and the L5 pedicle resected.

The L5 and S1 nerve roots are carefully mobilized. If the roots join proximally, they may be adherent to the side of the vertebra, but can generally be retracted enough to allow removal of the vertebra. With medial retraction of the S1 root and either medial or lateral retraction of L5, the L4–L5 and L5–S1 discs can be drilled out, and the L5 vertebra removed as discussed above. Instrumentation is as indicated, and anterior and posterior fusion is then performed. During closure, reapproximation of the muscles detached from the iliac crest is important.

Postoperative Care and Complications

Historically, patients were kept in the intensive care unit following this operation. In recent years, we have found this to be usually unnecessary because of improved intraoperative hemodynamic control. Patients are mobilized on the day of surgery. An external orthosis is used for 3 to 4 months until the bone graft appears to be healed.

The most common complications are the same as those of most major spine procedures. Blood loss and poor replacement may lead to coagulopathy as well as continuing anemia. Ileus may occur for one to two days after the procedure. Infection rates are low; in our series less than 2% of patients had superficial skin infections, and less than 0.5% had deep infections. Anterior fusion nonunion rates approached 6% overall and were primarily seen in those undergoing redo procedures, in smokers, and in patients who have been irradiated. We have found that performing posterior fusion during posterior fixation decreases this risk. Dural lacerations may occur or be encountered in the trauma patient: closure should be attempted, but fibrin gluing is rarely successful because of the cavity created by the decompression.

Results

The authors have performed more than 400 extracavitary decompressions and fusions in the lumbar spine between 1975 and 1997, for tumor, trauma, infection, and degenerative disease. Reoperation rate for complications (including instrumentation failure) and non-union is less than 5%. This is certainly comparable to or better than most alternatives.

Blood loss has decreased from an average of four liters in the early 1980s to 1200 ml now, including tumor. Neurologic deterioration has occurred three times, all resolved.

Clearly, there is a steep learning curve for this procedure, and as a result, many surgeons hesitate to make the investment in learning how to do it. However, the logical sequence of the procedure, its flexibility, and its great utility make it an important and valuable part of the spine surgeon's skills.

Anterior Lumbar Fusion

Indications

The primary indication for the anterior approach to the lumbar spine is to achieve vertebral decompression for isolated anterior spinal canal compromise, as well as to achieve fusion.[62] Anterior lumbar procedures may range from biopsy or decompression of single vertebral masses,[93,94] and anterior interbody fusions (ALIF)[78] to large, multilevel corpectomies with grafts and plates.[31] We continue to avoid anterolateral procedures alone for "three-column" disease, although at times we feel quite quixotic arguing that posterior fixation should be incorporated for significant instability. In addition, we rarely perform anterior/posterior fusions for discogenic disease; if it is felt that a patient undergoing posterior decompression requires vertebral as well as transverse process fusion, we prefer PLIF.

In cases of nonunion of transverse process fusion, repeat posterior fusion may fail because the lamina and spinous processes are relatively avascular. The complications associated with dissecting and excising old scar are considerable. Direct vertebral approaches often represent a better option because they offer a fresh, broad, bony surface between the vertebral bodies and an increased chance of successful bony fusion. Furthermore, ALIF, especially when instrumented, offers a 95% fusion rate with minimal local morbidity. Relative contraindications for anterior lumbar fusion include osteopenia, severe peripheral vascular disease, active infection, and obesity.[3,19,23,28]

Preoperative Assessment

Radiographic evaluation is for the primary spinal disorder.

Selection of the proper operative approach is crucial. There are two main approaches to the anterior lumbar spine: transperitoneal and retroperitoneal. We generally reserve the transperitoneal approach for interbody fusions at L5–S1,[31] although recently we have occasionally performed midline retroperitoneal exposures here as well, with some trepidation vis-à-vis retraction of the iliac vessels. However, L4–L5 interbody fusions may be performed via a transperitoneal approach if preoperative assessment shows that the aortic bifurcation is well above the L4–L5 disc space.[45] MR angiography (MRA) and reconstructed contrast-enhanced computed tomography provide detailed three-dimensional visualization of the aorta and iliac vessels and their relation to the L4–L5 disc space.

For lesions above L4, a retroperitoneal exposure is optimal. It gives good access to the anterior lumbar spine and limits the amount of retraction of the vascular system.[50] Many have performed transperitoneal or anterior retroperitoneal approaches up to L2, with a vascular surgeon retracting the aorta and the iliac arteries and veins. In principle, we assiduously avoid vascular retraction. We do not employ a procedure with significant vascular risk for the treatment of spinal disorders that are manageable through other approaches.

Patients with previous abdominal problems should be thoroughly evaluated, including CT of the abdomen. Some surgeons prefer bowel cleansing prior to surgery; we recommend only usual surgical precautions.

Technique

Transperitoneal Exposure

The patient is positioned supine; some elevate the sacrum by creating hyperextension in the operating table or placing a pad under the buttocks or lumbosacral junction. A subumbilical incision several centimeters above the pubis allows adequate exposure of L5–S1 (Fig. 13–13A). As an alternative to a vertical incision, a transverse Pfannenstie incision 5 cm above the symphysis pubis allows adequate exposure of L5–S1 (Fig. 13–13B). A 20 cm incision centered just below the umbilicus exposes L3–L4. We usually obtain a preoperative localization film

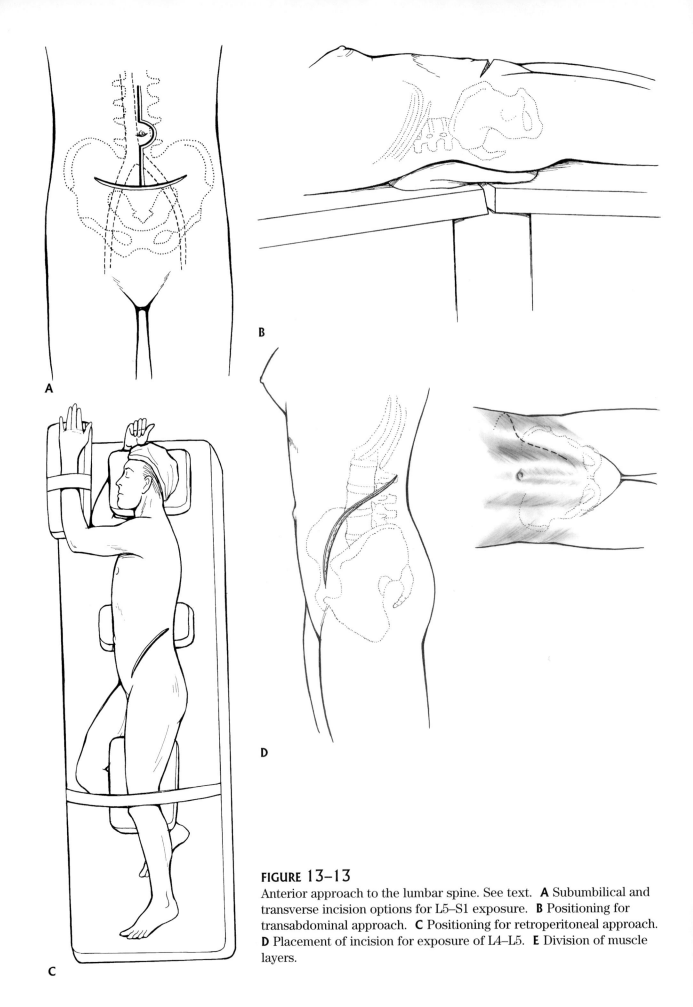

FIGURE 13-13
Anterior approach to the lumbar spine. See text. **A** Subumbilical and transverse incision options for L5–S1 exposure. **B** Positioning for transabdominal approach. **C** Positioning for retroperitoneal approach. **D** Placement of incision for exposure of L4–L5. **E** Division of muscle layers.

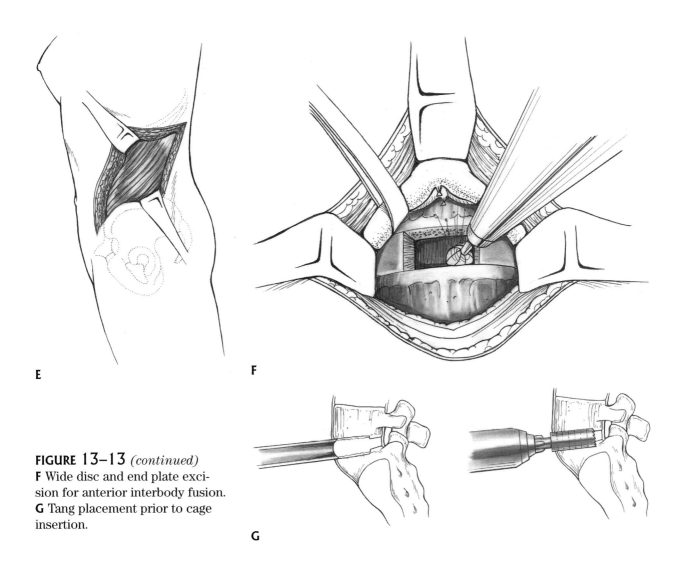

FIGURE 13-13 *(continued)*
F Wide disc and end plate excision for anterior interbody fusion.
G Tang placement prior to cage insertion.

before the incision is made. In addition, a separate incision is needed if iliac crest graft is to be obtained.

The abdominal wall fascia is incised in the midline, and the peritoneum is opened in a controlled manner. With the transperitoneal approach, the posterior peritoneum should be opened to the right of the midline above the aortic bifurcation, avoiding the sympathetic fibers to the left of the midline over the L5 vertebral body and L5–S1 disc. The prevertebral tissue should be incised longitudinally and retracted bluntly in a lateral to medial fashion. The intestines are kept in the upper abdomen by the Trendelenberg position. The redundant sigmoid, cecum, and small bowel are displaced superiorly in the upper portion of the abdomen with a self-retaining retractor if necessary, and the lower lumbar and pelvic portions of the posterior peritoneum may then be readily visualized. The pelvic portion of the colon and its mesentery are then retracted to the left. The ureters are identified and safely retracted. We have found that the Farley retractor enables excellent bowel mobilization and enhances visualization of the vertebral bodies and disc spaces anteriorly.

After the bowel is mobilized, we identify the aortic bifurcation, sacral promontory, inferior vena cava, and collateral vessels. Of particular importance is safe mobilization of the left common iliac vein.[48] Gentle dissection is required to strip the connective tissue and nerves from the vessel's friable wall: injury to the iliac vein results in potentially fatal hemorrhage. Steinman pins secured into the lateral vertebra can be used, if necessary, to aid in retraction of the iliac veins.

The superior hypogastric plexus overlies the L5–S1 disc, distal to the bifurcation of the abdominal aorta, over the sacral promontory. It is often not well visualized: damage to the superior hypogastric plexus, which may produce impotence or retrograde ejaculation, may be avoided by gently pushing the loosely adherent tissue away from the

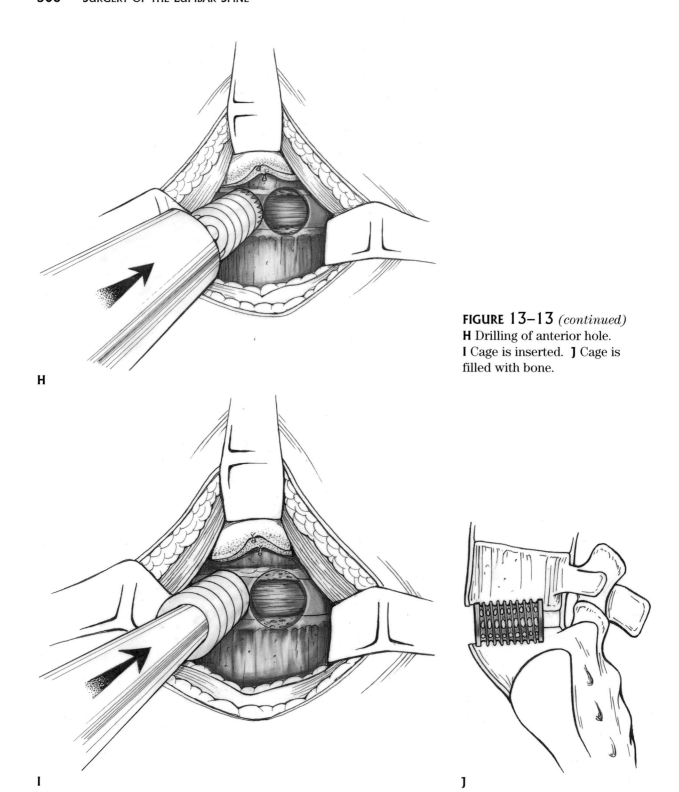

FIGURE 13–13 *(continued)*
H Drilling of anterior hole.
I Cage is inserted. **J** Cage is filled with bone.

L5–S1 disc. Indeed, the best way to protect the nerve may be to not see it at all: rather, soft tissue overlying the body is elevated together. Coagulation and division of the middle sacral artery may be necessary. Radiography is obtained to ensure accuracy of positioning.

Retroperitoneal Exposure

The retroperitoneal exposure is our anterior procedure of choice for visualization of the lumbar spine from L2–L5; it may be used for all anterior lumbar procedures in which a multilevel fusion or stabilization is needed. Our first choice of procedure, however, remains the extracavitary approach, from T11-L. A disadvantage of the retroperitoneal approach is that the vertebral bodies and intervertebral discs can be viewed from only one side: again, if bilateral exposure is necessary, the extracavitary approach should be used. Moreover, a right-sided approach to the upper lumbar spine may be hampered by the size and location of the liver.

The exposure is performed through a flank incision, with the patient positioned in the lateral decubitus position. Our general surgeon prefers a 20 degree angle off true lateral to facilitate exposure. However, if anterior instrumentation is to be used the patient should be in a true lateral position: this improves screw placement and radiography. As an alternative, the operating table—or, in our case, the Jackson spine frame—can be turned to a limited extent. The shoulder and hips are supported, with the arm on the operated side supported and held across the chest, and the knees and hip slightly flexed. The surgeon is on the ventral side of the patient (Fig. 13–13C).

We prefer approaching the patient from the left. This avoids retraction on the liver and—most important—the thin walled inferior vena cava, which is present on the right side. From a left-sided approach, the smaller spleen is easily retracted to expose the spine, and the larger, thick-walled aorta may be easily located because of its pulsations.

The incision varies according to the level of the spine that is approached, and a preoperative localizing film is routinely obtained. Several incisional guidelines may be readily applied. For L4–L5, the incision is placed above the iliac crest; for L3–L4, at the umbilicus; and for L2–L3, above the umbilicus (Fig. 13–13D).

The goal of the dissection is to obtain access to the anterior lumbar spine without entering the peritoneal cavity. The external oblique, internal oblique, and transversalis fasciae are divided (Fig. 13–13E), and the peritoneum is identified and mobilized. The dissection proceeds along the peritoneum and in the potential space between the renal fascia and the quadratus lumborum and psoas muscles. The peritoneum may then be mobilized medially to the midline, off the posterior abdominal wall from the inferior edge of the left kidney down to the sacrum. The anterior surfaces of the psoas muscle and the quadratus lumborum may now be easily visualized. Two smaller structures, the genitofemoral nerve (identified as a small nerve lying on top of the psoas muscle) and the ureter (identified as a cylindrical-shaped structure with rich, superficial vascular network and peristaltic movements) need to be mobilized.

Once this is completed, iliac crest bone can easily be taken, if desired. The periosteum is incised, and cortico-cancellous graft is taken. The fascia or periosteum is closed with interrupted sutures. We do not routinely drain the iliac crest separately from the main wound.

The lumbar vertebrae are now visible under their periosteum. Before dissecting this off the vertebrae, we again obtain a localizing x-ray to be certain that we are at the correct level. We then dissect the body free anteriorly to the anterior longitudinal ligament if the procedure is for trauma or anterior fusion. If for tumor or infection, the periosteum is reflected to the anterior midline.

The lateral surface of the psoas muscle must be retracted dorsally for true lateral exposure of the vertebra. However, the lumbosacral plexus is located within this muscle: with retraction of the psoas muscle, the yellow-white sympathetic trunk, with its periodic ganglionic enlargements, may be seen as it traverses the lateral aspect of the vertebral bodies. The ascending lumbar venous system, which drains blood from the extraspinal venous plexuses, is located on the lateral aspect of the vertebral bodies at the level of the neural foramen. These should be carefully mobilized and retracted with the muscle. Our preference is to retract the psoas enough to allow us to palpate the foramina but not expose them unless necessary. This minimizes the risk of neurological injury as well as blood loss from the foraminal venous plexus.

Anterior Interbody Fusion

We generally outline the disc space from the adjacent end plate and vertebral body using a knife. The monopolar is avoided at the L5–S1 interspace to prevent thermal injury to the sympathetic plexus. The disc is partially removed using biopsy forceps. We use a D'Errico or high-speed drill to make a hole through the disc space and to disrupt the end plates, exposing cancellous bone. The bony surfaces of the vertebral bodies above and below the disc space are further curretted to ensure a bleeding bone surface (Fig. 13–13F). Interbody fusion is then performed using iliac crest or bank bone in various configurations, synthetic interbody spacers, or, most recently, titanium cages. Radiography should be performed repeatedly because the angle of the L5–S1 disc will confuse the surgeon regarding graft or cage placement. The patient is mobilized in a TLSO brace postoperatively.

Instrumented ALIF

The exposure is the same as that described earlier for the anterior lumbar interbody fusion; similarly, the cage technique is similar to that of the instrumented posterior lumbar interbody fusion. In transabdominal anterior fusion, the cage diameter is determined by disc diameter, as for PLIF. Cage length must be carefully measured for anterior interbody fusion, again as for PLIF. Especially during retroperitoneal approaches to L5–S1, using a cage that is too long may injure neural elements, such as the contralateral L5 nerve root. At L1–L5, for retroperitoneal placement, we use the longest cages available.

First, a scalpel is used to make a generous hole in the annulus anteriorly, or—in the retroperitoneal approach—from the side. In transperitoneal anterior lumbar fusion, it is important to be lateral enough of the midline to allow placement of two cages that are not touching (Fig. 13–13G). The largest tang or distracter that will fit is pounded into the disc space. Following radiographic confirmation of correct tang placement, the hole is drilled (Fig. 13–13H). The vertebral tap is then used to make the threads in the cancellous bone, and the cage is inserted (Fig. 13–13I). Local or autologous bone is used to fill the cage (Fig. 13–13J). The second cage is placed in a similar manner.

Retroperitoneal ALIF

Following the exposure as discussed above, anterior fusion is quite straightforward, except at L5–S1. The disc space is incised using a scalpel; generally, we recommend staying dorsal to the anterior longitudinal ligament (Fig. 13–14A). The end plates are roughened: we generally use a D'Errico drill to make a hole in both end plates simultaneously. We then impact bone (Fig. 13–14B). Although tricortical bone is easily used at most levels, at L5–S1 we usually find ourselves placing small fragments of bone and impacting them, because of the angles present. At least some autologous bone is recommended, since many of these are performed for nonunion of posterior fusions.

In recent years, we have become enthusiastic proponents of the use of intervertebral cages in ALIF. In our experience, a size 18 Ray cage can be used in most retroperitoneal approaches, unless there are other structures near the end plate. For example, if patients have undergone previous posterior fixation, pedicle screws near the end plate may make it necessary to use smaller cages.

Patients are in the true lateral decubitus position, as discussed above. This is important for the radiography to be performed later. The standard retroperitoneal incision is made as inferior and medial as possible to facilitate exposure to L5–S1. The iliolumbar vein is divided, again to facilitate exposure. The psoas muscle must be mobilized more dorsally than is usually the case for the retroperitoneal approach if L5–S1 is to be included.

Above L5–S1, we prefer to place the cages immediately dorsal to the lateral border of the anterior longitudinal ligament.[112] After opening the annulus with a scalpel and removing a generous amount of disc material, the largest distracter—in the case of multilevel fusion—or tang that will fit is placed, ideally at a true lateral trajectory. We attempt to place distracters at multiple levels before placing the cage so that one radiograph can be used to check the placement of all of them, saving time, money, and radiation exposure. (Fig. 13–14C).

The disc spaces are then drilled and tapped as discussed above. Since most vertebrae are significantly wider than 26 mm, we overdrill and overtap to countersink the cage. We also typically pack bone into the drilled hole before placing the cage.

L5–S1 Cage Placement Performing fusion via a retroperitoneal approach at L5–S1 has long been challenging. True lateral cage placement is not possible, in part because of the exposure, and because the border of the sacrum aligns poorly with L5. Some surgeons have advocated converting the retroperitoneal approach to a transabdominal one: following fusion at levels above L5, the patient is repositioned supine, and the peritoneum opened as discussed above. Others have accepted less robust bone placement, packing small bone fragments into a curetted disc space, rather than using bi- or tricortical grafts. However, this may be associated with disc space collapse or nonunion.

We have developed, and regularly use, instrumented ALIF to solve this dilemma.[110] Oblique cage placement is optimal. First of all, cage diameter is determined from the CT using templates, or by "eyeballing" the disc diameter. Ideal cage length is determined by measuring the oblique diameter through the L5–S1 disc space from CT. Most often, the 21-mm-long cage is ideal.

The annulus of the disc is cut using a scalpel, this time straddling the lateral border of the anterior longitudinal ligament. The disc is removed using a biopsy forceps and curette. The appropriate tang is impacted into the disc space at an angle of 35 to 45 degrees from true lateral (Fig. 13–14C); this is confirmed radiographically. Ideally, the tang approaches the disc from an anterior and medial trajectory, and the shaft presents immediately superior to the anterior iliac spine. The disc is then drilled, and the hole carefully probed to ensure that the annulus has not been violated. Following vertebral tapping, the cage is countersunk into the hole and filled with bone. We usually confirm the position of cages with radiography (Fig. 13–14D, E). To date, we have had excellent success with this approach: we have had no instrument- or cage-related complications, and have noted excellent fixation and fusion in all cases. In addition, we have avoided the complications and technical difficulties of combined transabdominal and retroperitoneal approaches.

Vertebrectomy

The performance of vertebrectomy, particularly for thecal sac decompression (Fig. 13–15A), is far more difficult than discectomy. For single-level vertebrectomy, two discs are exposed: for tumor, we may actually take an additional level to be certain that total resection is possible. The discs are removed as described in the previous section (Fig. 13–15B). We first perform discectomy, as opposed to removal of the mass itself, to maintain anatomic orientation.

We resect and drill the intervening vertebral body, staying ventral to a line extending across the ventral aspect of the foramina and dorsal of the anterior longitudinal ligament, except in surgery for tumor removal. It is important to extend the bone removal across the spinal canal away from the surgeon, as in the extracavitary approach (Fig. 13–15C). This can be facilitated by drilling more ventrally in the vertebra and turning the patient away from the surgeon.

Pedicle removal can be accomplished through this procedure; generally, this is done through a combination of thinning across the pedicle and working from the ventral surface in the cavity where the body has been removed.

The thin dorsal plate still compressing the thecal sac is now removed (Fig. 13–15D). In the lateral extracavitary approach, the bone is pushed *away* from the thecal sac because of its lateral exposure via pedicle removal. In the anterior lumbar fusion, the surgeon carefully thins and bites away the residual bone until the dural sac is exposed. As is true for the extracavitary approach, the most critical technical error is incomplete decompression because of inadequate initial vertebral removal. Following full decompression, a bone is inserted (Fig. 13–15E). We prefer bank bone to methylmethacrylate, even in instances of tumor.

Postoperatively, patients are mobilized in a thoracolumbar orthosis the day of surgery. They are allowed to begin drinking as soon as they are thirsty, and are fed when hungry or when bowel sounds are present. Usually, they are on liquid diets within 24 hours.

Anterior Plating Devices

It is beyond the context of this chapter to discuss in detail the merits and disadvantages of the various anterior plating systems available on the market today. There are two main types of systems: those based on anterior locking plates, and those based on rods or screws. Advantages of the former include the contouring to the vertebra and ease of use, particularly with the locking plate systems. However, extending plates over more than three adjacent segments or into the sacrum is extremely difficult. Rod and screw systems, such as the Kaneda device, allow multisegment fixation, can be applied in exposures that do not allow for the width of the plate, and can sometimes provide sacral fixation.

Indications for anterior fixation may include burst fractures with mechanical compromise, particularly when there is neither deformity or posterior element injury; (Fig. 13–17); reconstruction after resection of local tumors not requiring multisegment fixation (for example, benign tumors and anterior column support after osteotomies for kyphosis); and deformity, but in conjunction with posterior fixation.[92] To repeat ad nauseum, anterior fixation generally does not obviate posterior instrumentation; it should be looked on as an adjunct in

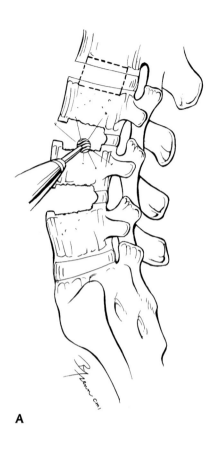
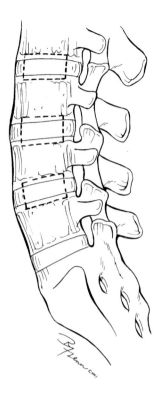
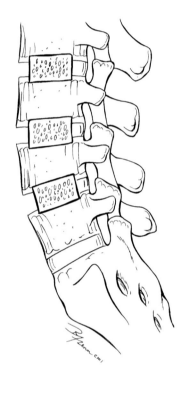

FIGURE 13–14
Interbody fusion via retroperitoneal approach. **A** Discectomy dorsal to anterior longitudinal ligament. **B** Bone impacted for fusion.

severe dislocation or deformity. Indeed many have suggested that anterior fixation is of little more value than a solid tricortical bone graft. A recent biomechanical study demonstrated anterior plating to be biomechanically inferior to posterior fixation following vertebrectomy.[103]

Contraindications for anterior plating include severe osteopenia, fixed scoliosis, and unreduced fracture dislocations.

Surgical Considerations In placing anterior plates, we have found proper anatomical identification to be critical. Nerve roots exiting from the involved levels or in the iliopsoas muscle and the sensory nerves anterior to the psoas muscle (genitofemoral and ilioinguinal nerves) must be protected at all times.[114] Plates need to be located onto the lateral vertebral body surface for optimal screw purchase. The most common mistake is to place the plates too far anterior, which results in suboptimal screw purchase and plate placement. Moreover, since screw length is measured for lateral placement and not for an anterior one, erroneous placement may lead to violation of the spinal canal. Accurate identification of the intervertebral foramen, as well as the posterior border of the anterior longitudinal ligament, orients the surgeon to the lateral aspect of the spine and properly locates the plate anterior to the foramen.

Another common error is to misinterpret intraoperative x-rays because of patient positioning. We have found that preoperative positioning of the

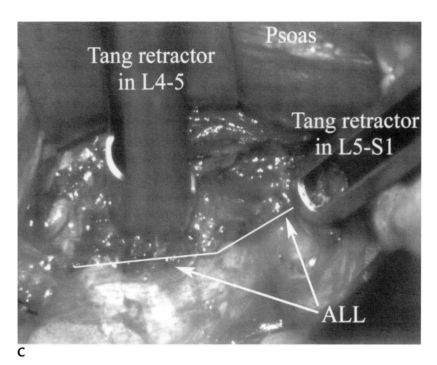

FIGURE 13-14 *(continued)* **C** placement of multiple tangs during retroperitoneal fusion of lumbar spine; note especially angle of tang at L5–S1. **D and E** Retroperitoneal cage placement.

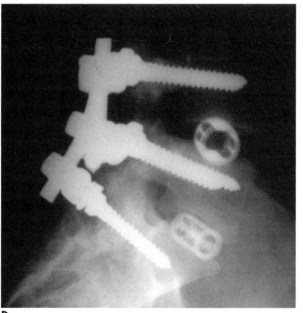
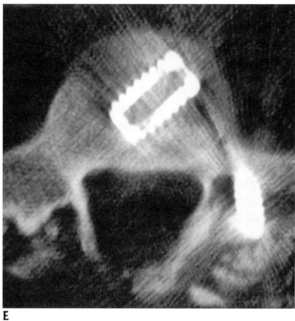

patient as close to lateral as possible is the most optimal way to ensure proper interpretation of x-ray orientation to ensure lateral placement of the screws.

We currently use the Synthes AO titanium anterior thoracolumbar plating system (ATLP); thus its appearance in the technical drawings. However, placement principles are the same for all systems, although others may require bicortical purchase.

The ATLP is MRI and tissue compatible. It comes in a variety of plate sizes and is fixated to the vertebral body using triangulated screw tips and screws countersunk in the plate. The ATLP is biomechanically comparable to other anterior plate constructs, including the Z-plate and the Kaneda device.[115] Overall, the locking screw plate design of the ATLP and the Z-plate is probably better biomechanically than that of the nonlocking plates (TSRH, Kenda), although all are acceptable.[22]

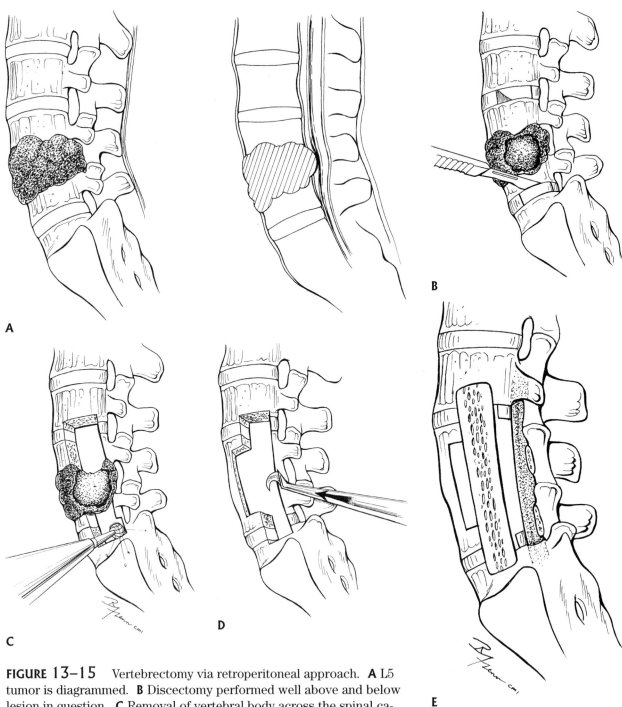

FIGURE 13–15 Vertebrectomy via retroperitoneal approach. **A** L5 tumor is diagrammed. **B** Discectomy performed well above and below lesion in question. **C** Removal of vertebral body across the spinal canal. **D** Dorsal bone or tumor still compressing the thecal sac is removed. **E** Bone graft is placed.

Surgical Technique Following decompression, as described in the previous section, the vertebral body spreader (Fig. 13–16A) can be used to reduce kyphosis at the vertebrectomy site, allowing a longer graft.[54] This is usually only effective in total vertebrectomy or when the surgeon fractures the anterior cortex. We rarely find this step useful. However, distraction can occasionally be used as in the figure to allow optimal placement of the bone graft.

Plate size is then determined. The manufacturer recommends using templates to determine plate size; we have not found this to be useful. Using the threaded drill guide, which also functions as the plate holder, a plate felt to be appropriate is picked. The longest portion of the plate (the dorsal surface) should be several millimeters ventral to the dorsal surface of the vertebral body (Fig. 13–16B). It is imperative that the plate be placed on the true lateral vertebral surface so that the screws do not go into the spinal canal. A lateral radiograph is recommended to ensure this.

The plate should be just long enough so that all screws are well within the vertebral body. Avoid the temptation to use the longest plate possible, since this may result in placing screws into adjacent disc spaces; conversely, a plate that is too short will lead to screw placement in the graft or the graft/vertebra interface rather than into the adjacent vertebral body. Furthermore, we currently do not recommend using this plate over more than three adjacent vertebral segments. If multilevel fixation is necessary, other techniques, such as multilevel anterior vertebral screw fixation, should be performed.

While the assistant holds the plate in place, a medial temporary fixation hole is drilled using the 2.5-mm guide and drill bit as diagrammed. The guide will help direct the screw. Be certain that the arrow on the barrel points toward the graft (Fig. 13–16C). The hole is probed to verify bone throughout its extent, and a 4-mm temporary cancellous bone screw is gently hand-tightened. The opposite temporary screw is then placed. Both temporary screws are then tightened down sequentially (Fig. 13–16D) and the plate holder removed.

The permanent screws are then placed. Screw length is best measured from the computed tomogram. The threaded drill guides are placed in the dorsal holes at the long corners of the plate (see Fig. 13–16E). Although some drill the permanent holes freehand, we strongly recommend using the guides to ensure that the screws are placed perpendicular to the plate, a requirement of effective locking. The posterior holes are then drilled with the 5-mm flexible drill bit. Several types of drill bits and handles are now manufactured: these can either be rigid or flexible to allow bending around the retroperitoneal cavity. The stop prevents drilling the hole more than 30 mm (Fig. 13–16F).

Once the two holes at the ends of the plate are drilled, 7.5-mm locking screws are inserted (Fig. 13–16G). The holes must be probed prior to placing the screws to ascertain that the hole is well within the vertebra and that the canal is not violated. Especially if the patient is not in true lateral position for this part of the procedure, x-rays can be deceiving. The surgeon then seats the 7.5-mm anterior locking screw. Do not terminally tighten the screws at this point.

The more medial temporary screws placed earlier are now removed (Fig. 13–16H). Some have tried to leave the temporary screws in place; these prevent good positioning of the permanent locking screws in the anterior part of the plate.

The threaded drill guides are now inserted into the anterior holes. As discussed earlier, holes are drilled using the 5-mm flexible drill bit and 7.5-mm locking screws that are placed and tightened. Again, probe each hole to be certain that the entire path of the hole is within the vertebra (see Fig. 13–16I). While terminally tightening the screws, be certain they are completely seated into the plate so that true locking has occurred (see Fig. 13–16J).

Complications We had one known complication in our series: in one early case, the plate and screws were placed with the patient rotated for the approach. Although plate position seemed good on intraoperative radiography, subsequent CT showed the screws to violate the spinal canal. Fortunately, no deficit resulted, and the device was repositioned without difficulty. In Thalgott et al's series, complications were primarily related to broken screws, with no sequelae.[99,100]

We have heard anecdotes of screws loosening from the plate. We suspect this is due to inadequate locking of the screws into the plate. Alternatively, as mentioned earlier, anterior fixation does not effectively substitute for posterior fixation in the unstable spine; plates will loosen and deformity occur in the presence of significant posterior element instability.

Complications of Anterior Lumbar Fusion

The two main surgical complications are vascular and neurological.

Vascular Complications

Injury of the aorta may be minimized by selecting the proper approach.[75] In lesions below the aortic bifurcation, the transperitoneal approach allows direct access without vascular retraction. In lesions above the bifurcation, transperitoneal approaches may involve manipulation of the aorta and iliac arteries, leading to arterial injury and the possibil-

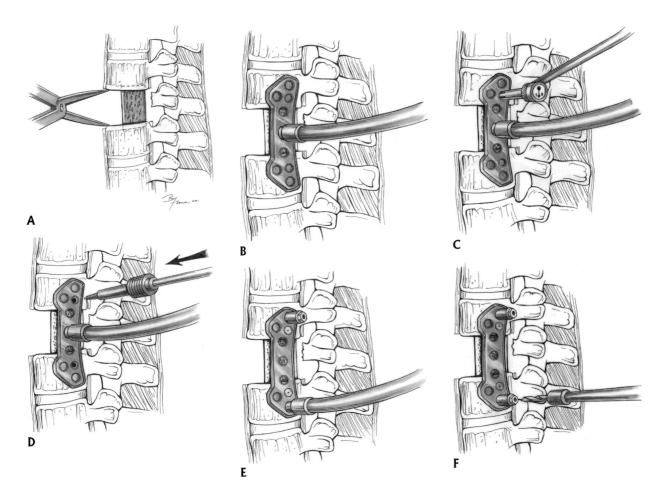

FIGURE 13–16 Technique for placement of anterior lumbar plates, described more fully in text. **A** Vertebral body spreader. **B** Plate sizing and positioning. **C** Drilling of temporary screw holes. **D** Both temporary screws are tightened. **E** Permanent screw drill guide placed, and **F** hole drilled.

ity of emboli in patients with peripheral vascular disease.[104]

Injury to the venous system is potentially more devastating: the inferior vena cava and iliac veins are thin-walled, and inadvertent injury is extremely difficult to repair. The iliolumbar vein, a tributary of the inferior vena cava or left iliac vein, may be avulsed, resulting in a tear of the inferior vena cava. Baker et al have evaluated the incidence of vascular injury in 102 patients undergoing anterior lumbar spinal procedures. They found that the overall rate of vascular complications in the hands of two experienced vascular surgeons was 15.6%. Although all the injuries were repaired and did not result in long-term sequelae, venous injuries are serious, resulting in significant blood loss and potential catastrophe.[3]

Neurological Complications

Injury may occur to the sympathetic plexus or the cauda equina itself.[81] The superior hypogastric plexus forms the sympathetic chain and is responsible for bladder neck closure during ejaculation; injury may lead to retrograde ejaculation.[101] It is located beneath the parietal peritoneum and overlies L5–S1, just distal to the bifurcation of the abdominal aorta and over the sacral promontory. It should be noted that retrograde ejaculation probably occurs in only a very small percentage of anterior lumbar fusions. Flynn et al in a survey of 4,500 cases of anterior lumbar fusions found sterility in 0.42% of patients, with a quarter of these

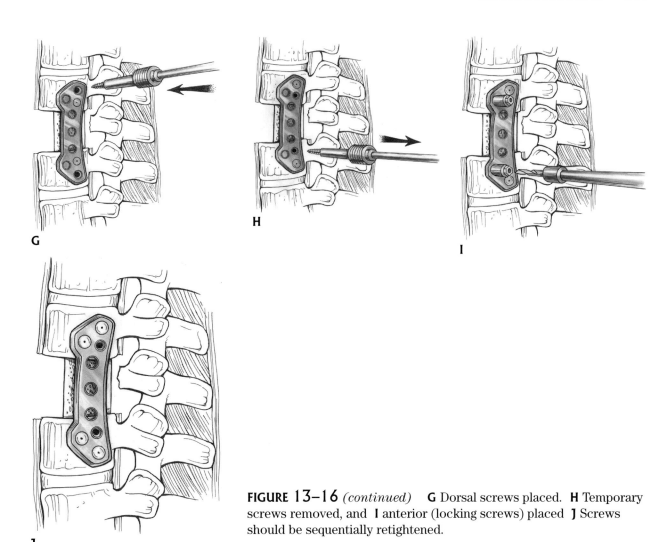

FIGURE 13-16 *(continued)* **G** Dorsal screws placed. **H** Temporary screws removed, and **I** anterior (locking screws) placed **J** Screws should be sequentially retightened.

patients spontaneously resolving.[30] Hypogastric plexus injury does not result in inability to maintain an erection, because this is a parasympathetic function (S2–S4 is located within the pelvis, which is almost never injured from an anterior approach).

Electrocautery should be avoided at the L5–S1 bifurcation, since heat transmission may damage the hypogastric plexus. The L5–S1 disc should not be cut in a transverse fashion until all prevertebral tissue is removed. The paraspinous lumbar plexus may also be damaged from overretraction of the psoas muscle, leading to ipsilateral foot vasodilation and contralateral lower extremity coldness. Injury to the femoral nerve, presumably from overretraction of the psoas muscle, has also been reported. Direct injury to the nerve root, cauda equina, or thecal sac may also occur during decompression or placement of anterior plates. Inappropriate placement of bone grafts or cages has been reported to induce iatrogenic spinal canal compromise with neural compression.

Other Complications

Other complications from the approach include peritoneal perforation during the retroperitoneal approach. These tears in the peritoneum are not uncommon and should be repaired. Peritoneal hernias secondary to entrapment of bowel from peritoneal tears may also occur. Damage to the ureter is more likely from a retroperitoneal approach.[46] The ureter is normally reflected anteriorly and is identified on the undersurface of the peritoneum. It is located immediately lateral to the aorta on a left-sided retroperitoneal approach and to the right of the inferior vena cava on a right-sided approach, and is adjacent to the anterolateral aspect

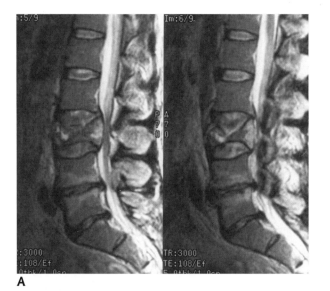
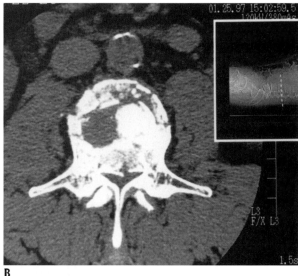
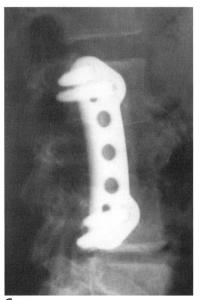
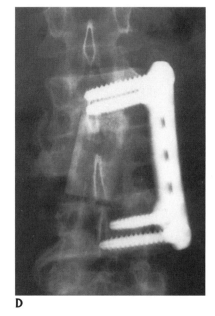

FIGURE 13-17
Fifty-year-old male with L3 fracture and severe neurological deficit, but no posterior element injury. Sagittal MRI **A** and axial computed tomogram **B** with severe canal compromise and thecal sac compression. **C and D** Lateral and anteroposterior postoperative radiographs. Although bone graft is angled, it is well fixated. Note that the decompression extends across the spinal canal.

of the L4–L5 disc space. In the transperitoneal approach, the ureter is usually quite lateral and not routinely seen. Damage to the ureter should be suspected in a patient with an abdominal fluid collection, low-grade fever, and leukocytosis. Other reported complications include rectus sheath hematoma from avulsion of the inferior epigastric artery, infections, and bone graft donor site complications.

Results

We are not aware of any large randomized series comparing the different interbody fusion or plating procedures. Successful fusion rates should be greater than 90% for single-level disease. Two-level constructs are slightly less likely to heal. On the whole, fusion results are good, with minimal mortality.

Crock has published a series of 1,000 anterior lumbar fusions performed with autogenous iliac crest grafts with an incidence of three perioperative mortalities (two related to heart attacks, one from suicide), no urological complications, and two possible cases of sterility.[19] Faciszewski et al reviewed 1,223 anterior thoracic and lumbar procedures performed from 1969 through 1992. Although the patients that had thoracic versus lumbar procedures were not clearly defined, the incidence of clinically significant complications (death—0.3%, paraplegia—0.2%, deep wound infection—0.6%) was low.[28]

In our recent series for all disorders, we have had one wound infection, no nonunions, and one patient who required reoperation for inadequate initial vertebral decompression. One patient had temporary, but severe, neurological deficit from coexisting vascular disease; this largely resolved within six months.

Endoscopic Lumbar Fusion

The authors have little experience with endoscopic fusion. Indeed, this author has only performed them since 1996, in part because of the resistance of his patients to consider new approaches. Furthermore, few of our patients require isolated L5–S1 fusion, often all that is safe through the transperitoneal approach. Recently, we have begun performing retroperitoneal endoscopic surgery; our experience is quite preliminary and really therefore represents only our theoretical impressions.

We find vertebrectomy, fusion, and fixation to be quite cumbersome through the endoscopic retroperitoneal approach. Particularly in multilevel lesions, the time and effort involved and the number of small incisions required limit the value of endoscopy. For two- to three-level discectomy and fusion, particularly using dowels or cages, results seem to be comparable. Our patients typically begin drinking in 24 hours, which is not as quick as with endoscopy, but length of stay is comparable. Open procedures do not require the expensive equipment and extra time of endoscopy; thus the open procedure may actually be more cost-effective.

The techniques discussed have emerged as promising areas of future investigation for anterior lumbar interbody fusion. Onimus et al described a video-assisted two-incision technique for anterior fusion at both L4–L5 and L5–S1. In their procedure, the peritoneum is dissected from lateral to medial, allowing anterior spinal exposure through a retroperitoneal approach. Although iliac vessel retraction is simplified, there are still risks in manipulating them.[80] This is not a true endoscopic approach, in that the peritoneum is not insufflated but uses video to supplement standard instrumentation.

Mayer uses microsurgical technique and fluoroscopic localization to perform both retroperitoneal (L2–L3, L3–L4, L4–L5) and transperitoneal approaches (L5–S1) for interbody fusions with autologous iliac crest grafts. He reports minimal blood loss with good visualization and no significant increase in surgical time.[72] However, performing, for example, an L3–S1 fusion requires changing the patient's position intraoperatively. The open retroperitoneal approach we have described allows one exposure and dissection to approach and instrument L2–S1. Mathews et al also have reported excellent results with anterior interbody fusion performed endoscopically on five patients using autologous bone at the L5–S1 level. One patient had an iliac vein tear, requiring conversion to an open procedure.[71]

Zucherman et al reported on 17 patients who underwent laparoscopic spinal fusion using BAK cages. Fourteen single-level and three two-level fusions, all involving L4–S1 levels, were performed. Two patients required conversions to open procedures; two patients had donor site wound infections, and one patient required subsequent posterior spinal decompression because of a displaced end plate fracture.[117] Of the patients without complications, the length of hospital stay was 2 days, the same as our average for open PLIF.

In an early series, Regan et al successfully performed thirty transperitoneal laparoscopic lumbar fusions at L4–L5 and L5–S1. Four had to be converted to open procedures, two due to iliac vein injuries and two due to poor visualization. The average operative time was 3.5 hours and hospitalization 3.7 days. This is slightly longer than our average hospitalization for open L5–S1 fusion, but the endoscopic procedure has been refined since then.[87]

The ultimate utility of endoscopy for fusion remains to be determined. Although accepted by some with wild enthusiasm and deprecated by many others with equal disdain, further experience may decrease the technical difficulties, and, more importantly better define the appropriate use of these procedures. The key, of course, is that endoscopy is not a new operation; rather, it represents the modification of accepted exposures, and still requires surgeons who understand the anatomy of the region and the surgical principles of lumbar fusion.[73] It is not an area to be adopted by the "occasional" spine surgeon following a two-day course. If anything will destroy the potential of this field, it will be those who choose to use it inappropriately.

REFERENCES

1. Allen BL, Ferguson RL: The Galveston technique of pelvic fixation with L rod instrumentation of the spine. Spine 9:388–394, 1984.
2. Bagby G: Arthrodesis by the distraction-compression method using a stainless-steel implant. Orthopedics 11:931–934, 1988.
3. Baker JK, Reardon PR, Reardon MJ, et al: Vascular injury in anterior lumbar surgery. Spine 18:2227–2230, 1993.
4. Bennett GJ, Serhan HA, Sorini PM, et al: An experimental study of lumbar stabilization: Restabilization and bone density. Spine 22:1448–1453, 1997.
5. Benzel EC: The lateral extracavitary approach to the spine using the three-quarter prone position. J Neurosurg 71:837–841, 1989.
6. Benzel EC, Larson SJ: Postoperative stabilization of the posttraumatic thoracic and lumbar spine: A review of concepts and orthotic techniques. J Spinal Disord 2:47–51, 1989.
7. Blumenthal SL, Gill K: Can lumbar spine radiographs accurately determine fusion in postoperative patients? Spine 18:1186–1189, 1993.
8. Bogdanffy GM, Ohmeiss DD, Guyer RD: Early changes in bone mineral density above a combined anteroposterior L4–S1 lumbar spinal fusion. Spine 20:1674–1678, 1955.
9. Bosworth DM: Techniques of spinal fusion: Pseudoarthrosis and method of repair. American Academy of Orthopedic Surgeons Instructional Course V, pp 295–313, 1948.
10. Breslau J, Eskridge JM: Preoperative embolization of spinal tumors. J Vasc Interven Radiol 6:871–875, 1995.
11. Brodke DS, Dick JC, Kunz DN, et al: Posterior lumbar interbody fusion: A biomechanical comparison, including a new threaded cage. Spine 22:26–31, 1997.
12. Brodsky AE, Evan SK, Momtaz AK: Correlation of radiologic assessment of lumbar spine fusions with surgical exploration. Spine 16:S261–265, 1991.
13. Carlson GD, Abitbol JJ, Anderson DR, et al: Screw fixation in the human sacrum. Spine 17: S196–203, 1992.
14. Cervellati S, Bettini N, Bianco T, et al: Neurological complications in segmental spinal instrumentation: Analysis of 750 patients. Eur Spine J 5(3):161–166, 1996.
15. Christoferson LA, Selland B: Intervertebral bone implants following excision of protruded lumbar discs. J Neurosurg 42:401–405, 1975.
16. Cloward RB: The treatment of ruptured lumbar intervertebral discs by vertebral body fusion: Indications, operative technique and aftercare. J Neurosurg 10:154–168, 1953.
17. Collis JS: Total disc replacement: A modified posterior lumbar interbody fusion. Clin Orthop 193: 64–67, 1985.
18. Cotrel Y, Dubousset J, Guillaumat M: New universal instrumentation in spinal surgery. Clin Orthop 227:10–23, 1988.
19. Crock H: Anterior lumbar interbody fusion: indications for its use and notes on surgical technique. Clin Orthop 165:157–163, 1982.
20. Cybulski GR, Von Roenn KA, D'Angelo CM, et al: Luque rod stabilization for metastatic disease of the spine. Surg Neurol 28:277–283, 1987.
21. DeWald RL, Bridwell KL, Prodromas C, et al: Reconstructive surgery as palliation for metastatic malignancies of the spine. Spine 10:21–26, 1985.
22. Dick JC, Brodke DS, Zdeblick TA, et al: Anterior instrumentation of the thoracolumbar spine: A biomechanical comparison. Spine 22:744–750, 1997.
23. Dossett A: Anterior lumbar fusion. Semin Spine Surg 8:235–249, 1996.
24. Dove J. Segmental wiring for spinal deformity: A morbidity report. Spine 14:229–231, 1989.
25. Emery SE, Fuller DA, Stevenson S: Ceramic anterior spinal fusion: Biologic and biomechanical comparison in a canine model. Spine 21:2713–2719, 1996.
26. Esses SI, Botsford DJ, Wright T, et al: Operative treatment of spine fractures with the AO internal fixator. Spine 16:146S–150, 1991.
27. Esses SI, Sachs BL, Dreyzin V: Complications associated with the technique of pedicle screw fixation. Spine 18:2231–2239, 1993.
28. Faciszewski T, Winter RB, Lonstein JE, et al: The surgical and medical perioperative complications of anterior spinal fusion surgery in the thoracic and lumbar spine in adults. Spine 20:1592–1599, 1995.
29. Faraj AA, Webb JK: Early complications of spinal pedicle screw. Eur Spine J 6:324–326, 1997.
30. Flynn JC, Price CT: Sexual complications of anterior fusion of the lumbar spine. Spine 9:489–492, 1983.
31. Freebody D, Bendall R, Taylor RD: Anterior transperitoneal lumbar fusion. J Bone Joint Surg 53B:617–627, 1971.
32. Fuller DA, Stevenson S, Emery SE: The effects of internal fixation on calcium carbonate: Ceramic anterior spinal fusion in dogs. Spine 21:2131–2136, 1996.
33. Gertzbein SD, Robbins SE: Accuracy of pedicular screw placement in vivo. Spine 15:11–14, 1990.
34. Glazer PA, Colliou O, Klisch SM: Biomechanical analysis of multilevel fixation methods in the lumbar spine. Spine 22:171–182, 1997.

35. Greenough CG, Peterson MD, Hadlow S, et al: Instrumented posterolateral lumbar fusion: Results and comparison with anterior interbody fusion. Spine 23(4):479–486, 1998.
36. Guanciale AF, Dinsay JM, Watkins RG: Lumbar lordosis in spinal fusion: A comparison of intraoperative results of patient positioning on two different operative table frame types. Spine 21:964–969, 1996.
37. Gurr KR, McAfee PC: Cotrel-Dubousset instrumentation in adults: A preliminary report. Spine 13:510–520, 1988.
38. Hacker RJ: Comparison of interbody fusion approaches for disabling low back pain. Spine 22:660–666, 1997.
39. Hadra BE: Wiring of the vertebrae as a means of immobilization in fracture and Potts' disease. Med Times Reg 22:423, 1901.
40. Harrington PR: The history and development of Harrington instrumentation. Clin Orthop 93:110–112, 1973.
41. Hinkley BS, Jaremko ME: Effects of 360 degree lumbar fusion in a workers' compensation population. Spine 22:312–322, 1997.
42. Hollowell JP, Vollmer DG, Wilson C,R, et al: Biomechanical analysis of thoracolumbar interbody constructs: How important is the endplate? Spine 21:1032–1036, 1996.
43. Horowitch A, Peck RD, Thomas JC, et al: The Wiltse pedicle screw fixation system: Early clinical results. Spine 14:461–467, 1989.
44. Hoshijima K, Nightingale RW, Yu JR, et al: Strength and stability of posterior lumbar interbody fusion: Comparison of titanium fiber mesh implant and tricortical bone graft. Spine 22:1181–1188, 1997.
45. Inoue SI, Watanabe T, Hirose A, et al: Anterior discectomy and interbody fusion for lumbar disc herniation: A review of 350 cases. Clin Orthop 183:22–31, 1984.
46. Isiklar ZU, Lindsey RW, Coburn M: Ureteral injury after anterior lumbar interbody fusion: A case report. Spine 20: 2379–2382, 1996.
47. Kanayama M, Cunningham BW, Weis JC, et al: The effects of rigid spinal instrumentation and solid bony fusion on spinal kinematics: A posterolateral spinal arthrodesis model. Spine 23:767–773, 1998.
48. Kawahara N, Tomita K, Baba H, et al: Cadaveric vascular anatomy for total en bloc spondylectomy in malignant vertebral tumors. Spine 21:1401–1407, 1996.
49. Kim S, Michelsen C: Revision surgery for failed back surgery syndrome. Spine 17:957–960, 1992.
50. Kozak JA, Heilman AE, O'Brien JP. Anterior lumbar fusion options: Technique and graft materials. Clin Orthop 300:45–51, 1994.
51. Krag MH, Beynnon BD, Pope MH, et al: An internal fixator for posterior application to short segments of the thoracic, lumbar, or lumbosacral spine: Design and testing. Clin Orthop 203:75–81, 1986.
52. Krag MH, Beynnon BD, Pope MH, et al: Depth of insertion of transpedicular vertebral screws into human vertebrae: Effect upon screw-vertebra interface strength. J Spinal Disord 1:287:–294, 1989.
53. Krag MH, Van Hal ME, Beynnon BD: Placement of transpedicular vertebral screws close to the anterior vertebral cortex: Description of methods. Spine 14: 879–883, 1989.
54. Kumar A, Kozak JA, Doherty BJ: Interspace distraction and graft subsidence after anterior lumbar fusion with femoral strut allograft. Spine 18: 2393–2400, 1993.
55. Laine T, Makitalo K, Schlenzka D, et al: Accuracy of pedicle screw insertion: A prospective CT study in 30 low back patients. Eur Spine J 6:402–405, 1997.
56. Larson SJ: Lateral extracavitary approach to the spine: Indications and operative technique. Contemp Neurosurg 15:1–16, 1993.
57. Larson SJ: Thoracolumbar trauma. Clin Neurosurg 40:416–426, 1993.
58. Larson SJ, Holst RA, Hemmy DC, et al: Lateral extracavitary approach to traumatic lesions of the thoracic and lumbar spine. J Neurosurg 45:628–637, 1976.
59. Lee CK, DeBari A: Lumbosacral spinal fusion with Knodt distraction rods. Spine 11:373–375, 1986.
60. Lin PM, Cautilli RA, Joyce MF: Posterior lumbar interbody fusion. Clin Orthop 180:154–168, 1983.
61. Lindsey RW, Dick W: The fixateur interne in the reduction and stabilization of thoracolumbar spine fractures with neurological deficit. Spine 16:140S–145S, 1991.
62. Loguidice VA, Johnson RG, Guyer RD, et al: Anterior lumbar interbody fusion. Spine 13: 366–369, 1988.
63. Luque ER: Anatomic basis and development of segmental spinal instrumentation. Spine 7:256–259, 1982.
64. Luque LR, ISF: Surgical technique. Memphis, TN: Danek Medical, Inc., 1988.
65. MacNab I: The blood supply of the lumbar spine and its application to the technique of intertransverse lumbar fusion. J Bone Joint Surg 53B: 628–638, 1971.
66. Maiman DJ, Larson SJ, Benzel EC: Neurological improvement associated with late decompression of the thoracolumbar spinal cord. Neurosurgery 14:302–307, 1984.
67. Maiman DJ, Larson SJ, Luck E, et al: Lateral extracavitary approach to the spine for thoracic disc

herniation: Report of 23 cases. Neurosurgery 14:178–182, 1984.

68. Maiman DJ, Larson SJ: The lateral extracavitary approach to the thoracic and lumbar spine: Indications and technique. In: Atlas of operative neurosurgical techniques, American Association of Neurological Surgeons 2:153–161, 1992.

69. Maiman DJ, Pintar FA, Yoganandan N, et al: Effects of anterior vertebral grafting on the traumatized lumbar spine following pedicle screw-plate fixation. Spine 18:2423–2430, 1993.

70. Maiman DJ, Sances A Jr, Larson SJ, et al: Comparison of the failure of biomechanics of spinal fixation devices. Neurosurgery 17:574–580, 1985.

71. Mathews HH, Evans MT, Molligan HJ, et al: Laparoscopic discectomy with anterior lumbar interbody fusion: A preliminary review. Spine 20:1797–1802, 1995.

72. Mayer H: A new microsurgical technique for minimally invasive anterior lumbar interbody fusion. Spine 22:691–700, 1997.

73. McAfee PC: Laparoscopic fusion and BAK stabilization of the lumbar spine. In: Regan JJ, McAfee PC, Mack MJ, (eds.) Atlas of endoscopic spine surgery. St. Louis: Quality Medical Publishing Inc. 1995, pp. 306–320.

74. McCormick PC: Surgical treatment of dumbbell and paraspinal tumors of the thoracic and lumbar spine. Neurosurgery 38:67–74, 1996.

75. McDonnell MF, Glassman SD, Dimar JR II, et al: Perioperative complications of anterior procedures on the spine. J Bone Joint Surg 78:839–847, 1996.

76. Mirkovic S, Abitbol J, Steinman J, et al: Anatomic considerations for sacral screw placement. Spine 16:S289–294, 1991.

77. Misenheimer GR, Peek RD, Wiltse LL, et al: Anatomic analysis of pedicle cortical and cancellous diameter as related to screw size. Spine 14:367–372, 1989.

78. Newman MH, Grinstead GL: Anterior lumbar interbody fusion for internal disc disruption. Spine 17:831–837, 1992.

79. Odgers CJ IV, Vacaro AR, Pollack ME, et al: Accuracy of pedicle screw placement with the assistance of lateral plain radiography. J Spinal Disord 9:334–338, 1996.

80. Onimus M, Papin P, Gangloff S: Extraperitoneal approach to the lumbar spine with video assistance. Spine 21:2491–2494, 1996.

81. Papastefanou SL, Stevens K, Mulholland RC: Femoral nerve palsy: An unusual complication of anterior lumbar interbody fusion. Spine 19:2842–2844, 1994.

82. Pihlajamaki H, Bostman O, Ruuskanen M, et al: Posterolateral lumbosacral fusion with transpedicular fixation: 63 consecutive cases followed for 4 (2–6) years. Acta Orthop Scand 67:63–68, 1996.

83. Pihlajamaki H, Myllynen P, Bostman O: Complications of transpedicular lumbosacral fixation for nontraumatic disorders. J Bone Joint Surg 79(B):183–189, 1997.

84. Ray C: Threaded fusion cages for lumbar interbody fusions: An economic comparison with 360 fusions. Spine 22:681–685, 1997.

85. Ray C: Threaded titanium cages for lumbar interbody fusions. Spine 22:667–679, 1997.

86. Rechtine GR, Sutterlin CE, Wood GW, et al: The efficacy of pedicle screw/plate fixation on lumbar autogenous bone graft fusion in adult patients with degenerative spondylolisthesis. J Spinal Disord 9:382–391, 1996.

87. Regan JJ, McAfee PC, Guyer RD, et al: Laparoscopic fusion of the lumbar spine in a multicenter series of the first 34 consecutive patients. Surg Laporsc Endosc 6:459–468, 1996.

88. Roy-Camille R, Saillant G, Mazel C: Internal fixation of the lumbar spine with pedicle screw plating. Clin Orthop 203:7–17, 1986.

89. Rudisch A, Kremser C, Peer S, et al: Metallic artifacts in magnetic resonance imaging of patients with spinal fusion: A comparison of implant materials and imaging sequences. Spine 2:692–699, 1998.

90. Sandhu HS, Turner S, Kabo JM, et al: Distractive properties of a threaded interbody fusion device: An in vivo model. Spine 21:1201–1210, 1996.

91. Selby D: Internal fixation with Knodt's rods. Clin Orthop 203:179–184, 1986.

92. Shirado O, Zdeblick TA, McAfee PC, et al: Quantitative histologic study of the influence of anterior spinal instrumentation and biodegradable polymer on lumbar interbody fusion after corpectomy: A canine model. Spine 17:795–803, 1992.

93. Siegal T, Siegal T: Current considerations in the management of neoplastic spinal cord compression. Spine 14:223–228, 1989.

94. Siegal TZ, Siegal T: Vertebral body resection for epidural compression by malignant tumors. J Bone Joint Surg 67A:375–382, 1985.

95. Simmons JW: Posterior lumbar interbody fusion with posterior elements as chip grafts. Clin Orthop 193:85–89, 1985.

96. Sjostrom L, Jacobsson O, Karlstrom G, et al: CT analysis of pedicles and screw tracts after implant removal in thoracolumbar fractures. J Spinal Disord 6:225–231, 1993.

97. Steffee AD, Biscup RS: Segmental spine plates with pedicle screw fixation. Clin Orthop 203:45–53, 1986.

98. Steffee AD, Biscup RS, Sitkowski DJ: Segmental spine plates with pedicle screw fixation: A new internal fixation device for disorders of the lumbar and thoracolumbar spine. Clin Orthop 203:45–53, 1986.

99. Thalgott JS, Kabins MB, Timlin M, et al: Four year experience with the AO anterior thoracolumbar locking plate. Spinal Cord 35:286–291, 1997.

100. Thalgott JS, LaRocca H, Aebi M, et al: Reconstruction of the lumbar spine using AO DCP plate internal fixation. Spine 14:91–95, 1989.

101. Tiusanen H, Seitsalo S, Osterman K, Soini J: Retrograde ejaculation after anterior interbody lumbar fusion. Euro Spine J 4:339–342, 1995.

102. Vaccaro AR, Garfin SR: Internal fixation (pedicle screw fixation) for fusions of the lumbar spine. Spine 20:57S–165S, 1995.

103. Vahldiek MJ, Panjabi MM: Stability potential of spinal instrumentations in tumor vertebral body replacement surgery. Spine 23:543–550, 1998.

104. Watkins R: Anterior lumbar interbody fusion: Surgical complications. Clin Orthop 284:47–53, 1992.

105. Weiner BK, Fraser RD: Spine update: Lumbar interbody cages. Spine 23: 634–640, 1997.

106. Weinstein JN, Spratt KF, Spengler D, et al: Spinal pedicle fixation: Reliability and validity of roentgenogram-based assessment and surgical factors on successful screw placement. Spine 13:1012–1018, 1988.

107. Whitecloud TS, Butler JC, Cohen JL, et al: Complications with the variable spinal plating system. Spine 14:472–476, 1989.

108. Wiltberger BR: Intervertebral body fusion by the use of posterior bone dowel. Clin Orthop 35: 69–79, 1964.

109. Wolfla CE, Maiman DJ: The lateral extracavitary approach to the spine. Tech Neurosurg (in press).

110. Wolfla CE, Maiman DJ: Retroperitoneal anterior lumbar interbody fusion using threaded titanium fusion cage (unpublished data).

111. Wood GW, Boyd R, Carothers TA, et al: The effect of pedicle screw/plate fixation on lumbar autogenous bone graft fusions in patients with degenerative disc disease. Spine 20:819–830, 1995.

112. Wu H, Yao R: Mechanical behavior of the human annulus fibrosis. J Biomech 9:1–7, 1976.

113. Yoganandan N, Maiman DJ, Pintar F, et al: Kinematics of the lumbar spine following pedicle screw-plate fixation. Spine 18: 504–512, 1993.

114. Yuan HA, Mann KA, Found EM, et al: Early clinical experience with the Syracuse I plate: An anterior spinal fixation device. Spine 12:278–285, 1988.

115. Zdeblick TA, Warden KE, Zou D, et al: Anterior spinal fixators: A biomechanical in vitro study. Spine 18:513–517, 1993.

116. Zindrick MR, Wiltse LL, Widel EH, et al: A biomechanical study of interpeduncular screw fixation in the lumbosacral spine. Clin Orthop 203:99–112, 1986.

117. Zuckerman J, Hsu K, White A, et al: Early results of spinal fusion using variable spine plating technique. Spine 13:570–579, 1988.

118. Zhucherman JF, Zdeblick TA, Bailey SA, et al: Instrumented laparoscopic spinal fusion. Spine 20:2029–2034, 1995.

Index

Page numbers followed by "f" indicate figures. Page numbers followed by "t" indicate tables.

Abscess, epidural, 153
Allergies, to metal, disc fusion, 121–123
Aneurysmal bone cysts, 195–197
   clinical presentation, 196
   diagnosis, 196–197
   radiographic evaluation, 196–197
   surgical management, 197
Ankylosing spondylitis of lumbar spine, 66–74
   clinical presentation, 68
   diagnosis, 68–69, 69f
   management, 69–74
     drug therapy, 69
     exercise, 69
     nonoperative treatment of fractures, 70
     physical therapy, exercise, 69
     surgical treatment, 70–74
       ankylosing spondylitis, 70–72, 71f
       complications, 74
       fractures, 70
       lumbar wedge osteotomy, 72–74, 73f
   pathology, 68
Annulus fibrosis, 7–8, 8f
Anterior grafting studies, pedicular fixation, 28–29
Anterior lumbar fusion, 305–319
   anterior interbody fusion, 309–310
   anterior plating devices, 311–315
   complications, 315–319
     neurological complications, 316–317
     peritoneal hernias secondary, 317
     peritoneal perforation, 317
     ureter, damage to, 317
     vascular complications, 315–316
   indications, 305
   instrumented ALIF, 310
   preoperative assessment, 305
   results, 318–319
   retroperitoneal ALIF, 310–311
     L5-S1 cage placement, 310–311
   retroperitoneal exposure, 308–309
   technique, 305–315
   transperitoneal exposure, 305–308
   vertebrectomy, 311
Apophyseal joints, lumbar, 6
Arteries, vertebral, 2–3
Autogenous graft *vs.* allograft, for fusion surgery, 257–258
   allografts in posterior fusion, 257–258

Benign tumors of spine, 185–199
   aneurysmal bone cysts, 195–197
     clinical presentation, 196
     radiographic evaluation, 196–197
     surgical management, 197
   giant cell tumors, 188–191
     adjunctive therapy, 191
     clinical presentation, 188–189
     management, 189–191
     pathology, 188
     radiographic evaluation, 189
     surgical treatment, 189–191
   hemangiomas, 191–195
     clinical presentation, 192
     drug therapy, 193
     embolization, 193
     management, 193–195
     pathology, 195–196
     radiographic evaluation, 193
     radiotherapy, 193
     surgical treatment, 193–195
   osteoblastomas, 186–188
     clinical presentation, 188
     radiographic evaluation, 188
     surgical management, 188
   osteochondromas, 186
   osteoid osteomas, 184–186
     clinical presentation, 184–185
     management, 186
     pathology, 184
     radiographic evaluation, 185–186

Benign tumors of spine (*continued*)
  vascular tumors, 191–195
    clinical presentation, 192
    drug therapy, 193
    embolization, 193
    management, 193–195
    pathology, 195–196
    radiographic evaluation, 193
    radiotherapy, 193
    surgical treatment, 193–195
Biomechanics, 13–33
  in fixation, 24–29
  intervertebral fusion, 25
  motion, lumbar spine, 22
  pedicular fixation
    in degenerative disease, 29
    in trauma, 26–29
      anterior grafting studies, 28–29
      construct, 27–28
      geometry, pedicle fixation, 26–27
      instrumentation testing methods, 28
      studies, 28
  research, 18–19
    loading variables, 18–19
      complex loading, 18–19
      dynamic loading, 19
      pure moment, 18–19
      quasistatic loading, 19
  spinal elements, 19–22
    intervertebral disc, 20
    spinal ligaments, 20–22
      capsular ligaments, 21
      instability, 21–22
      interspinous ligaments, 21
      intertransverse ligaments, 21
      ligamentum flavum, 21
      longitudinal ligament
        anterior, 20
        posterior, 21
      supraspinous ligaments, 21
    vertebra, 19–20
  spinal stability, 14–18
    column theories, 15–17
      three-column theory, 16f, 16–17
      two-column theory, 15–16, 16f
    continuum concept, 17f, 17–18
    elastic zone, 15
    neutral zone theory, 14–15, 15f
  thoracic spine trauma, 22–24
    burst fracture, 22–23
    chance fractures, 23–24
    flexion-compression injuries, 23
    osteoporotic fractures, 24
  trauma, lumbar spine, 22–24
  in treatment, 24–29
  "universal" instrumentation, 25–26
Blood supply to vertebrae, 2–4
  arteries, 2–3
  veins, 4
Bone, metabolic diseases of, 51–77
  ankylosing spondylitis of lumbar spine, 66–74

    clinical presentation, 68
    diagnosis, 68–69, 69f
    management, 69–74
      drug therapy, 69
      exercise, 69
      nonoperative treatment of fractures, 70
      physical therapy, 69
      surgical treatment, 70–74
        ankylosing spondylitis, 70–72, 71f
        complications, 74
        fractures, 70
        lumbar wedge osteotomy, 72–74, 73f
    pathology, 68
  osteitis deformans, 52–61
    clinical presentation, 52–53, 54–59f
    diagnosis, 53–55, 60–61f
    management, 55–61
      drug therapy, 55–57
      surgical treatment, 57–61
    pathology, 52
  osteoporosis, 61–66
    clinical presentation, 62
    diagnosis, 63
    management, 63–66
      dietary supplements, 63–64
      drug therapy, 64–65
      surgical treatment, 65–66, 67f
    pathology, 62
Bone cysts, aneurysmal, 195–197
  clinical presentation, 196
  radiographic evaluation, 196–197
  surgical management, 197
Bone fusion, enhancement of, 259–261
  bone morphogenetic protein, 260–261
  electrical stimulation, 259–260
  external stimulation, 260
  implanted stimulation, 260
  magnetic fields, 259–260
Bone graft
  autogenous graft, *versus* allograft for fusion surgery, 257–258
    allografts in posterior fusion, 257–258
    tumor surgery, 258
  fusion, 256–257
    cell types, 256
    surgical considerations, 256–257
Bone morphogenetic protein, 260–261
Bone substitutes, 258–261
Burst fracture, thoracic spine trauma, biomechanics, 22–23

Capsular ligaments, biomechanics, 21
Cell types, bone grafts, 256
Chance fractures, thoracic spine trauma, biomechanics, 23–24
Chondrosarcomas, 213
Chordomas, 207–212
  clinical characteristics, 207–208
  histologic characteristics, 207–208
  radiographic evaluation, 208–209
    computed tomography, 208

        magnetic resonance imaging, 208–209
        plain radiography, 208
    treatment, 209–212
        adjunctive therapy, 211
        patient preparation, 209–210
        prognosis, 211
        sacral tumors, 210
Coccygeal-sacral tumors, 213–215
Column theories, biomechanics, 15–17
    three-column theory, 16f, 16–17
    two-column theory, 15–16, 16f
Continuum concept, spinal stability biomechanics, 17f, 17–18
Cysts, bone, aneurysmal, 195–197
    clinical presentation, 196
    radiographic evaluation, 196–197
    surgical management, 197

Degenerative disease, pedicular fixation with, 29
Degenerative scoliosis, 99–103, 102–103f
    clinical presentation, 100, 104f
    diagnosis, 100, 104f
    surgical management, 100–103, 103–105f
Degenerative spondylolisthesis, 96–98
    clinical presentation, 97
    diagnosis, 97
    management, 98
    pathology, 96, 98–100f
    surgical treatment, 98
        fusion, 98, 101f
Disc degeneration, 79–132
    degenerative scoliosis, 99–103, 102–103f
        clinical presentation, 100, 104f
        surgical management, 100–103, 103–105f
    degenerative spondylolisthesis, 96–98
        clinical presentation, 97
        management, 98
        pathology, 96, 98–100f
        surgical treatment, 98
            fusion, 98, 101f
    discogenic pain, 91–92
        discography, 91–92
        internal disc disruption, 92
    fusion, 112–123
        anterior fusion, 118
        circumferential fusion, 118
        complications, 120–123
            infection, 120–121
            metal allergies, 121–123
            stress on motion segments, 121, 124f
        instrumentation, 118–123, 119–124f, 123t
        midline fusion, 115, 116f
        posterior lumbar interbody fusion, 91f, 115–118, 117f
        transverse process fusion, 118
    intervertebral disc herniation, 80–91
        clinical presentation, 80–82
        diagnosis, 81–82, 82f, 84f, 124f
        management, 83
        nonsurgical treatment, 83
        surgical treatment, 83–91

        central protrusion, 84f, 84–85
        disc removal, 85
        fusion, 89–91, 90–92f
        other herniation, 85–86f, 85–87
        pain, 83f, 83–84
        patient selection for surgery, 89
        percutaneous techniques, 87
        recurrent pain, 87–89, 88f
    lumbar stenosis, 104–112
        acquired lumbar stenosis, 106
        clinical presentation, 106, 108f
        developmental lumbar stenosis, 104–105, 105f
        facetectomy, postfacetectomy instability, 107f, 109–110, 112–115f
        fusion, 110–112
        idiopathic lumbar stenosis, 106
        laminectomy, 110
        pathology, 106, 108–110f
        surgical treatment, 106–112, 111f
    raised intraosseous pressure, 92–93
        clinical presentation, 93
        diagnosis, 93
        management, 93, 94–95f
        pathology, 92–93
    zygapophyseal "facet" joints, 93–96
        clinical presentation, 95
        hip/spine syndrome, 96
        injection, management by, 95–96, 97f
        pathology, 93–95
Disc space infection, 151–153
    clinical presentation, 151–152
    diagnosis, 151–152
    management, 152–153
Discogenic pain, 91–92
    discography, 91–92
    internal disc disruption, 92

Elastic zone, spinal stability, 15
Electrical stimulation, bone fusion, 259–260
Embolization, metastatic tumors of lumbar spine, 246
End plates, 8, 9f
Endoscopic lumbar fusion, 319
Epidural abscess, 153
    clinical presentation, 153
    diagnosis, 153
    management, 153
External stimulation, bone fusion, 260
Extracavitary surgical approach, 296–305
    anterior graft, 303
    complications, 304
    dumbbell lesions, 304
    exposure, 297–302
    incision location, 297
    L5 corpectomy, 304
    paraspinal lesions, 304
    patient preparation, 296–297
    postoperative care, 304
    results, 304–305
    technique, 297–303
    trauma, 171
    vertebral resection, 302–303

Facet joints, zygapophyseal, 93–96
　clinical presentation, 95
　hip/spine syndrome, 96
　injection, management by, 95–96, 97f
　pathology, 93–95
Fixation, biomechanics of, 24–29
Flexion-compression injuries, thoracic spine trauma, biomechanics, 23
Foraminotomy, isthmic spondylolisthesis, secondary to fracture of pars interarticularis, 138–140
Fusion
　bone, enhancement of, 259–261
　　bone morphogenetic protein, 260–261
　　electrical stimulation, 259–260
　　external stimulation, 260
　　implanted stimulation, 260
　　magnetic fields, 259–260
　disc, 112–123
　　anterior fusion, 118
　　circumferential fusion, 118
　　complications, 120–123
　　　infection, 120–121
　　　metal allergies, 121–123
　　　stress on motion segments, 121, 124f
　　instrumentation, 118–123, 119–124f, 123t
　　midline fusion, 115, 116f
　　posterior lumbar interbody fusion, 91f, 115–118, 117f
　　transverse process fusion, 118

Galveston fixation, 281–283
　results, 283
　technique, 281–283
Geometry, pedicular fixation, 26–27
Giant cell tumors, 188–191
　adjunctive therapy, 191
　clinical presentation, 188–189
　diagnosis, 189
　management, 189–191
　pathology, 188
　radiographic evaluation, 189
　surgical treatment, 189–191
Gunshot wounds of spine, 177

Hemangiomas, 191–195
　clinical presentation, 192
　drug therapy, 193
　embolization, 193
　management, 193–195
　pathology, 195–196
　radiographic evaluation, 193
　radiotherapy, 193
　surgical treatment, 193–195
Hematogenous osteomyelitis, pyogenic, 146–151
　clinical presentation, 146
　diagnosis, 146
　drug therapy, 146–147
　management, 146–151
　surgical treatment, 147–151
　　immobilization, 148–151
　　instrumentation, 148–151
Herniation, intervertebral disc, 80–91

　clinical presentation, 80–82
　diagnosis, 81–82, 82f, 84f, 124f
　management, 83
　nonsurgical treatment, 83
　surgical treatment, 83–91
　　central protrusion, 84f, 84–85
　　disc removal, 85
　　fusion, 89–91, 90–92f
　　other herniation, 85–86f, 85–87
　　pain, 83f, 83–84
　　patient selection for surgery, 89
　　percutaneous techniques, 87
　　recurrent pain, 87–89, 88f
Hook-rod fixation. *See* Universal fixation

Implanted stimulation, bone fusion, 260
Infection, 145–156
　with disc degeneration, 120–121
　disc space, 151–153
　　clinical presentation, 151–152
　　management, 152–153
　epidural abscess, 153
　　clinical presentation, 153
　　management, 153
　pyogenic hematogenous osteomyelitis, 146–151
　　clinical presentation, 146
　　diagnosis, 146
　　drug therapy, 146–147
　　management, 146–151
　　surgical treatment, 147–151
　　　immobilization, 148–151
　　　instrumentation, 148–151
　tuberculous vertebral osteomyelitis, 153–156
　　clinical presentation, 153–155
　　management, 155
Injection, zygapophyseal "facet" joints, 95–96, 97f
Instability
　spinal elements, 21–22
　vertebral column, 35–49
　　abnormal functioning, 37–38, 37–40f
　　chronic vertebral trauma, instability, 38–42
　　　acute vertebral trauma, 42–46, 43–47f
　　　radiographic evaluation, 41–42, 42f
　　　　limitations, 41–42
　　normal functioning, 36–37
Instrumentation testing methods, pedicular fixation, 28
Interbody fusion, posterior lumbar, 286–296
Intertransverse lumbar fusion, posterior, 270–274
Intervertebral disc, 7–10
　annulus fibrosis, 7–8, 8f
　collagen, 8–9
　end plates, 8, 9f
　herniation, 80–91
　　clinical presentation, 80–82
　　diagnosis, 80–82, 82f, 84f, 124f
　　management, 83
　　nonsurgical treatment, 83
　　surgical treatment, 83–91
　　　central protrusion, 84f, 84–85
　　　disc removal, 85
　　　fusion, 89–91, 90–92f

        other herniation, 85–86f, 85–87
        pain, 83f, 83–84
        patient selection for surgery, 89
        percutaneous techniques, 87
        recurrent pain, 87–89, 88f
      microfractures, 9–10
      nucleus pulposus, 7
      ossification, 9–10
      proteoglycans, 8–9
      vertical loads, 10
Intraosseous pressure, raised, 92–93
    clinical presentation, 93
    diagnosis, 93
    management, 93, 94–95f
    pathology, 92–93
Isthmic spondylolisthesis, 134–144
    congenital, 134
      clinical presentation, 134
      diagnosis, 134
      management, 134
    pars interarticularis, secondary to fracture of, 134–143
      clinical presentation, 135–138
      diagnosis, 135–138
      foraminotomy, 138–140
      fusion, 140–143

Laminectomy, 268–270
    lumbar discectomy, 268–269
    lumbar laminectomy, 269–270
    metastatic tumors, 242
    transpedicular approaches, 270
Ligamentotaxis, trauma, 170–171
Ligaments, 6–7
Loading variables
    pure moment, research, 18–19
    quasistatic loading, research, 19
    research, 18–19
Lumbar anatomy, 1–12
    apophyseal joints, 6
    blood supply, to vertebrae, 2–4
      arteries, 2–3
      veins, 4
    intervertebral disc, 7–10
      annulus fibrosis, 7–8, 8f
      collagen, 8–9
      end plates, 8, 9f
      microfractures, 9–10
      nucleus pulposus, 7
      ossification, 9–10
      proteoglycans, 8–9
      vertical loads, 10
    ligaments, 6–7
    nerve supply, to vertebrae, 4–6, 5f
    vertebral body, 2, 3–4f
Lumbar ankylosing spondylitis of, 66–74
    clinical presentation, 68
    diagnosis, 68–69, 69f
    management, 69–74
      drug therapy, 69
      exercise, 69
      nonoperative treatment of fractures, 70

      physical therapy, exercise, 69
      surgical treatment, 70–74
        ankylosing spondylitis, 70–72, 71f
        complications, 74
        fractures, 70
        lumbar wedge osteotomy, 72–74, 73f
    pathology, 68
Lumbar apophyseal joints, 6
Lumbar discectomy, 268–269
Lumbar laminectomy, 269–270
Lumbar metastatic tumors, 232–255
    anterior lumbar approaches, 243
    clinical presentation, 233–234
    diagnostic biopsy, 236
    drug therapy, 240–241
    embolization, 246
    epidemiology, 232
    factors affecting treatment outcomes, 236–239
      biology, 236–237
      location, 239
      neurological status prior to treatment, 237–239
    indications, 241
    laminectomy, 242
    lateral extracavitary approaches, 243–246
    management, 239–248
    pathophysiology, 232–233
    presurgical planning, 246
    prognosis, 241–242
    radiography, 234–236
      magnetic resonance imaging, 235–236
      myelography, 234–235
      plain radiography, 234
      radionuclide studies, 234
    radiotherapy, 246–247
    surgical treatment, 241
    techniques, 242–246
    transpedicular approaches, 242–243
    vertebroplasty, 242
Lumbar motion, biomechanics, 22
Lumbar stenosis, 104–112
    acquired lumbar stenosis, 106
    clinical presentation, 106, 108f
    developmental lumbar stenosis, 104–105, 105f
    diagnosis, 106, 108f
    facetectomy, 109–110
      postfacetectomy instability, 107f, 109–110, 112–115f
    fusion, 110–112
    idiopathic lumbar stenosis, 106
    laminectomy, 110
    pathology, 106, 108–110f
    surgical treatment, 106–112, 111f
Lumbar trauma, biomechanics, 22–24

Magnetic resonance imaging, with trauma, 160–161
Malignant tumors, primary, 202–229
    chordomas, 207–212
      histologic characteristics, 207–208
      radiographic evaluation, 208–209
        computed tomography, 208
        magnetic resonance imaging, 208–209
        plain radiography, 208

Malignant tumors, primary (continued)
    treatment, 209–212
        adjunctive therapy, 211
        chordomas of mobile spine, 210–211
        patient preparation, 209–210
        prognosis, 211
        sacral tumors, 210
    diagnostic biopsy, 202–203
    multiple myeloma, 205–207
        histologic characteristics, 205
        radiographic evaluation, 205–206
        treatment, 206–207
    plasma cell lesions, 203–205
        solitary plasmacytomas, 203–205
            histologic characteristics, 203
            prognosis, 205
            radiation therapy, 205
            radiographic evaluation, 203
            surgery, 205
            treatment, 203–205
    sacral-coccygeal tumors, 213–215
    sacrum, malignant tumors of, 215–224
        anterior/posterior resection, 219–224
        high sacral resection, via anterior/posterior approach, 224
        low sacral resection, 217
        paramedian tumors, 217–219
        posterior approaches, 216–219
        sarcomas of sacrum, 215–216
        surgical treatment of sacral tumors, 216
    sarcomas, 212–213
        adjunctive therapy, 213
        chondrosarcomas, 213
        osteosarcomas, 212
        radiographic evaluation, 212, 213
        treatment, 212–213
Metabolic diseases of bone, 51–77
    ankylosing spondylitis of lumbar spine, 66–74
        clinical presentation, 68
        diagnosis, 68–69, 69f
        management, 69–74
            drug therapy, 69
            exercise, 69
            nonoperative treatment of fractures, 70
            physical therapy, 69
            surgical treatment, 70–74
                ankylosing spondylitis, 70–72, 71f
                complications, 74
                fractures, 70
                lumbar wedge osteotomy, 72–74, 73f
        pathology, 68
    osteitis deformans, 52–61
        clinical presentation, 52–53, 54–59f
        diagnosis, 53–55, 60–61f
        management, 55–61
            drug therapy, 55–57
            surgical treatment, 57–61
        pathology, 52
    osteoporosis, 61–66
        clinical presentation, 62
        diagnosis, 63

        management, 63–66
            dietary supplements, 63–64
            drug therapy, 64–65
            surgical treatment, 65–66, 67f
        pathology, 62
Metal allergies, disc fusion, 121–123
Metastatic tumors, lumbar spine, 232–255
    anterior lumbar approaches, 243
    clinical presentation, 233–234
    diagnostic biopsy, 236
    drug therapy, 240–241
    embolization, 246
    epidemiology, 232
    factors affecting treatment outcomes, 236–239
        biology, 236–237
        location, 239
        neurological status prior to treatment, 237–239
    indications, 241
    laminectomy, 242
    lateral extracavitary approaches, 243–246
    management, 239–248
    pathophysiology, 232–233
    presurgical planning, 246
    prognosis, 241–242
    radiography, 234–236
        magnetic resonance imaging, 235–236
        myelography, 234–235
        plain radiography, 234
        radionuclide studies, 234
    radiotherapy, 246–247
    surgical treatment, 241
    techniques, 242–246
    transpedicular approaches, 242–243
    vertebroplasty, 242
Mobile spine, chordomas of, 210–211
Morphogenetic protein, bone, 260–261
Motion segments, stress on, with disc degeneration, 121, 124f
Multiple myeloma, clinical characteristics, 205
Myelography, metastatic tumors of lumbar spine, 234–235

Nerve supply, to vertebrae, 4–6, 5f
Neurological status, evaluation of, with trauma, 161–163
Neutral zone theory, spinal stability, 14–15, 15f
Nucleus pulposus, 7

Orthoses, 261–262
    biomechanics, 261
    indications for use, 261–262
Ossification, intervertebral disc, 9–10
Osteitis deformans, 52–61
    clinical presentation, 52–53, 54–59f
    diagnosis, 53–55, 60–61f
    management, 55–61
        drug therapy, 55–57
        surgical treatment, 57–61
    pathology, 52
Osteoblastomas, 186–188
    clinical presentation, 188
    diagnosis, 188

radiographic evaluation, 188
surgical management, 188
Osteochondromas, 186
Osteoid osteomas, 184–186
   clinical presentation, 184–185
   diagnosis, 185–186
   management, 186
   pathology, 184
   radiographic evaluation, 185–186
Osteomyelitis
   pyogenic hematogenous, 146–151
      clinical presentation, 146
      diagnosis, 146
      drug therapy, 146–147
      management, 146–151
      surgical treatment, 147–151
         immobilization, 148–151
         instrumentation, 148–151
   tuberculous vertebral, 153–156
      clinical presentation, 153–155
      management, 155
Osteoporosis, 61–66
   clinical presentation, 62
   diagnosis, 63
   fracture, thoracic spine trauma, biomechanics, 24
   management, 63–66
      dietary supplements, 63–64
      drug therapy, 64–65
      surgical treatment, 65–66, 67f
   pathology, 62
Osteosarcomas, 212

Pain
   discogenic, 91–92
      discography, 91–92
      internal disc disruption, 92
   recurrent, intervertebral disc herniation, 87–89, 88f
Pars interarticularis, isthmic spondylolisthesis secondary
      to fracture of, 134–143
   clinical presentation, 135–138
   diagnosis, 135–138
   foraminotomy, 138–140
   fusion, 140–143
Pedicular fixation, 26–29
   in degenerative disease, biomechanics, 29
   in trauma, biomechanics, 26–29
      anterior grafting studies, 28–29
      construct, 27–28
      geometry, pedicle fixation, 26–27
      instrumentation testing methods, 28
      studies, 28
Pelvic fixation. *See* Galveston fixation
Plain radiographs, with trauma, 159
Plasma cell lesions, solitary plasmacytomas
   chemotherapy, 205
   clinical characteristics, 203
PLIF. *See* Posterior lumbar interbody fusion
Posterior intertransverse lumbar fusion, 270–274
   postoperative care, 271–274
   results, 274
   technique, 270–271

Posterior lumbar interbody fusion, 286–296
   complications, 293–296
   indications, 286–287
   intervertebral cages in, 291–293
   results, 288–290, 296
   risks, 293–296
   technical considerations, 287
   technique, 287–288
Pressure, intraosseous, raised, 92–93
   clinical presentation, 93
   diagnosis, 93
   management, 93, 94–95f
   pathology, 92–93
Primary malignant tumors, 202–229
   chordomas, 207–212
      histologic characteristics, 207–208
      radiographic evaluation, 208–209
         computed tomography, 208
         magnetic resonance imaging, 208–209
         plain radiography, 208
      treatment, 209–212
         adjunctive therapy, 211
         chordomas of mobile spine, 210–211
         patient preparation, 209–210
         prognosis, 211
         sacral tumors, 210
   diagnostic biopsy, 202–203
   multiple myeloma, 205–207
      histologic characteristics, 205
      radiographic evaluation, 205–206
      treatment, 206–207
   plasma cell lesions, 203–205
      solitary plasmacytomas, 203–205
         histologic characteristics, 203
         prognosis, 205
         radiation therapy, 205
         radiographic evaluation, 203
         surgery, 205
         treatment, 203–205
   sacral-coccygeal tumors, 213–215
   sacrum, malignant tumors of, 215–224
      anterior/posterior resection, 219–224
      high sacral resection, via anterior/posterior approach,
            224
      low sacral resection, 217
      paramedian tumors, 217–219
      posterior approaches, 216–219
      sarcomas of sacrum, 215–216
      surgical treatment of sacral tumors, 216
   sarcomas, 212–213
      adjunctive therapy, 213
      chondrosarcomas, 213
      osteosarcomas, 212
      radiographic evaluation, 212, 213
      treatment, 212–213, 213
Protein, morphogenetic, bone, 260–261
Proteoglycans, 8–9
Pyogenic hematogenous osteomyelitis, 146–151
   clinical presentation, 146
   diagnosis, 146
   drug therapy, 146–147

Pyogenic hematogenous osteomyelitis (continued)
    management, 146–151
        surgical treatment, 147–151
            immobilization, 148–151
            instrumentation, 148–151

Radionuclide studies, metastatic tumors of lumbar spine, 234
Raised intraosseous pressure, 92–93
    clinical presentation, 93
    diagnosis, 93
    management, 93, 94–95f
    pathology, 92–93
Research, biomechanics, 18–19
    loading variables, 18–19
        pure moment, 18–19
        quasistatic loading, 19
Retroperitoneal decompression, trauma, 171

Sacral-coccygeal tumors, 213–215
Sacrum
    fractures, 175–177
    tumors
        malignant, 215–224
            anterior/posterior resection, 219–224
            high sacral resection, via anterior/posterior approach, 224
            low sacral resection, 217
            paramedian tumors, 217–219
            posterior approaches, 216–219
            sarcomas of sacrum, 215–216
            surgical treatment, 216
        treatment, 210
Sarcomas, 212–213
    adjunctive therapy, 213
    chondrosarcomas, 213
    osteosarcomas, 212
    radiographic evaluation, 212, 213
    sacrum, 215–216
    treatment, 212–213, 213
Scoliosis, degenerative, 99–103, 102–103f
    clinical presentation, 100, 104f
    diagnosis, 100, 104f
    surgical management, 100–103, 103–105f
Seat belt fractures, thoracic spine trauma, biomechanics, 23–24
Smoking, bone grafts and, 259
Spinal elements
    biomechanics, 19–22
        intervertebral disc, 20
        spinal ligaments, 20–22
            capsular ligaments, 21
            instability, 21–22
            interspinous ligaments, 21
            intertransverse ligaments, 21
            ligamentum flavum, 21
            longitudinal ligament
                anterior, 20
                posterior, 21
            supraspinous ligaments, 21
        vertebra, 19–20

    intervertebral disc, biomechanics, 20
Spinal ligaments
    interspinous ligaments, biomechanics, 21
    intertransverse ligaments, biomechanics, 21
    ligamentum flavum, biomechanics, 21
    longitudinal ligament
        anterior, biomechanics, 20
        posterior, anterior, 21
    supraspinous ligaments, biomechanics, 21
Spinal stability, biomechanics, 14–18
    column theories, 15–17
        three-column theory, 16f, 16–17
        two-column theory, 15–16, 16f
    continuum concept, 17f, 17–18
    elastic zone, 15
    neutral zone theory, 14–15, 15f
Spine fractures, classification, 156–157
Spondylitis, ankylosing, of lumbar spine, 66–74
    clinical presentation, 68
    diagnosis, 68–69, 69f
    management, 69–74
        drug therapy, 69
        exercise, 69
        nonoperative treatment of fractures, 70
        physical therapy, exercise, 69
        surgical treatment, 70–74
            ankylosing spondylitis, 70–72, 71f
            complications, 74
            fractures, 70
            lumbar wedge osteotomy, 72–74, 73f
    pathology, 68
Spondylolisthesis
    degenerative, 96–98
        clinical presentation, 97
        diagnosis, 97
        management, 98
        pathology, 96, 98–100f
        surgical treatment, 98
            fusion, 98, 101f
    isthmic, 134–144
        congenital, 134
            clinical presentation, 134
            diagnosis, 134
            management, 134
        pars interarticularis, secondary to fracture of, 134–143
            clinical presentation, 135–138
            diagnosis, 135–138
            foraminotomy, 138–140
            fusion, 140–143
Stability, biomechanics, clinical evaluation of, 24
Stenosis, lumbar, 104–112
    acquired lumbar stenosis, 106
    clinical presentation, 106, 108f
    developmental lumbar stenosis, 104–105, 105f
    diagnosis, 106, 108f
    facetectomy, 109–110
        postfacetectomy instability, 107f, 109–110, 112–115f
    fusion, 110–112
    idiopathic lumbar stenosis, 106
    laminectomy, 110

pathology, 106, 108–110f
surgical treatment, 106–112, 111f
Stress, on motion segments, with disc degeneration, 121, 124f
Sublaminar wiring, 280–281
technique, 280–281
Substitutes, bone, 258–261
Surgical approaches
anterior lumbar fusion, 305–319
endoscopic lumbar fusion, 319
extracavitary approach, 296–305
Galveston fixation, 281–283
laminectomy-based approaches, 268–270
posterior intertransverse lumbar fusion, 270–274
posterior lumbar interbody fusion, 286–296
sublaminar wiring, 280–281
transpedicular fixation, 274–280
universal fixation, 283–286

Thoracic spine trauma, biomechanics, 22–24
burst fracture, 22–23
chance fractures, 23–24
flexion-compression injuries, 23
osteoporotic fractures, 24
Transpedicular fixation, 274–280
complications, 277–279
patient selection, 275
preparation, 275
results, 279–280
technical considerations, 275–276
technique, 276–277
Trauma, 157–182
gunshot wounds of spine, 177
management, 163–175
non-surgical treatment, 163–165
protocol, 165
surgical treatment, 165–167
techniques, 169–174
extracavitary approach, 171
instrumentation, 171–174
ligamentotaxis, 170–171
retroperitoneal decompression, 171
timing, 167–169
pathology, 156
pedicular fixation, 26–29
pedicle fixation construct, 27–28
prognosis, 178
radiographic evaluation, 159–162
computed tomography, 161
evaluation of neurological status, 161–163
magnetic resonance imaging, 160–161
plain radiographs, 159
rehabilitation, 178
sacral fractures, 175–177
spine fractures, classification, 156–157
Tuberculous vertebral osteomyelitis, 153–156
clinical presentation, 153–155
diagnosis, 153–155
management, 155
Tumors
benign, 185–199

aneurysmal bone cysts, 195–197
clinical presentation, 196
radiographic evaluation, 196–197
surgical management, 197
giant cell tumors, 188–191
adjunctive therapy, 191
clinical presentation, 188–189
management, 189–191
pathology, 188
radiographic evaluation, 189
surgical treatment, 189–191
hemangiomas, 191–195
clinical presentation, 192
drug therapy, 193
embolization, 193
management, 193–195
pathology, 195–196
radiographic evaluation, 193
radiotherapy, 193
surgical treatment, 193–195
osteoblastomas, 186–188
clinical presentation, 188
radiographic evaluation, 188
surgical management, 188
osteochondromas, 186
osteoid osteomas, 184–186
clinical presentation, 184–185
management, 186
pathology, 184
radiographic evaluation, 185–186
vascular tumors, 191–195
clinical presentation, 192
drug therapy, 193
embolization, 193
management, 193–195
pathology, 195–196
radiographic evaluation, 193
radiotherapy, 193
surgical treatment, 193–195
metastatic, lumbar spine, 232–255
anterior lumbar approaches, 243
clinical presentation, 233–234
diagnostic biopsy, 236
drug therapy, 240–241
embolization, 246
epidemiology, 232
factors affecting treatment outcomes, 236–239
biology, 236–237
location, 239
neurological status prior to treatment, 237–239
indications, 241
laminectomy, 242
lateral extracavitary approaches, 243–246
management, 239–248
pathophysiology, 232–233
presurgical planning, 246
prognosis, 241–242
radiography, 234–236
magnetic resonance imaging, 235–236
myelography, 234–235
plain radiography, 234

Tumors (continued)
    radionuclide studies, 234
    radiotherapy, 246–247
    surgical treatment, 241
    techniques, 242–246
    transpedicular approaches, 242–243
    vertebroplasty, 242
  primary malignant, 202–229
    chordomas, 207–212
      histologic characteristics, 207–208
      radiographic evaluation, 208–209
        computed tomography, 208
        magnetic resonance imaging, 208–209
        plain radiography, 208
      treatment, 209–212
        adjunctive therapy, 211
        chordomas of mobile spine, 210–211
        patient preparation, 209–210
        prognosis, 211
        sacral tumors, 210
    diagnostic biopsy, 202–203
    multiple myeloma, 205–207
      histologic characteristics, 205
      radiographic evaluation, 205–206
      treatment, 206–207
    plasma cell lesions, 203–205
      solitary plasmacytomas, 203–205
        histologic characteristics, 203
        prognosis, 205
        radiation therapy, 205
        radiographic evaluation, 203
        surgery, 205
        treatment, 203–205
    sacral-coccygeal tumors, 213–215
    sacrum, malignant tumors of, 215–224
      anterior/posterior resection, 219–224
      high sacral resection, via anterior/posterior approach, 224
      low sacral resection, 217
      paramedian tumors, 217–219
      posterior approaches, 216–219
      sarcomas of sacrum, 215–216
      surgical treatment of sacral tumors, 216
    sarcomas, 212–213
      adjunctive therapy, 213
      chondrosarcomas, 213
      osteosarcomas, 212
      radiographic evaluation, 212, 213
      treatment, 212–213

Universal fixation, 283–286
  technique, 285
"Universal" instrumentation, biomechanics, 25–26
Ureter, damage to, with anterior lumbar fusion, 317

Vascular tumors, 191–195
  clinical presentation, 192
  diagnosis, 193
  drug therapy, 193
  embolization, 193
  immobilization, 193
  management, 193–195
  pathology, 195–196
  radiographic evaluation, 193
  radiotherapy, 193
  surgical treatment, 193–195
Veins, vertebral, 4
Vertebrae
  biomechanics, 19–20
  blood supply to, 2–4
    arteries, 2–3
    veins, 4
  nerve supply to, 4–6, 5f
Vertebral body, 2, 3–4f
  anatomy, 2, 3–4f
Vertebral column instability, 35–49
  abnormal functioning, 37–38, 37–40f
  chronic vertebral trauma, instability, 38–42
    acute vertebral trauma, 42–46, 43–47f
    radiographic evaluation, 41–42, 42f
      limitations, 41–42
  normal functioning, 36–37
Vertebral osteomyelitis, tuberculous, 153–156
  clinical presentation, 153–155
  management, 155
Vertebrectomy, anterior lumbar fusion, 311
Vertebroplasty, metastatic tumors, lumbar spine, 242
Vertical loads, intervertebral disc, 10

Wiring, sublaminar, 280–281
  technique, 280–281

Zygapophyseal "facet" joints, 93–96
  clinical presentation, 95
  diagnosis, 95
  hip/spine syndrome, 96
  injection, management by, 95–96, 97f
  pathology, 93–95